Health in Hard Times

Austerity and Health Inequalities

Edited by
Clare Bambra

First published in Great Britain in 2019 by

Policy Press
University of Bristol
1-9 Old Park Hill
Bristol
BS2 8BB
UK
t: +44 (0)117 954 5940
pp-info@bristol.ac.uk
www.policypress.co.uk

North America office:
Policy Press
c/o The University of Chicago Press
1427 East 60th Street
Chicago, IL 60637, USA
t: +1 773 702 7700
f: +1 773-702-9756
sales@press.uchicago.edu
www.press.uchicago.edu

British Library Cataloguing in Publication Data
A catalogue record for this book is available from the British Library

Library of Congress Cataloging-in-Publication Data
A catalog record for this book has been requested

978–1-4473-4485-8 hardback
978-1-4473-4486-5 ePdf
978-1-4473-4487-2 ePub
978-1-4473-4488-9 Mobi
978-1-4473-4486-5 OA PDF

The right of Clare Bambra to be identified as editor of this work has been asserted by her in
accordance with the Copyright, Designs and Patents Act 1988.

Cover design by Hayes Design
Front cover image: 'Industrial landscape', © Connor Guy 2019
Printed and bound in Great Britain by CPI Group (UK) Ltd,
Croydon, CR0 4YY
Policy Press uses environmentally responsible print partners

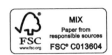

Contents

List of tables, figures and boxes   iv
About the authors   vii
Acknowledgements   xi
Foreword by Jamie Pearce   xiii
Preface   xvii

one   Introduction: Local Health Inequalities in an   1
           Age of Austerity
           Clare Bambra

two   Austerity Then and Now   35
           Mike Langthorne

three   Placing Health in Austerity   77
           Ramjee Bhandari

four   How the Other Half Live   109
           Kayleigh Garthwaite

five   Divided Lives   141
           Kate Mattheys

six   Minding the Gap   171
           *Nasima Akhter, Kate Mattheys, Jon Warren
           and Adetayo Kasim*

seven   Mothers in Austerity   201
           Amy Greer Murphy

eight   Conclusion: Health in Hard Times   233
           Clare Bambra

Index   255

List of tables, figures and boxes

Tables

1.1   Welfare reform in the UK, 2010–15   14
2.1   Unemployment Benefit before and after the cuts   39
3.1   Total number of survey participants before and after data cleaning   85
3.2   Sociodemographic characteristics of the baseline sample   87
3.3   Characteristics of the baseline sample: compositional characteristics   88
3.4   Characteristics of the baseline sample: contextual factors   89
3.5   Trend of health inequalities in Stockton-on-Tees: estimates of fixed effects   90
3.6   Association between health outcome measures and the explanatory variables (shaded blocks indicate the presence of significant association)   92
3.7   Relative contribution of different categories standardised to the total explained percentage of the full model for the gap in general and physical health measures   94
6.1   Summary statistics (mean, standard deviation or %, n/N) for outcome and demographic indicators for least and most deprived areas in Stockton-on-Tees across waves   183
6.2   Summary statistics (%, n/N and median) for material socioeconomic indicators across waves for most deprived and least deprived areas of Stockton-on-Tees   184
6.3   Summary statistics (%, n/N) for material physical environmental indicators among households from most deprived and least deprived areas in Stockton-on-Tees across waves   185
6.4   Profile of psychosocial indicators (%, n/N or mean, standard deviation) for households in most and least deprived areas of Stockton-on-Tees across waves   186
6.5   Summary statistics for behavioural factors (%, n/mean, SD) among most and least deprived areas of Stockton-on-Tees   187
6.6   Percentage contribution of direct and indirect effects SF8-MCS and WEMWBS   188

Figures

1.1	Map of per-head welfare reductions for local authorities, England, 2010–15	16
1.2	Map of per-head reductions in local authority budgets, England, 2010–15	17
1.3	Location of Stockton-on-Tees	22
2.1	UK unemployment 1929–39, yearly average	38
2.2	Unemployment in Stockton, 1929–38	40
2.3	Constables Yard, Stockton, circa 1925	42
2.4	1930s Stockton – approximate locations of old housing (King Street; Queen Street; Bay Street) and new housing (Manor House Terrace; Brisbane Grove)	43
2.5	Overcrowding by ward, private housing only, 1935	47
2.6	Stockton, 1936 – slum clearance areas; doctors; midwives; health care facilities	49
2.7	Overall death rate, 1929–39 (per 1,000 population)	54
2.8	Infant mortality rate, 1929–38 (per 1,000 births)	55
2.9	Overall death rate by ward, 1936	56
2.10	Infant mortality by ward, 1935	56
2.11	Combined infant mortality and stillbirth rates, 1935	57
2.12	Stockton 1930s – 'slum' wards (circled area)	60
2.13	Stockton-on-Tees, 2015, with 1930s 'slum' areas circled	61
2.14	Unemployment in Stockton, 2008–17	62
3.1	Sampling strategy for the survey	84
3.2	Trend of estimated inequality gap in EQ5D-VAS and SF8PCS scores between most and least deprived areas with 95% confidence interval	91
3.3	Understanding geographical inequalities in health	94
6.1	Maps of Stockton-on-Tees including most and least deprived survey neighbourhoods	178
6.2	Sampling strategy for the survey	179
6.3	Mean Warwick Edinburgh Mental Wellbeing Score (WEMWBS) and SF8 Mental Component Summary (SF8MCS) for study participants in most and least deprived areas across waves	188
6.4	Longitudinal analysis of association between psychosocial factors and mental health outcomes, estimates from multilevel models	189
6.5	Unemployment prevalence in Stockton-on-Tees 2004–17 in comparison to North East England and Britain	192
7.1	Home baking from women's group	207

7.2   Row of terraced housing in Town Centre ward   221
7.3   Town centre on market day   224

Boxes

6.1   Mental health   173

About the authors

Nasima Akhter is Assistant Professor (Research) in the Wolfson Research Institute for Health and Wellbeing and the Department of Anthropology, Durham University. She has a PhD in child health from University College London. Her research focuses on health inequalities, particularly in terms of ethnicity and nutrition in the UK and in the global south (particularly Bangladesh). She has over 15 years' experience in evaluation, monitoring and data analysis. She works across many projects in applied health research, including evaluation of interventions and advanced data analysis.

Clare Bambra is Professor of Public Health at the Institute of Health and Society, Newcastle University. Her research focuses on understanding and reducing health inequalities. She has published extensively including *Work, Worklessness and the Political Economy of Health* (Oxford University Press, 2011), *How Politics Makes Us Sick: Neoliberal Epidemics* (Palgrave, 2015), *Health Inequalities: Critical Perspectives* (Oxford University Press, 2016) and *Health Divides: Where You Live Can Kill You* (Policy Press, 2016). She was previously Executive Director of the Wolfson Research Institute for Health and Wellbeing, Durham University.

Ramjee Bhandari is a Postdoctoral Research Fellow in the GCRF Centre for Sustainable, Healthy and Learning Cities and Neighbourhoods at University of Glasgow. His research examines the relationship between health and place in the UK and in the global south. He holds an MA and PhD in geography (Durham University) and a Master in public health (Tribhuvan University, Nepal). He was previously a Postgraduate Fellow of the Wolfson Research Institute for Health and Wellbeing, Durham University.

Kayleigh Garthwaite is a Birmingham Fellow in the Department of Social Policy, Sociology and Criminology, University of Birmingham. She has a PhD in human geography from Durham University. Her research interests focus on poverty and inequality, foodbank use and welfare reform, with a particular focus on stigma. She has published extensively in these fields including *Hunger Pains: Life inside Foodbank Britain* (Policy Press, 2016). She was previously a Research Associate in the Institute of Health and Society, Newcastle University, and a

Fellow of the Wolfson Research Institute for Health and Wellbeing, Durham University.

Amy Greer Murphy is an independent researcher in Ireland. She has a PhD from the Department of Geography and School of Applied Social Sciences, Durham University. Her research focuses on qualitative methods, formal and informal care, health inequalities and gender equity. She was previously a Postgraduate Fellow at the Wolfson Research Institute for Health and Wellbeing, Durham University.

Adetayo Kasim is Associate Professor (Research) in the Wolfson Research Institute for Health and Wellbeing, Durham University. He holds a Master's degree and PhD in biostatistics from Hasselt University, Belgium. He leads statistical input into large educational evaluations, epidemiological surveys and clinical trials. His research interests include generalised linear models, longitudinal data analysis and Bayesian modelling framework. He has published extensively on the development of statistical methods including *Applied Biclustering Methods for Big and High-Dimensional Data Using R* (CRC Press, 2016).

Mike Langthorne is a historian focusing on the social history of health and poverty. He is an Honorary Research Associate of the Institute of Health and Society, Newcastle University. He has a BA and PhD in history and an MA in museum studies from Newcastle University. He was previously a Postgraduate Fellow of the Wolfson Research Institute for Health and Wellbeing, Durham University.

Kate Mattheys is Research Fellow in the Faculty of Health Sciences at Stirling University. Her background is in social care and social work, previously working as a frontline social worker in the North East of England. She holds an MA in sociology from the University of Glasgow, and a Master of social work and a PhD in geography from Durham University. Her research interests focus on inequalities in mental health, participatory methods, learning disabilities and dementia. She was previously a Postgraduate Fellow of the Wolfson Research Institute for Health and Wellbeing, Durham University.

Jon Warren is Vice Principal of St Cuthbert's Society, Durham University. He has a PhD in sociology from Durham University. His research focuses on work, employment, social policy and the industrial history of the North East of England. He has published widely, including *Industrial Teesside, Lives and Legacies: A Post-Industrial Geography* (Palgrave, 2018). He was previously a Senior Research Associate, Institute of Health and Society, Newcastle University, and in the Department of Geography and the Wolfson Research Institute for Health and Wellbeing, Durham University.

Acknowledgements

This book was funded by a Research Leadership grant from the Leverhulme Trust to investigate local health inequalities in an age of austerity (awarded to Clare Bambra, reference RL-2012–006). We would also like to thank our project steering group members: Professor Ray Hudson (chair), Dr Phil Edwards, Helen Hardcastle, Professor Dave Byrne, Mike Robinson, Dr Peter Collins, Dr Sinclair Sutherland, Andrea Edwards, Dr Paul Williams and Professor Peter Kelly. We would also like to thank Jayne Kenworthy, Suzanne Boyd, Jen Cook, Freda Denby and Victoria Morgan who provided administrative support to the project. We would also like to thank Michelle Allan and Chris Orton of the Durham Cartography Unit at Durham University. Thanks are also given to QA Research for their support in delivering the survey, to the Stockton Citizens Advice Bureau, Trussell Trust Stockton, and Thrive Teesside who provided access to their services. Last but by no means least, we would like to thank the research participants from Stockton-on-Tees who made this project possible.

Foreword

Jamie Pearce

Over the past decade there has been growing unease among researchers and policy makers about the long-term health implications of the global economic recession following the financial crisis in 2007, and the subsequent austerity measures implemented in many countries. National responses to this major economic downturn varied substantially but in many cases led to extensive reductions in public expenditure, including cuts to central and local government budgets, welfare services and benefits. While it may take many years to document and understand the full extent of the health implications of the 'Great Recession' and the resulting austerity measures, the early international evidence suggests they have been extremely harmful to physical and mental health. In the UK for example, there is concern that the austerity measures in particular have been instrumental in the observed slowing down in the rate of improvement in life expectancy and an increase in mortality rates at older ages (Hiam et al., 2018).

Although there is emerging evidence that the events of the past decade have had detrimental impacts on physical and particularly mental health outcomes, the implications for health inequalities have received much less attention. This lacuna is despite consistent evidence in the UK showing that austerity measures have resulted in greater socioeconomic inequalities between regions, cities and towns across the country. In particular fiscal retrenchment through changes to benefit entitlements and tax credits as well as reductions in local government expenditure have exerted a far greater impact on some regions of the country, including the North of England. Clearly there is an urgent need to document and understand these spatially uneven processes and to understand the impacts for health and inequalities.

It is for these reasons that this new collection of essays edited by Clare Bambra on the nature of health inequalities in a period of austerity is a welcome and timely contribution to the literature. The book brings together a multidisciplinary team of researchers who turn their collective expertise to examine the impact of the Great Recession and the UK's programme of austerity. The focus is the town of Stockton-on-Tees in Northern England, which provides an exemplary site to study the health impacts of the recent economic, social and political changes in the UK. We learn that Stockton-on-Tees has a long track record of revealing and addressing health inequalities which dates back to the early 20th century. It is also apparent that the local economy has long been reliant on public expenditure and was therefore particularly badly hit by the financial crisis and the UK government's ensuing deficit reduction programme. It is also a highly unequal part of the country with areas of extreme poverty in close proximity to areas of affluence, and there is a 15-year gap in life expectancy between the most and least deprived areas of the town. Stockton-on-Tees therefore provides the ideal setting for a detailed and in-depth multi-method study of the implications of austerity for local health and wellbeing.

The authors of the chapters make a number of important contributions that deepen our understanding of the breadth and depth of the health impacts of the substantial economic and social changes in the UK over the past decade, as well as provide novel insights into the interconnections between health and place. Two contributions in particular stand out. First, the authors' work demonstrates that understanding the extent to which local populations are vulnerable or resilient to the 'shocks' of large structural changes such as those recently seen in the UK requires a long-term historical perspective which examines the changing social, economic and physical resources in these areas. This multigenerational longitudinal perspective on health and place relations has been operationalised in the health geography literature using a 'life course of place' framework, an approach that is having increasing traction among researchers (Lekkas et al., 2017; Cherrie et al., 2018; Pearce et al., 2018)importantly, also that there can be critical periods where the effects of exposure can be greater. Yet few researchers have applied a life-course perspective to the study of health and place, which has resulted in a partial understanding of the dynamics of person-health-place relations. By explicitly recognising that places are spatial-temporal products, and applying a novel longitudinal life-course approach, this study examines the opportunities for incorporating aspects of place into a life-course framework. The focus is the influence of neighbourhood social deprivation and provision of local green space on mental health (particularly anxiety and depression. Various components of the research presented in this edited collection demonstrates the value of considering the historical development of places in revealing underlying social, economic and political drivers of contemporary health trajectories. Second, an important collective contribution of the work presented in the book is demonstrating the vital importance of political drivers in not only affecting population health but also shaping the relations between health and place. The austerity agenda adopted in the UK from 2010 onwards was a political response to the financial crisis of the proceeding period. The research team's work reveals how top-down political decision making profoundly affects the health and wellbeing of many residents of Stockton-on-Tees, and also how place-based factors can mediate these political drivers. Examples include how the local experiences of social connectedness, feelings of exclusion and stigma, and the nature of family life may mediate the pernicious influence of many austerity-related concerns.

In a period of significant global disruption characterised by rapid social, political and demographic changes, health inequalities are almost certain to remain a major challenge in a number of nation states. Developing successful pro-equity approaches to improving population health are likely to remain on the policy agenda of national and local policy makers for the foreseeable future. To make progress in addressing geographical inequalities across the UK and elsewhere there is an urgent need to develop a better understanding how the interconnections between structural changes, political prioritisation and place-based processes operate to shape local health and inequalities. This edited collection is a very welcome entry into these debates and will be of great interest to researchers and practitioners working in fields of health inequalities, public health, social policy, and a range of health-related social science disciplines including political science, sociology and geography. The findings provide a number of important insights into how experiences of place can increase vulnerability or promote resilience to structural changes. Importantly, though, the research presented in the *Health in Hard Times* collection provides a vivid illustration of how health inequalities are largely the result of political choices, including those made in the immediate aftermath of the financial crisis. Therefore, this book should mobilise our political leaders into taking action to address the UK's unenviable track record in health inequalities. Securing equitable and long-term enhancements to population health will require a sustained political commitment to addressing the social and economic divisions expertly exemplified in this important book.

Jamie Pearce is Professor of Health Geography in the Centre for Research on Environment Society and Health, University of Edinburgh.

References

Cherrie, M. P. C., Shortt, N. K., Mitchell, R. J., Taylor, A. M., Redmond, P., Thompson, C. W., Starr, J. M., Deary, I. J., Pearce, J. R. (2018) Green space and cognitive ageing: A retrospective life course analysis in the Lothian Birth Cohort 1936. *Soc. Sci. Med.* 196, 56–65. doi:10.1016/j.socscimed.2017.10.038

Hiam, L., Harrison, D., McKee, M., Dorling, D. (2018) Why is life expectancy in England and Wales 'stalling'? *J. Epidemiol. Community Health* 72, 404LP–408.

Lekkas, P., Paquet, C., Howard, N. J., Daniel, M. (2017) Illuminating the lifecourse of place in the longitudinal study of neighbourhoods and health. *Soc. Sci. Med.* 177, 239–47. doi:10.1016/j.socscimed.2016.09.025

Pearce, J., Cherrie, M., Shortt, N., Deary, I., Ward Thompson, C. 2018. Life course of place: A longitudinal study of mental health and place. *Trans. Inst. Br. Geogr.* doi:10.1111/tran.12246

Preface

The financial crisis of 2007 led to a massive collapse in financial markets across the world. Banks increasingly required state bailouts, stock markets posted massive falls and unemployment rates increased. In 2009, the International Monetary Fund announced that the global economy was experiencing its worst period for 60 years. The global economic recession continued throughout 2009 and 2010, and while many wealthy governments injected liquidity into their economies (so-called quantitative easing) it was also accompanied in many countries, including the UK, by escalating public expenditure cuts: austerity. In the UK, no time was wasted in 'making the most of a crisis' with the 2010–15 coalition government, and then the Conservative majority government elected in 2015, enacting large-scale cuts to central and local government budgets, increasing NHS privatisation and steeply reducing welfare services and benefits. It is estimated that the UK welfare reforms will take nearly £19 billion a year out of the economy (Beatty and Fothergill, 2014). This is equivalent to around £470 a year for every adult of working age in the country. However, despite the claim by prime minister David Cameron (2010–16) that 'we are all in it together', the financial impact of the welfare 'reforms' varies greatly across the country: more than two-thirds of the 50 local authority districts worst affected by the reforms are the northern 'old industrial areas' – places like Liverpool, Stoke and Teesside.

There is an emerging literature that examines the repercussions of austerity for population health. In a wide-ranging and well publicised analysis of the health effects of austerity, for example, Stuckler and Basu (2013) concluded that the overall effects of recessions on health vary significantly by political and policy context, with those countries (such as Iceland or the US) who responded to the financial crisis of 2007/08 with an economic stimulus faring much better – particularly in terms of mental health and suicides – than those countries (for example, Spain, Greece or the UK) who *chose* to pursue a policy of austerity: austerity kills. However, the effects on health inequalities have been less explored – although there are early indications that it is serving to increase existing divides such as that between the North and the South of England and having a negative effect on the health of vulnerable groups, especially those individuals and families, including children and people with disabilities, on the lowest incomes.

It is in this context, that this edited book brings together the findings of a five-year Leverhulme Trust funded research project conducted by researchers based at the Institute for Health and Society, Newcastle University, and the Wolfson Research Institute for Health and Wellbeing, Durham University. The intention of this edited volume is to provide a definitive, detailed examination of the effects of austerity on health inequalities by providing an overview of the historical and contemporary nature of austerity and its impacts on local health inequalities. The book also takes a case study approach, combining methods from across the social sciences (ethnographic and qualitative; epidemiological and quantitative; archival and oral history) to provide a holistic, in-depth, interdisciplinary, mixed methods analysis of the experiences of austerity and the impact on local health inequalities in a specific place: Stockton-on-Tees in the North East of England. Stockton-on-Tees has some of the highest health inequalities of any English local authority with a life expectancy gap of 15 years for men and 12 years for women between the most and least deprived neighbourhoods. Stockton is also a de-industrialised, northern borough, disproportionately affected by the public sector and welfare cuts enacted under austerity. Drawing on insights from epidemiology, public health, geography, sociology, anthropology, history and social policy, this book examines this large health divide in a period of economic constraint and austerity, thereby engaging with, advancing and influencing several key debates around the causes, development and localised experience of health inequalities.

References

Beatty, C. and Fothergill, S. (2014) The local and regional impact of the UK's welfare reforms. *Cambridge Journal of Regions Economy and Society*, 7(1): 63–79

Stuckler, D. and Basu, S. (2013) *The Body Economic: Why Austerity Kills*, London: Allen Lane

ONE

Introduction: Local Health Inequalities in an Age of Austerity

Clare Bambra

This introductory chapter provides the academic and policy/political context of the project. It starts by outlining geographical inequalities in health and some of the debates from the wider academic literature that are important foundations for the following chapters. It then outlines the financial crisis and the austerity measures that have been undertaken in the UK, and provides an overview of the wider literature on the effects of recessions, austerity and welfare cuts on health and health inequalities. The Leverhulme study is then introduced and situated it within this body of work, providing an introduction to the case study method, the case study location (Stockton-on-Tees) and the project as a whole. It concludes by providing an overview of the main chapters in this edited collection, highlighting their themes and connections.

Place matters: geographical inequalities in health

People in the North of England live two years less than those in the South of England and boys born in the most deprived neighbourhoods of England can expect to live nine years less than those born in the most affluent wards (ONS, 2015). For baby girls, the gap is seven years. In our case study town of Stockton-on-Tees in the North East of England, the gaps in life expectancy are even greater – some of the largest in the world – as there is a 15-year gap in life expectancy between men living in the most affluent suburbs such as Hartburn and those living in the most deprived such as Town Centre ward (PHE, 2017). For women the gap is 11 years. Perhaps most shocking of all is that these two neighbourhoods are only two miles apart.

Understanding place helps in terms of thinking of why these stark geographical inequalities in health exist and how our health is inextricably linked to our geographies (Gatrell and Elliot, 2009). Place can be seen either in simple geometric terms as 'a portion of space in which people dwell together' (for example, latitude, longitude, elevation and so on) or in a more experiential (phenomenological) sense as 'a milieux that exercises a mediating role on physical, social and economic processes and which effects how such process operate' or put more concisely 'a distinctive coming together in space' (Agnew, 2011: 318). Places are not though bounded and static (as is often assumed within statistical spatial analysis) but fluid and relational – nodes within social, economic and political networks (Cummins et al., 2007). Place does though require membership, for example, of communities, cities or states. Place both creates and contains social, economic and political relations as well as physical resources. Spatial inequalities in health are therefore a result of a complex mix of economic, social, environmental and political processes – coming together in particular places. Places can be health-promoting (salutogenic) or health-damaging (pathogenic) (Bambra, 2016).

Research has conventionally presented two main explanations as to why these geographical inequalities in health exist: compositional and contextual (Macintyre et al., 2002). The compositional explanation argues that the health of a given area, such as a ward, town or region, is a result of the individual characteristics of the people who live there. Whereas, the contextual explanation argues that area-level health is also in part determined by the nature of the place itself in terms of its economic, social and physical environmental – the nature of the neighbourhood. The relationship between health and place has therefore been thought of in terms of 'who lives here' (compositional/individual) and 'what is this place like' (contextual/neighbourhood). More recently though, drawing on political economy approaches, the political determinants of health (the macro/societal context) have also been examined – how our political choices shape the relationship between health and place (Bambra, 2016). It is also acknowledged though that these approaches are not mutually exclusive and that the health of places results from the interaction of people with the wider local and macro environment (Cummins et al., 2007). The characteristics of individuals are influenced by the characteristics of the area; for example, occupational class can be determined by local school quality and the availability of jobs in the local labour market, while these contextual factors are in turn influenced by the wider political and economic environment. Health is influenced by individual (compositional), collective (contextual)and political-economic (macro) factors.

Who lives here: The compositional approach

The compositional view argues that *who lives here* – primarily the health behaviours (smoking, alcohol, physical activity, diet, drugs) and socioeconomic (income, education, occupation) characteristics of the people living within a particular area (neighbourhood, city, region, country) determines its health outcomes: that *poor people* result in *poor places*. Smoking, alcohol, physical activity, diet and drugs – the five so-called lifestyle factors or risky health behaviours, all influence health significantly. Smoking remains the most important preventable cause of mortality in the wealthy world and is causally linked to most major diseases such as cancer and cardiovascular disease (Jarvis and Wardle, 2006). Likewise, excessive alcohol consumption is related to some cancers as well as other key risks such as high blood pressure. Alcohol-related deaths and diseases are on the increase. Poor diet and low exercise rates can lead to obesity which is a major risk factor for poorer health and longevity. Drug abuse is an increasingly important determinant of death among the young (Bambra et al., 2010). People who do not smoke, have only moderate alcohol intake, consume a large amount of fruit and vegetable and engage regularly in physical activity will on average have a 14-year higher life expectancy than individuals achieving no healthy behaviours (Khaw et al., 2008). So, on average, areas (countries, regions, cities, neighbourhoods) with higher rates of these unhealthy behaviours among their populations would have worse health than others, all things being equal.

The socioeconomic status of people living in an area is also of huge health significance. Socioeconomic status is a term that refers to occupational class, income or educational level (Bambra, 2011). People with higher occupational status (for example, professionals such as teachers or lawyers) have better health outcomes than non-professional workers (for example, manual workers). By way of example, data shows that infant mortality rates were 16% higher in children of routine and manual workers as compared with professional and managerial workers (Marmot, 2010). Having a higher income or being educated to degree level can also have a protective health effect, where as having a lower income or no educational qualifications can have a negative health impact. The poorer someone is, the less likely they are to live in good quality housing, have time and money for leisure activities, feel secure at home or work, have good quality work or a job at all, or afford to eat healthy food – the social determinants of health (Marmot, 2010).

There are three main *pathways* linking socioeconomic status and health: materialist, psychosocial and behavioural/cultural (Skalická et al., 2009; Bartley, 2016). The materialist explanation focuses on income and on what income enables – access to goods and services and exposures to material (physical) risk factors (for example, poor housing, inadequate diet, physical hazards at work, environmental exposures). Psychosocial explanations focus on how social inequality makes people feel – domination/subordination, superiority/inferiority, social support, demands and control – and the effects of the biological consequences of these feelings on health. The behavioural explanation considers the association between socioeconomic status and health to be a result of health-related behaviours as a result of adverse personal/ psychological characteristics or because unhealthy behaviours may be more culturally acceptable among lower socioeconomic groups (Skalická et al., 2009; Bartley, 2016).

What is this place like: the contextual approach

So while the compositional view argues that it is *who lives here* that matters for area health – and that essentially *poor people make poor health*, the contextual approach instead highlights the fact that *what is this place like* also matters for health. Health differs by place because it is also determined by the economic, social and physical environment of a *place*: that *poor places lead to poor health*. Place mediates the way in which individuals experience social, economic and physical processes on their health: places can be salutogenic (health promoting) or pathogenic (health damaging) environments – place acts as a health ecosystem. These place-based effects can also be seen as the *collective* effects of the social determinants of health. There are three contextual aspects to place that have traditionally been considered as important to health: economic, social and physical.

The compositional view takes into account the effects of individual socioeconomic position on health status. Area-level economics instead looks at the health effects of the local economic environment, independent of individual socioeconomic position. Area-economic factors that influence health are often summarised as economic deprivation. They include area poverty rates, unemployment rates, wages, and types of work and employment in the area. The mechanisms whereby the economic profile of a local area affects health are multiple. For example, it affects the nature of work that an individual can access in that place (regardless of their own socioeconomic position). It also has an impact on the services available in a local area, as more affluent areas will attract different services (such as food available locally or physical activity opportunities) than more deprived areas as businesses adapt to the different consumer demands in each area (see access to services in the opportunity structures section below). Area-level economic factors such as poverty are a key predictor of health including cardiovascular disease, all-cause mortality, limiting long-term illness and health-related behaviours (Macintyre, 2007).

Places also have social aspects which affect health. Opportunity structures are the socially constructed and patterned features of the area which may promote health through the possibilities they provide (Macintyre et al., 2002). These include the services provided, publicly or privately, to support people in their daily lives such as child care, transport, food availability or access to a general practitioner or hospital, as well as the availability of health promoting environments at home (for example, good housing quality, access and affordability), work (good quality work) and education (such as high quality schools). For example, local environments can shape our access to healthy – and unhealthy – goods and services thus enhancing or reducing our opportunities to engage in healthy or unhealthy behaviours such as smoking, alcohol consumption, fruit and vegetable consumption or physical activity. One example is the obesogenic environment. The local food environment – such as the availability of healthy and unhealthy foods in the neighbourhood – as well as opportunities for physical activity – are there parks or gyms, is the outside space safe and walkable – are both central components of the obesogenic environment. Research has shown that in some low-income areas food deserts exist where there is a paucity of supermarkets and shops selling affordable fresh food on the one hand, alongside an abundance of convenience stores and fast food outlets selling energy dense junk food and ready meals (Pearce et al., 2007). Low-income neighbourhoods – particularly urban ones – may also inhibit opportunities for physical activity. Associations have been found between neighbourhood availability of fast food and obesity rates in a number of wealthy countries including the UK, the US and New Zealand (Pearce et al., 2007; Burgoine et al., 2011).

A second social aspect of place is collective social functioning. Collective social functioning and practices that are beneficial to health include high levels of social cohesion and social capital within the community. Social capital – 'the features of social organisation such as trust, norms and networks that can improve the efficiency of society by facilitating coordinated actions' (Putnam, 1993: 167) – has been put forward as a social mechanism through which place mediates the relationship between individual socioeconomic status and health outcomes (Hawe and Shiell, 2000). Some studies have found that areas with higher levels of social capital have better health such as lower mortality rates, self-rated health, mental health and health behaviours. More negative collective effects can also come from the reputation of an area (for example, stigmatised places can result in feelings of alienation and worthlessness) or the history of an area (for example, if there has been a history of racial oppression). Place attachment (an emotional bond that individuals or groups have with specific places) in contrast can have a protective health effect (Gatrell and Elliot, 2009). Certain places become marginalised by obtaining a spoiled identity and subsequently become stigmatised and discredited. This can be as a result of environment factors such as air pollution or dirt as well as from social stigma – such as being labelled the obesity capital of Britain as happened with Copeland in West Cumbria (North West England), or economic stigma such as low property prices (Bush et al., 2001). Residents of stigmatised places can also be discredited by association with these place characteristics. A notable case of such placed-based stigma is Love Canal, New York – the location of a toxic waste dump. Research has shown that such place-based stigma can result in psychosocial stress and associated ill health alongside feelings of shame, on top of the physical health effects of air pollution such as respiratory disease (Airey, 2003). Local attitudes, say around smoking, can also influence health and health behaviours either negatively or positively (Thompson et al., 2007).

The physical environment is widely recognised as an important determinant of health and health inequalities (WHO , 2008). There is a sizeable literature on the positive health effects of access to green space, as well as the negative health effects of waste facilities, brownfield or contaminated land as well as air pollution (Bambra, 2016). A (in) famous example of the latter is the so-called 'Cancer Alley' – the 87-mile stretch in the US state of Mississippi between Baton Rouge and New Orleans, the home of the largest petrochemicals site in the country (Markowitz and Rosner, 2003). In 2016 it was estimated that air pollution levels in London accounted for up to 10,000 unnecessary deaths per year (Walton et al., 2015). Another example of how the physical environment of areas varies is in respect to land pollution. A study found that in the US city of Baltimore, mortality rates from cancer, lung cancer and respiratory diseases were significantly higher in neighbourhoods with larger amounts of brownfield land (Litt et al., 2002). Similarly, an English study of differences in exposure to brownfield land found that neighbourhoods with larger amounts of brownfield land have higher rates of poor health and limiting long-term illness (Bambra et al., 2014).

The literature has also established the role of natural or green spaces as therapeutic or health-promoting landscapes. So for example, studies have found that walking in natural, rather than urban, settings reduce stress levels and people residing in green areas report less poor health than those with less green surroundings (Maas et al., 2005). Research also indicates that green space can have an impact on health by attention restoration, stress reduction and/or the evocation of positive emotions (Abraham et al., 2010). Awareness of how such factors differ by place has led to the development of the concept of 'environmental deprivation' – the extent of exposure to key characteristics of the physical environment that are either health promoting or health damaging (Pearce et al., 2010). Environmental deprivation is associated with all-cause mortality: mortality was lowest in areas with the least environmental deprivation and highest in the most environmentally deprived. The unequal socio-spatial distribution of the environmental deprivation has also led to commentators developing the concept of environmental justice (Pearce et al., 2010). The fact that more deprived neighbourhoods are more likely to have air and land pollution and less likely to have green space can be seen as an aspect of social injustice (Pearce et al., 2010).

Poor people and poor places: the relational approach

The contextual and compositional explanations for how place relates to health are not mutually exclusive and to separate them is an over simplification and ignores the interactions between these two levels (Macintyre et al., 2002). The characteristics of individuals are influenced by the characteristics of the area. For example, occupational class can be determined by local school quality and the availability of jobs in the local labour market or, children might not play outside due to not having a private garden (a *compositional* resource), because there are no public parks or transport to get to them (a *contextual* resource) or because it might not be seen as appropriate for them to do so (*contextual* social functioning) (Macintyre et al., 2002). Similarly, areas with more successful economies (for example, more high-paid jobs) will have lower proportions of lower socioeconomic status residents.

Further, the collective resources model suggests that all residents, and particularly those on a low income, enjoy better health when they live in areas characterised by more/better social and economic collective resources. This may be especially important for those on low incomes as they are usually more reliant on local services. Conversely, the health of poorer people may suffer more in deprived areas where collective resources and social structures are limited, a concept known as deprivation amplification: that the health effects of individual deprivation, such as lower socioeconomic status, can therefore be *amplified* by area deprivation (Macintyre, 2007).

Composition and context should not therefore be seen as separate or competing explanations – but entwined. Both contribute to the complex relationship between health and place – an ecosystem made up of people, systems and structures. As Cummins and colleagues (2007: 1826) argue, 'there is a mutually reinforcing and reciprocal relationship between people and place' – a relational approach should therefore be taken to understanding how compositional and contextual factors interact to produce geographical inequalities in health.

Politics matters: the political economy approach

The political economy approach to explaining health inequalities focuses on the social, political and economic structures and relations that may be, and often are, outside the control of the individuals or the local areas they affect (Bambra et al., 2005; Krieger, 2003). Individual and collective social and economic factors such as housing, income and employment – indeed many of the issues that dominate political life – are key determinants of health and wellbeing (Bambra et al., 2015). Why some places and people are consistently privileged while others are consistently marginalised is a political choice – it is about where the power lies and in whose interests that power is exercised. Political choices can thereby be seen as the *causes of the causes of the causes* of geographical inequalities in health (Bambra, 2016).

By way of example, we can examine the causes of stroke or heart disease (Bambra, 2016). The immediate clinical *cause* could be hypertension (high blood pressure). The *proximal cause* of the hypertension itself could be compositional lifestyle factors such as poor diet, of which the contextual cause might be living in a low-income neighbourhood. The causes of the latter are political – low-income neighbourhoods exist because the political and economic system allows them to exist. Wages could be regulated so that they are higher (an example being the living wage), or food prices could be controlled/subsidised (for example, in the US it is meat and corn oil that receive government subsidies, not fruit and vegetables; likewise in the European Union, farmers are encouraged to produce dairy) and neighbourhood food provision does not have to be left to the vagaries of the market (which leads to clustering of poor food availability in poor neighbourhoods).

In this sense, geographical patterns of health and disease are produced by the structures, values and priorities of political and economic systems (Krieger, 2003). Area-level health – be it local, regional or national – is determined, at least in part, by the wider political, social and economic system and the actions of the state (government) and international-level actors (supra-national government bodies such as the European Union, international trade agreements such as the Transatlantic Trade and Investment Partnership, as well as the actions of large corporations): politics can make us sick – or healthy (Schrecker and Bambra, 2015). Politics and the balance of power between key political groups – notably labour and capital – determine the role of the state and other agencies in relation to health and whether there are collective interventions to improve health and reduce health inequalities, and also whether these interventions are individually, environmentally or structurally focused. In this way, politics (broadly understood) is the fundamental determinant of our health inequalities because it shapes the wider social, economic and physical environment and the social and spatial distribution of salutogenic and pathogenic factors both collectively and individually (Bambra, 2016). The effects of recessions and austerity on the social determinants of health and resulting effects on health inequalities is an example of the importance of macro political and economic factors – an example that is the focus of this edited collection.

The Great Recession: implications for health

The financial crisis of 2007 was a result of a downturn in the US housing market, which led to a massive collapse in financial markets across the world. Banks increasingly required state bailouts (for example, in the UK the retail bank Northern Rock was nationalised while in the US Lehmann Brothers investment bank filed for bankruptcy and the mortgage companies Freddie Mac and Fannie Mae were given major government bailouts). Stock markets posted massive falls which continued as the effects in the 'real' economy began to be felt with unemployment rates of over 10% in the US and the Eurozone. In 2009, the International Monetary Fund announced that the global economy was experiencing its worst period for 60 years (Gamble, 2009). The global economic recession continued throughout 2009 and 2010 (leading to the moniker the 'Great Recession') and while many wealthy governments injected liquidity into their economies (so-called quantitative easing), youth unemployment remained high across Europe particularly in the periphery economies of the Eurozone with rates of over 40% (Greece and Spain) and over 30% (Italy and Portugal). General unemployment levels in Greece amounted to 25% of those aged 16–65 in 2015 while poverty rates doubled since the financial crisis of 2007 to 40%. Government debt stood at 177% of gross domestic product (GDP) in 2015.

Recessions, health and health inequalities

National economic wealth (that is, GDP) has long been considered as the major global determinant of population health, with the vast differences in mortality between the developed and developing countries accounted for in terms of differences in economic growth. Changes in the economy therefore potentially have important implications for population health and inequalities in health. Recessions are globally defined as two successive quarters of negative growth in GDP (Gamble, 2009). They are characterised by instability (in terms of inflation and interest rates) and sudden reductions in production and consumption with corresponding increases in unemployment. For example, the Great Recession has been characterised by unemployment rates of around 8.5% in the UK and the US, 10% in France and more than 20% in Spain. The economic downturn since 2008 is popularly referred to as the Great Recession as it has been longer, wider and deeper than any previous economic downturns including the Great Depression of the 1930s.

The short term overall population health effects of recessions are rather mixed with the majority of international studies concluding that all-cause mortality, deaths from cardiovascular disease and from motor vehicle accidents and hazardous health behaviours *decrease* during economic downturns, while deaths from suicides, rates of mental ill health and chronic illnesses *increase* (Bambra, 2011). Studies suggesting that recessions are 'good for health' include Gerdtham and Ruhm's (2006) study of 23 OECD countries from 1960 to 1997 which found that mortality rates actually rose during periods of economic growth. Tapia Granados's (2005) study of mortality trends in the US also found that the overall decline in mortality rates in the 20th century actually reversed during periods of recession. One potential explanation of this inverse relationship between mortality rates and recession is given by Adams (1981), who suggests higher unemployment rates leads to a decrease in business activity and therefore a reduction in work-related deaths, combined with a reduction in alcohol and tobacco consumption as incomes reduce, resulting in a reduction in mortality risks. A number of studies also found road traffic accidents decreased during periods of recession, as people have less need to – and are less able to afford to – drive (Ruhm, 1995, 2000; Tapia Granados, 2005).

In contrast, in terms of mental illness, the literature suggests that recessions are in fact 'bad for health'. For instance, Katikireddi et al.'s (2012) study using Health Survey for England data found that the self-reported mental health of men in England, measured by the General

Health Questionnaire (GHQ12) scores, deteriorated over the two years following recession. Mental health problems such as stress and depression were also found to increase during periods of recession in studies in Spain (Gili et al., 2013), Greece (Economou et al., 2011) and Northern Ireland (Houdmont et al., 2012). In a number of studies this was found to lead to an increase in mortality rates during periods of recession, particularly from suicide (Barr et al., 2012).For example, following the 2007/08 crisis, worldwide an excess of 4884 suicides were observed in 2009 (Corcoran et al., 2015) and over the next three years (2008–10) an excess of 4,750 suicides occurred in the US, 1,000 suicides in England and 680 suicides in Spain. Areas of the UK with higher unemployment rates had greater increases in suicide rates (Hawton et al., 2016). There is also evidence of other increases in poor mental health and wellbeing after the Great Recession including self-harm and psychiatric morbidity (Vizard and Obolenskaya, 2015; Barnes et al., 2017). However, it is not just the mental health of individuals that is affected by recessions, as a number of studies worldwide have found the self-related health status of individuals worsened during times of recession (Zavras et al., 2013).

In many ways it is still too early to be conclusive about the effects of the current Great Recession on health inequalities as few studies have been conducted to date and because it will take time to see the longer-term health impacts, for example on mortality. However, we can look back on data from past economic downturns to gain insights in to what to expect. There were post-war economic downturns in the 1970s, 1980s and 1990s in the UK and other Western countries. Studies of these events suggest that the health effects of economic downturns are unequally distributed across the population thereby exacerbating health inequalities – in some countries but not others (Kondo et al., 2008).

For example, a study of the Japanese working-age population found that economic downturn increased inequalities in self-rated health among men (Kondo et al., 2008), while a Finnish study found that the economic downturn slowed down the trend towards increased inequalities in mortality (Valkonen et al., 2000). Similarly, a comparative study of working age (16–64) morbidity conducted in Finland (Manderbacka et al., 2001), Norway (Dahl and Elstad, 2000), Sweden (Lundberg et al., 2001) and Denmark (Lahlema et al., 2002) found that inequalities in self-reported health remained stable during the 1980s and 1990s. A more recent comparative study of self-reported health from 1991–2010 found that there was a more negative impact on the health of the most vulnerable in England than in Sweden during recessions (Copeland et al., 2013). These findings are also supported by a study of inequalities in pre-term births in the Scandinavian countries which remained broadly stable from 1981 to 2000 despite economic downturn (Petersen et al., 2009).

Studies that have examined whether the health effects of recessions vary by gender have been few and the results varied. For example, Gerdtham and Johannesson (2005) found that recessions increased all-cause mortality in Swedish men, but there was no significant increase in Swedish women. However, Novo and colleagues (2000) study of young adults in Japan found that in fact women suffered worse self-reported health than men during recessions. They also replicated these findings in a similar study in Sweden (Novo et al., 2001). Copeland and colleagues' study (2013) of health inequalities in England and Sweden found that while overall, recessions had a significant positive effect on the health of women – but not men – in both England and Sweden, in England, this improvement was only enjoyed by the most educated women with the health of less educated women declining during recession. In contrast, in Sweden, the health of all women improved significantly during recession regardless of their educational status, although the most educated benefitted the most.

The health inequalities effects of recessions may well therefore be experienced quite differently by otherwise similar individuals and communities due to national policy variation (Whitehead et al., 2000; Burstrom et al., 2010) with more generous welfare systems protecting the health of the population and especially the most vulnerable (Copeland et al., 2013). This may be because the comparatively strong social safety nets they provide buffer against the structural pressures towards widening health inequalities (Lahelma et al., 2002). The welfare states of the social democratic countries – in contrast to others – seem to protect the health of the most vulnerable during economic downturns. These findings are also in keeping with the wider political economy literature which has shown that population health indicators (including self-reported health, life expectancy as well as infant mortality rates) vary by type of welfare state (Bambra, 2011, 2016; Schrecker and Bambra, 2015) with the more generous and encompassing Scandinavian welfare states enhancing population health (especially infant mortality rates).

Austerity: all in it together?

Unlike previous recent recessions of the 1980s and 1990s, the Great Recession was accompanied in many European countries (including the UK, but most notably in Greece and Spain) by escalating public expenditure cuts: austerity. Austerity – reducing budget deficits in economic downturns by decreasing public expenditure and/or increasing taxes – has arguably exacerbated the recession in some European countries, most notably in Greece, Spain, Italy and Portugal. The UK, while not as affected as the Eurozone by the financial crisis and subsequent recession, still embarked on a programme of austerity. Here, no time was wasted in 'making the most of a crisis' with the 2010–15 coalition government (of Conservatives and Liberal Democrats) and then the Conservative government elected in 2015 (and re-elected in 2017), enacting large-scale cuts to central and local government budgets, NHS privatisation as well as steep reductions in welfare services and benefits. In a comparative European study, Reeves et al. (2013) found that the UK austerity policy was the third was most extensive.

Austerity in the UK

It is estimated that the UK welfare reforms enacted up to 2015 will take nearly £19 billion a year out of the economy. This is equivalent to around £470 a year for every adult of working age in the country. The reforms are detailed in Table 1.1. The biggest financial losses arise from reforms to incapacity-related benefits (£4.3 billion a year), changes to tax credits (£3.6 billion a year) and the 1% uprating of most working-age benefits (£3.4 billion a year) (Beatty and Fothergill, 2014). The 2010–15 Housing Benefit reforms result in more modest losses – an estimated £490 million a year arising from the under occupancy charge (most commonly referred to as 'bedroom tax'), for example – but for the households affected the sums are nevertheless still large (for example, £12 per week reductions per 'spare room' for those on benefits that are only around £65 per week).

Despite the claim by the UK Prime Minister David Cameron that 'we are all in it together' (Cameron, 2010), the financial impact of the welfare reforms varies greatly across the country. Tina Beatty and Steven Fothergill of Sheffield Hallam University have shown that austerity will widen the gaps in prosperity between the best and worst local economies across England, increasing the socioeconomic divide between the most and least deprived areas of towns and cities and between richer and poorer parts of the country (Beatty and Fothergill, 2014). Britain's older industrial areas, a number of seaside towns and some London boroughs were hit hardest. Much of the South and East of England (outside London) escaped comparatively lightly. Up

Table 1.1: Welfare reform in the UK, 2010–15

Date	Measure
January 2011	Child Trust Fund abolished
April 2011	Child benefit frozen until 2015
April 2012	A one year time limit to the receipt of contributory ESA for people in the Work Related Activity Group
	Tax credits withdrawn from 'middle income' families
May 2012	Lone Parent Obligations introduced
October 2012	Conditionality, sanctions and hardship payments introduced
January 2013	Child Benefit withdrawn from individuals earning more than £50,000
March 2013	Housing Benefit/Local Housing Allowance restricted to the Consumer Prices Index – as are other benefits
April 2013	Childcare costs covered by Working Tax Credit cut from 80% to 70%
	Council Tax Benefit – 10% reduction for welfare recipients in total payments to local authorities
	Up-rating of working-age benefits not related to disability restricted to 1% (inflation 3.5%)
	Household Benefit Cap (set at £26,000 maximum)
	Social Fund replaced by locally determined schemes for crisis loans and community care grants
	Under occupancy charge or 'Bedroom Tax' if claimant has one spare bedroom (14% reduction) or more (25% reduction)
	Restrictions in access to legal aid
April 2013–October 2017	Migration of all existing working-age Disability Living Allowance (DLA) claimants onto Personal Independence Payment (PIP)
June 2013	Replacement of DLA by PIP for all new claimants
October 2013	Universal Credit – new claims and changes
December 2013	PIP reassessment of DLA claims
April 2014	Universal Credit – transfer existing claims
February 2015	Roll out of Universal Credit
July 2015	Tax credits and family benefits under Universal Credit limited to the first two children only
	Working age benefits frozen for four years from 2016
	Working element of Employment and Support Allowance (ESA) payments reduced to Job Seeker's Allowance (JSA) levels
	The benefit cap reduced to £20,000
	Housing Benefit entitlement restricted for those aged between 18 and 21
	Those earning more than £30,000 pay more if they rent social housing

Source: Based on Bambra and Garthwaite (2015)

to 2015, Blackpool, in the North West of England, was hit worst of all – an estimated loss of more than £900 a year for every adult of working age in the town. The three regions of Northern England alone can expect to lose around £5.2 billion a year in benefit income by 2017. More than two-thirds of the 50 local authority districts worst affected by the reforms are the northern 'old industrial areas' – places like Knowsley, Liverpool, Middlesbrough, Hartlepool, Stoke, Burnley and Stockton-on-Tees. The higher reliance on benefits and tax credits in northern, post-industrial parts of England means that the failure to up-rate with inflation and the reductions to tax credits have a greater impact here (Beatty and Fothergill, 2014) The unequal spatial distribution of welfare cuts is shown in Figure 1.1. These 'reforms' have also disproportionately affected low-income households of working age (Browne and Levell, 2010) while, in contrast, pensioner households have been more protected by, for example, the universal state pension 'triple lock' (a guarantee to increase the state pension every year by whichever is the largest: the rate of inflation, average earnings growth or a minimum of 2.5%) and other universal allowances for older people such as the winter fuel allowance (Green et al., 2017).

Local government spending (excluding police, schools, Housing Benefit) fell by nearly 30% in real terms between 2008 and 2015 in England. In terms of the geographies of local authority budget cuts, a similar pattern to welfare reform emerges: as a general rule, the more deprived the local authority, the greater the financial hit (Beatty and Fothergill, 2014). At the extremes, the worst-hit local authority areas – mainly located in the North (for example, Middlesbrough) – lost around four times as much, per adult of working age, as the authorities least affected by the cuts – found exclusively in the South and East of England (for example, Hart, Hampshire). Here the cuts amounted to less than £50 per head in this period. In contrast, the loss per working age adult in the worst affected northern districts was £470 a year. The geographical distribution of cuts to local authority budgets is shown in Figure 1.2.

These 'upstream', politically driven changes of the UK government's austerity programme have already started to impact on the midstream and downstream determinants of health by unequally changing the social geographies of place and the social determinants of health (Pearce, 2013). For example, there have been spatially concentrated increases in poverty rates across the country – particularly in the North. In 2012, the regions with the lowest levels of poverty were the South East (17%) and East (18%). Rates were much higher in the northern regions with 22% in the North East, 23% in the North West

Figure 1.1: Map of per-head welfare reductions for local authorities, England, 2010–15

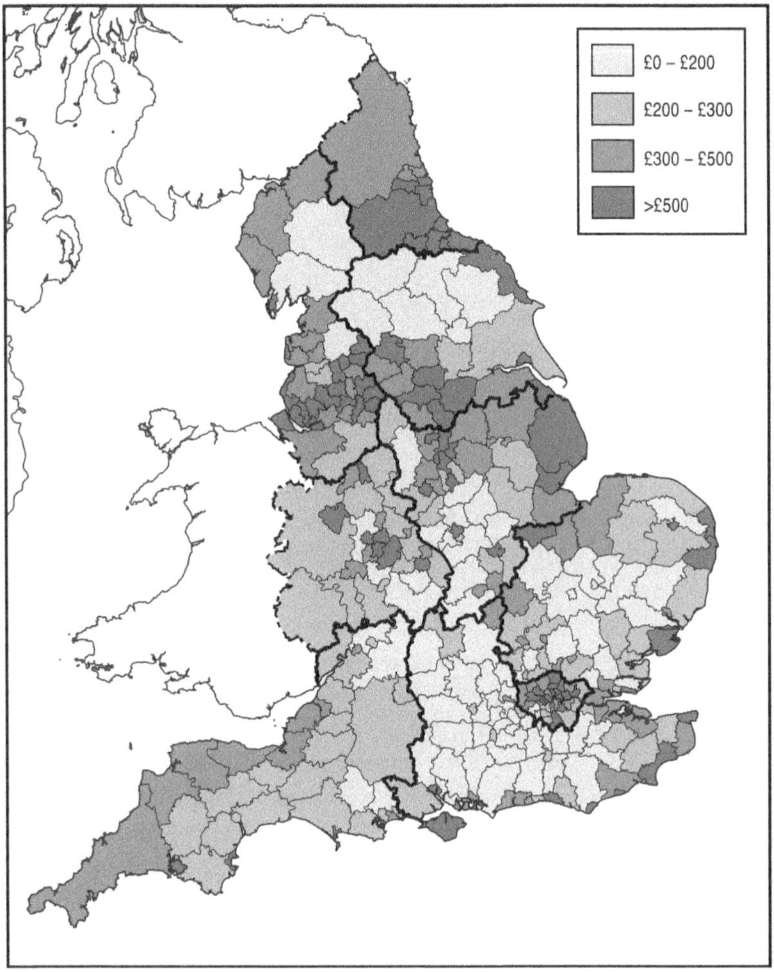

Legend:
- £0 – £200
- £200 – £300
- £300 – £500
- >£500

Source: Based on Whitehead et al (2014)

and 24% in Yorkshire and Humber. Child poverty rates follow similar geographies with rates much higher in the northern regions with 29% in the North East, 31% in the North West and 30% in Yorkshire and Humber, compared with the South East (21%). In certain areas of the North, the child poverty figure is over 35% (for example, 38% in Manchester and 37% in Middlesbrough) – although this is also the case in London (36%) (End Child Poverty, 2014).

Food poverty has also increased since the era of austerity with almost 1 million people accessing emergency food banks in the financial year

Figure 1.2: Map of per-head reductions in local authority budgets, England, 2010–15

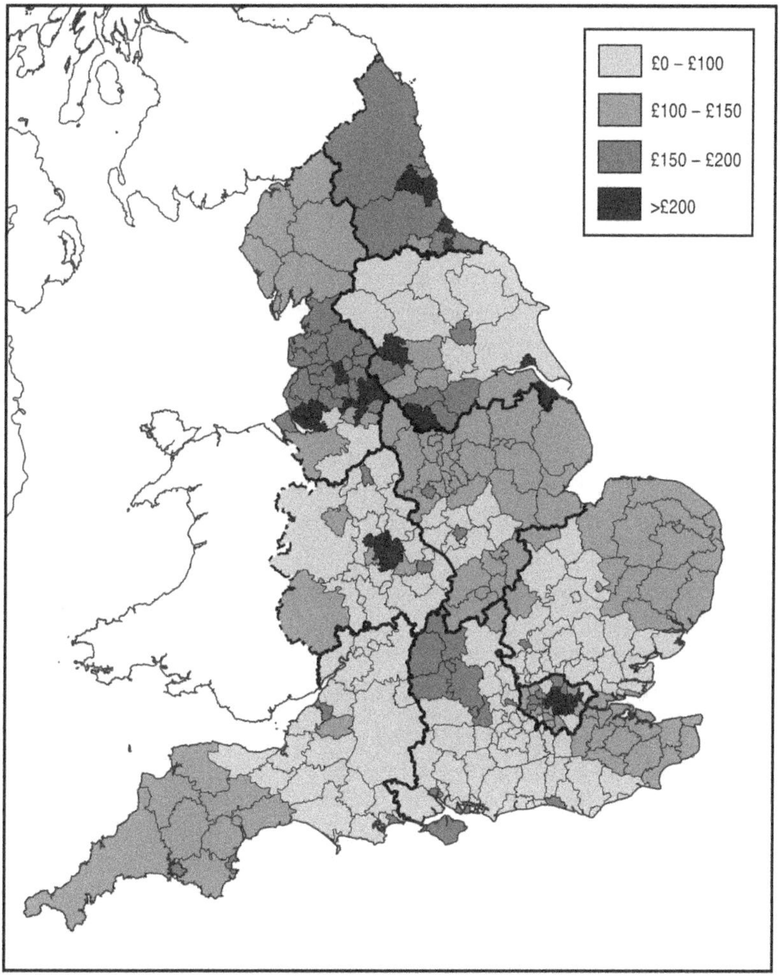

Source: Based on Whitehead et al (2014)

2013–14. In 2013, 83% of Trussell Trust foodbanks reported that benefits sanctions – when payments are temporarily stopped – had resulted in more people being referred for emergency food, and 30% of visits were put down to a delay in welfare payments (Trussell Trust, 2013). Alongside food poverty, many more are now also experiencing fuel poverty as energy costs rise. A household is defined as being in fuel poverty if it needs to spend more than 10% of its income on fuel to maintain a satisfactory heating regime (Bambra and Garthwaite, 2015). In 2011, the number of fuel poor households in England was estimated at around 2.39 million, representing approximately 11% of all English households (Department of Energy and Climate Change, 2013). The North East (21%) and North West (19%) have some of the highest levels of fuel poverty in England, while the South East (11%) has the lowest. Further, the number of children living in fuel poverty has risen to 1.6 million – 130,000 more than in 2010 (Levell and Oldfield, 2011).

Austerity, health and health inequalities

Studies have found that there are important variations in the effects of recessions and economic downturns on population health – depending on policy responses. In a wide-ranging and well publicised analysis of the health effects of austerity, Stuckler and Basu (2013) concluded that the overall effects of recessions on the health of different nations vary significantly by political and policy context with those countries (such as Iceland or the US) who responded to the financial crisis of 2007/08 with an economic stimulus, faring much better – particularly in terms of mental health and suicides – than those countries (for example, Spain, Greece or the UK) who chose to pursue a policy of austerity (public expenditure cuts to reduce government debt). Similarly, Karanikolos et al. (2013) found that across Europe, weak social protection systems increased the health and social crisis in Europe. While, previously, Hopkins (2006) found that in Thailand and Indonesia where social welfare spending was decreased during the Asian recession of the late 1990s, mortality rates increased. However, in Malaysia where no cut backs occurred, mortality rates were unchanged (Hopkins, 2006). Similarly, Stuckler et al.'s (2009) study of 26 European countries concluded that greater spending on social welfare could considerably reduce suicide rates during periods of economic downturn. In the UK, there is evidence that the pressures that austerity has placed on key social and health care services resulted in up to 10,000 additional deaths in 2018 compared with previous years (Dorling, 2018).

However, the effects on health inequalities have generally been less explored. Those studies that have been conducted suggest though that austerity has increased existing health inequalities such as that between the North and the South of England and between deprived and affluent neighbourhoods. For example, since 2007, suicide rates have increased across England – but at a greater rate in the North than the South: by 2012 they were 12.4 per 100,000 in the North West compared with 8.7 per 100,000 in London (ONS, 2014). Similarly, anti-depressant prescription rates have risen since 2007, again with the highest increases in the North: by 2012, anti-depressant prescription rates were highest in Blackpool (331 per 1,000) and lowest in Brent (71 per 1,000) (Spence, 2014). Foodbank use and malnutrition rates have also increased more in the North, with foodbanks in the South actually shipping food up to the North (Trussell Trust, 2013). Barr et al. (2015a) found that geographical inequalities in mental health and wellbeing increased at a higher rate between 2009 and 2013. Further, people living in more deprived areas have seen the largest increases in poor mental health (Barr et al., 2015b) and self-harm (Barnes et al., 2016). Recent data has also shown that there have been significant improvements in mortality rates among lower socioeconomic status women in the South (East, London and South East regions) but not in northern regions – where they have actually increased since 2002/03 (ONS, 2015). Spatially concentrated increases in unemployment over recent years have also led to an increase in the North–South divide for both morbidity and mortality (Moeller, 2013). It has also been shown that austerity is having a disproportionate impact on the health of vulnerable groups especially those individuals and families, including children, on the lowest incomes or in receipt of welfare benefits (MacLeavy, 2011). Internationally, Niedzwiedz et al. (2016) found that reductions in spending levels or increased conditionality may have adversely affected the mental health of disadvantaged social groups.

These early findings about the effects of austerity on health inequalities are in keeping with previous studies of the effects of public sector and welfare state contractions on increases in health inequalities in the UK, US and New Zealand in the 1980s and 1990s. Such prior research into austerity-style policies suggests that such geographically concentrated cuts to the social safety net will only serve to increase existing local divisions in health. Indeed, these studies from the 1980s and 1990s 'are almost certain to understate the scale and multitude of the health consequences' (Pearce, 2013: 2031) given the larger scale of the subsequent spending cuts this time around. Nonetheless, they provide the best available evidence at this stage of the effects on health inequalities of the 'austerity epidemic' (Schrecker and Bambra, 2015).

In terms of health inequalities between individuals of different socioeconomic status (compositional factors), for example, a US study found that while premature mortality (deaths under age 75) and infant mortality rates (deaths before age 1) declined overall in all income quintiles from 1960 to 2002, inequalities by income and ethnicity decreased only between 1966 and 1980, and then increased between 1980 and 2002 (Krieger et al., 2008). The reductions in inequalities

(1966–80) occurred during a period of welfare expansion in the US (the 'War on Poverty') and the enactment of civil rights legislation which increased access to welfare state services. The increases in health inequalities occurred during the Reagan-Bush period of neoliberalism when public welfare services (including health care insurance coverage) were cut, funding of social assistance was reduced, the minimum wage was frozen and the tax base was shifted from the rich to the poor leading to increased income polarisation.

These findings are mirrored in studies of welfare state reductions in New Zealand (Shaw et al., 2005; Blakely et al., 2008; Pearce and Dorling, 2006; Pearce et al., 2006) which found that while general mortality rates declined, socioeconomic inequalities among men, women and children in all-cause mortality increased in the 1980s and the 1990s then stabilised in the early 2000s. Likewise, spatial inequalities in health between local areas and regions increased. The increases in health inequality occurred during a period in which New Zealand underwent major structural reform (including a less redistributive tax system, targeted social benefits, regressive tax on consumption introduced, privatisation of major utilities and public housing, user charges for welfare services and a more deregulated labour market). The stabilisation of inequalities in mortality in the late 1990s and early 2000s was during a period in which the economy improved and there were some improvements in services (for example, better access to social housing, more generous social assistance and a decrease in health care costs).

Research into the health effects of Thatcherism (1979–90) has also concluded that the large-scale dismantling of the UK's social democratic institutions and the early pursuit of 'austerity-style' policies increased socioeconomic health inequalities. Thatcherism deregulated the labour and financial markets, privatised utilities and state enterprises, restricted social housing, curtailed trade union rights, marketised the public sector, significantly cut the social wage via welfare state retrenchment, accepted mass unemployment and implemented large tax cuts for the business sector and the most affluent (Scott-Samuel et al., 2014). In this period, while life expectancy increased and mortality rates decreased for all social groups, the increases were greater and more rapid among the highest social groups so that inequalities increased. Area inequalities also increased in this period with the North and Scotland falling behind the rest of the UK.

These historical increases in social and spatial health inequalities were not inevitable because in the UK – like the US and New Zealand – inequalities in mortality declined from the 1920s to the 1970s as income inequalities were reduced and the welfare state was expanded, showing the importance of social safety nets for health (Thomas et al., 2010). Nonetheless, this all suggests that the health of the poorest people and places suffer the most in times of welfare retrenchment. As northern towns such as Stockton-on-Tees have higher rates of poverty, unemployment and welfare receipt, they will disproportionately suffer the social and health consequences of austerity. This was explored in detail in the Leverhulme study of Stockton-on-Tees and the results are presented in the rest of this edited collection.

The Leverhulme study: local health inequalities in an age of austerity

The existing research literature on recessions, austerity and health inequalities therefore suggests: (1) health inequalities are linked to social and spatial inequalities; (2) the importance of social safety nets in mitigating health inequalities – particularly during recessions; and (3) that austerity is potentially increasing health inequalities by increasing social inequalities (Bambra et al., 2015). It is in this context that the Leverhulme study of local health inequalities in an age of austerity was conducted using Stockton-on-Tees in the North East of England as a case study.

Stockton-on-Tees

The borough of Stockton-on-Tees in the North East of England (Figure 1.3) provides an ideal microcosm for the interdisciplinary study of health inequalities in an age of austerity. It has high health inequalities with life expectancy gaps of 15 years between its most and least deprived wards. It is a highly differentiated place as it has areas with above average rates of poverty existing alongside areas that are very affluent. Stockton-on-Tees is also unusual in political terms as it has historically had a very shifting party political landscape with different political parties holding office at different times in the borough council and has recently been represented by both Conservative and Labour Members of Parliament.

Originally, Stockton-on-Tees was a market borough serving a largely rural and agricultural population. In the 19th century, the shipping and railway industries developed as well as manufacturing and engineering and, to a lesser extent, the chemical industry and iron and steel production. Throughout the 20th century, the borough experienced cyclical economic upheaval and since the 1970s, large-

Figure 1.3: Location of Stockton-on-Tees

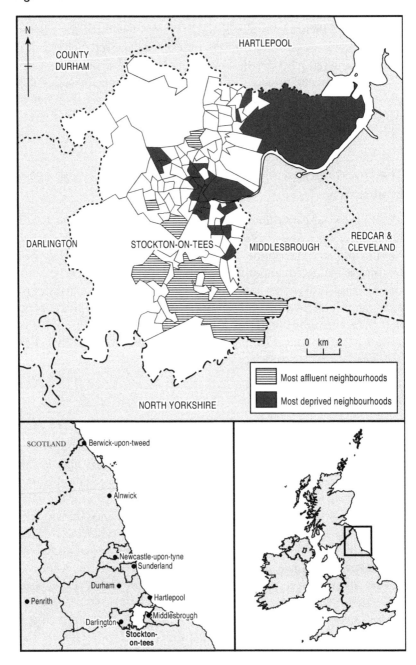

scale deindustrialisation has radically reshaped the character of the area. The shift to a post-industrial service economy in this area has only been partially successful as while most current employment is in the service sector, this is accompanied by well above average levels of long-term worklessness and structural unemployment. The Great Recession saw an above-average rise in unemployment alongside extensive local authority spending cuts and the removal of regional government structures in a local economy that has been historically highly dependent on public expenditure (Beynon et al., 1994). Stockton-on-Tees is thus a prime example of an area affected by economic downturn, the global relocation of primary industries, and which holds a marginal place in the new service based economy. It therefore provides a model contemporary location for case study research into health inequalities.

Further, Stockton-on-Tees was the location 75 years ago of one of the first studies of the effects of economic downturn and austerity on health. George M'Gonigle, the pre-war Medical Officer for Health in Stockton-on-Tees conducted a series of studies into unemployment, housing, income and health during the Great Depression of the 1930s (M'Gonigle, 1936). It also featured in J. B. Priestley's (1934) *English Journey* as well as in the classic commentary on post-industrial decline: *A Place Called Teesside* (Beynon et al., 1994). It was also the location of Margaret Thatcher's famous 1987 'walk in the wilderness'. The borough therefore provided a unique historical and research legacy within which a case study looking at health inequalities in a period of post-industrial economic decline and austerity could be conducted. The past attention paid to Stockton-on-Tees – and its current situation – presented an opportunity to look at continuity and discontinuity in the health and related experiences of a particular place using a case study approach.

Health in Hard Times: *edited collection overview*

This edited collection brings together the findings of a five-year Leverhulme Trust funded research project into the effects of austerity on local health inequalities in Stockton-on-Tees, thereby engaging with, advancing and influencing several key debates around the causes, development and experience of local health inequalities in an age of austerity. It provides a detailed overview of the historical and contemporary nature of austerity and its impacts on local health inequalities by taking a case study approach – using methods from across the social sciences (ethnographic qualitative; epidemiological and quantitative; visual, archival and oral history) and drawing on sociological, geographical, epidemiological, historical and social policy data. These aims are addressed through the following seven substantive empirical chapters that present findings of the key strands of Stockton-on-Tees study. Key overlapping themes include the extent and causes of spatial and socioeconomic inequalities in health in Stockton-on-Tees; the effects of austerity on people's lived experiences and the impact this has on their health; the wider historical context of Stockton-on-Tees within which the process of austerity operated; and the importance of social safety nets in protecting the health and wellbeing of deprived communities.

In Chapter Two, 'Austerity Then and Now', Mike Langthorne uses extensive archival research, to examine the political, economic and social determinants of health and health inequalities during the 1930s within the historical perspective of Stockton-on-Tees. This was the period of the Great Depression – another time in which severe economic downturn as a result of collapsing financial markets, was met with austerity by the UK government and the poor were blamed for their own diminished circumstances. This chapter outlines the effects of government spending cutbacks on unemployment, housing provision, and health care in 1930s Stockton-on-Tees, charting the detrimental consequences for health and health inequalities between neighbourhoods and social classes. It also highlights the pioneering work of Dr George M'Gonigle, medical officer of health for Stockton Borough from 1924–39. The parallels, consistencies, continuities and discontinuities between 1930s Stockton and Stockton today are also examined: austerity then and now. It thereby engages with contemporary debates about health and austerity as well as a long-running debate within historical research about the effects of the Great Depression on health and social inequalities.

In Chapter Three, 'Placing Health in Austerity', Ramjee Bhandari engages with a key debate within geographical research as to whether the health and wellbeing of an individual is determined by their own attributes (the *compositional* theory) and/or the political economy and environmental attributes of the area where the person lives (*contextual* approach). This chapter outlines this key debate and engages with it by using data from a longitudinal household survey conducted in the most and least deprived neighbourhoods of Stockton-on-Tees It examines the explanatory role of compositional and contextual factors and their interaction while longitudinal analysis also examines the effects of austerity and welfare reform as a unique explanatory factor. The survey results indicate that there is a significant gap in general and physical health in Stockton-on-Tees and that compositional-level material factors, contextual factors and their interaction appear to be the major explanations of the health gap. There were few changes in these relationships overtime. The findings are discussed in relation to geographical theories of health inequalities and the context of austerity. It further highlights the importance of 'relational approach' in understanding geographical inequalities in health.

In Chapter Four, 'How the Other Half Live', Kayleigh Garthwaite examines how people living in two socially contrasting areas of Stockton-on-Tees experience, explain and understand the stark health inequalities in their town. Drawing on extensive ethnographic observations and over 100 qualitative interviews, documentary research and photographic data with people living in one of the most and one of the least deprived neighbourhoods, this chapter emphasises the importance of stigma, place and, perception in people's everyday lives at a time of austerity. It focuses on three key themes: lay perspectives on inequalities, place and its meaning(s), and the relationship between austerity, family life and health. The chapter emphasises the importance of conducting ethnographic research across two socially contrasting neighbourhoods; explores how explanations for health inequalities, experiences of place, stigma, social networks and communities and family life are all affected by austerity and cuts to the social security safety net; and it concludes by arguing for a prioritisation of listening to, and working to understand, the experiences of communities experiencing the brunt of health inequalities; especially important at a time of austerity.

In Chapter Five, 'Divided Lives', Kate Mattheys considers how inequalities in mental health are affected by austerity, providing a qualitative account of the *human price* of government policy. Engaging with debates around inequalities in mental health, it uses interview data from people experiencing mental health problems in the most and the least deprived neighbourhoods of Stockton alongside interviews with key stakeholders and local service providers, to show how people experience austerity and inequality in their everyday lives. Austerity measures are shown to have a damaging impact on communities in the most deprived areas while leaving those from less deprived areas relatively unscathed. It documents how people's lived experiences have been shaped by austerity, and how long-standing structural inequalities have been compounded by deeply regressive policies which are shown to be having an incredibly damaging impact on the mental health of those affected by them, causing a chronic level of stress that has a relentless influence on their everyday lives. Although government rhetoric highlighted how we were 'all responsible' for fixing the national debt, this chapter shows how it is those on the lowest incomes and living in the most deprived communities who are paying the highest price.

In Chapter Six, 'Minding the Gap', Nasima Akhter, Kate Mattheys, Jon Warren and Adetayo Kasim examine mental health using survey data. They engage with key debates on the causes of socioeconomic inequalities in mental health by examining the extent and underpinning determinants of the gap in mental health and wellbeing between the most and least deprived neighbourhoods of Stockton-on-Tees. Using data from the longitudinal household survey, it establishes the extent of inequalities in mental health and wellbeing in Stockton-on-Tees and examines the explanatory role of behavioural, psychosocial and material factors in explaining this gap. Longitudinal time trend analysis also examines the effects of austerity and welfare reform on this gap and on the contribution of the underpinning determinants. The results indicate that there is a significant gap in mental health and wellbeing between the most and least deprived neighbourhoods of Stockton-on-Tees and, in contrast to the majority of public health practice and discourse, it is material and psychosocial factors that are the major explanations of the health gap – not to behavioural factors. There were few changes in these relationships overtime. The chapter discusses the implications of the findings for mental health policy and practice in the context of further likely exacerbation during prolonged austerity.

In Chapter Seven, 'Mothers in Austerity', Amy Greer Murphy uses the results of qualitative longitudinal research with mothers to understand the impact that austerity and welfare reform are having on mothers, families and their communities. Women, particularly mothers, face a set of distinct risks under austerity and the narratives presented in this chapter illustrate the detrimental impacts of austerity, as well as demonstrating the intersectional nature of inequalities. Three key themes are explored: first, the effects of austerity and what the continuation of it might mean for respondents' families, communities and livelihoods; second, the increasing devaluation of women's roles as mothers and carers; and third, that gender should be central to our reading of austerity. The chapter shows that mothers play a crucial role within families in insulating against many of the negative effects of austerity. It challenges articulations of austerity which ignore its gendered structure and argues that ongoing austerity measures are exacerbating the deeply gendered dynamics of the politics of inequality and austerity in the UK. The chapter concludes that the ongoing and intensifying pressures austerity is placing on mothers and their families is generating negative health consequences and increasing inequality.

In the concluding Chapter Eight, I bring together the main themes of the previous chapters highlighting the key contributions which the Stockton-on-Tees project has made to the wider social science and health inequalities literature, specifically our understanding of geographical inequalities in health during austerity. It discusses the case study, mixed methods approach, the contribution to understandings of health inequalities, and the effects of austerity on health inequalities. The chapter concludes by outlining the research, policy and practice implications of the project emphasising how our case study shows the need to integrate political economy perspectives into geographical research, the importance of universal social policy safety nets, and for public health practitioners to look beyond health behaviours when designing interventions.

Acknowledgement

Parts of this chapter are based on *Health Inequalities: Where You Live Can Kill You* (Clare Bambra, 2016, Policy Press), material reused with permission.

References

Abraham, A., Sommerhalder, K. and Abel, T. (2010) Landscape and well-being: a scoping study on the health-promoting impact of outdoor environments. *International Journal of Public Health*, 2010. 55(1): 59–69

Adams, O. (1981) Health and economic activity: A time-series analysis of Canadian mortality and unemployment rates. Health Division, Statistics Canada, Ottowa

Agnew, J. (2011) Space and place, in The SAGE handbook of geographical knowledge, J. Agnew and D. Livingstone, Editors. Sage: London, pp. 316–330

Airey, L. (2003) 'Nae as nice a scheme as it used to be': lay accounts of neighbourhood incivilities and well-being. *Health & Place.* 9(2): 129–137

Bambra, C., Fox, D. and Scott-Samuel, A. (2005) Towards a politics of health, *Health Promotion International*, 20: 187–193

Bambra, C. (2011) Work, worklessness and the political economy health. Oxford: Oxford University Press

Bambra, C. (2016) Health inequalities: Where you live can kill you, Bristol: Policy Press

Bambra, C. and Garthwaite, K. A. (2015) Austerity, welfare reform and the English health divide, *Area*, 47: 341–343

Bambra, C., Garthwaite, K., Copeland, A., and Barr, B. (2015) Chapter 12: All in it together? Health inequalities, welfare austerity and the 'Great Recession' in Smith, K. E., Hill, S. and Bambra, C. (eds) Health Inequalities: Critical Perspectives. OUP

Bambra, C., Joyce, K., Bellis, M., Greatley, A., Greengross, S., Hughes, S., Lincoln, P., Lobstein, T., Naylor, C., Salay, R., Wiseman, M., and Maryon-Davies, A. (2010) Reducing health inequalities in priority public health conditions: Developing an evidence based strategy? *Journal of Public Health*, 32: 496–505

Bambra, C., Robertson, S., Kasim, A., Smith, J., Cairns-Nagi, J., Copeland, A., Finlay, N., and Johnson., K. (2014) Healthy land? An examination of the area-level association between brownfield land and morbidity and mortality in England, *Environment and Planning A*, 46(2), pp. 433–54

Barnes, M. C., Gunnell, D., Davies, R., Hawton, K., Kapur, N., Potokar, J., and Donovan, J. L. (2016) Understanding vulnerability to self-harm in times of economic hardship and austerity: A qualitative study. *BMJ* Open 6:e010131

Barnes, M. C., Donovan, J. L., Wilson, C., Chatwin, J., Davies, R., Potokar, J., et al. (2017) Seeking help in times of economic hardship: access, experiences of services and unmet need. *BMC Psychiatry*, 17: 84

Barr, B., Taylor-Robinson, D., Scott-Samuel, A., McKee, M., and Stuckler, D. (2012) Suicides associated with the 2008–10 economic recession in England: time trend analysis. *BMJ: British Medical Journal,* 345

Barr, B. Kinderman, P. and Whitehead, P. (2015a) Trends in mental health inequalities in England during a period of recession, austerity and welfare reform 2004–2013. *Social Science and Medicine* 147: 324–331

Barr, B., Taylor-Robinson, D., Stuckler, D., Loodstra, R., Reeves, A., Whitehead, M. (2015b) 'First, do no harm': are disability assessments associated with adverse trends in mental health? A longitudinal ecological study. *Journal of Epidemiology and Community Health*, 0: 1–7

Bartley, M. (2016) Health inequality: An introduction to theories, concepts and methods. Cambridge: Polity Press

Beatty, C. and Fothergill, S. (2014) The local and regional impact of the UK's welfare reforms. *Cambridge Journal of Regions Economy and Society*. 7(1): 63–79

Beynon, H., Hudson, R. and Sadler, D. (1994) A place called Teesside. Edinburgh, Edinburgh University Press.

Blakely, T., Tobias, M. and Atkinson, J. (2008) Inequalities in mortality during and after restructuring of the New Zealand economy: repeated cohort studies. *British Medical Journal*. 336(7640): 371–375

Browne, J. and Levell, P. (2010) The distributional effect of tax and benefit reforms to be introduced between June 2010 and April 2014: A revised assessment. London: Institute for Fiscal Studies

Burgoine, T., Alvanides, S., and Lake., A. (2011) Assessing the obesogenic environment of North East England, *Health & Place*, 17(3): 738–47

Burstrom, B., Whitehead, M., Clayton, S., Fritzell, S., Vannoni, F., and Costa, G. (2010) Health inequalities between lone and couple mothers and policy under different welfare regimes–the example of Italy, Sweden and Britain. *Social Science and Medicine*, 70(6): 912–920

Bush, J., Moffatt, S., and Dunn, C. (2001) "Even the birds round here cough': stigma, air pollution and health in Teesside, *Health & Place*, 7(1): 47–56

Cameron, D. (2010) Big Society Speech, www.gov.uk/government/speeches/big-society-speech

Copeland A. et al., (2013) 'All in it together? Recessions, health and health inequalities in England and Sweden, 1991 to 2010', American Geographical Association Annual Conference, Los Angeles

Corcoran, P., Griffin, E., Arensman, E., Fitzgerald, A. P. and Perry, I. J. (2015) Impact of the economic recession and subsequent austerity on suicide and self-harm in Ireland: An interrupted time series analysis. *International Journal of Epidemiology*, 44: 969–977

Cummins, S., Curtis, S., Diez-Roux, A., and Macintyre, S. (2007) Understanding and representing 'place' in health research: A relational approach, *Social Science & Medicine*, 65(9): 1825–1838

Dahl, E., and Elstad, J. I. (2000) Recent changes in social structure and health inequalities in Norway. *Scandinavian Journal of Public Health*. Supplement, 55: 7–17

Department of Energy and Climate Change (2003) Fuel Poverty Report

Dorling, D. (2018) Rise in mortality in England and Wales in first seven weeks of 2018, *BMJ* 360: k1090

Economou M., Madianos M., Theleritis C., Peppou L., Stefanis C. (2011) Increased suicidality amid economic crisis in Greece. *Lancet*, 378: 1459

End Child Poverty (2014) Child Poverty map of the UK. www.endchildpoverty.org.uk/images/ecp/130212%20ECP%20local%20report%20final(2).pdf

Gamble, A. (2009) The spectre at the feast: Capitalist crisis and the politics of recession. Basingstoke: Palgrave

Gatrell, A. and Elliot, S. (2009) Geographies of health: An introduction. London: Wiley

Gerdtham, U. and Johannesson, M. (2005) Business cycles and mortality: results from Swedish microdata. *Social Science and Medicine*, 60: 205–218

Gerdtham, U. and Ruhm, C. (2006) Deaths rise in good economic times: Evidence from the OECD. *Economics and Human Biology*, 4: 298–316

Gili, M., Roca, M., Basu, S., McKee, M., and Stuckler, D. (2013) The mental health risks of economic crisis in Spain: evidence from primary care centres, 2006 and 2010. *The European Journal of Public Health*, 23(1), 103–108

Green, JM, Buckner, S., Milton, S., Powell, K., Salway, S and Moffatt, S. (2017) A model of how targeted and universal welfare entitlements impact on material, psycho-social and structural determinants of health in older adults. *Social Science & Medicine*, 187: 20–28

Hawe, P., and Shiell, A. (2000) Social capital and health promotion: a review. *Social Science & Medicine*, 51(6): 871–885

Hawton, K., Bergen, H., and Geulayov, G. (2016) Impact of the recent recession on self-harm: a longitudinal ecologic and patient level investigation from multicentre study of self-harm in England. *J Affect Disord*, 191, doi:10.1016/j.jad.2015.11.001

Hopkins, S. (2006) Economic stability and health status: Evidence from East Asia before and after the 1990s economic crisis. *Health Policy*, 75: 347–357

Houdmont, J., Kerr, R., and Addley, K. (2012) Psychosocial factors and economic recession: the Stormont Study. *Occupational medicine*, 62(2): 98–104

Jarvis, M., and Wardle, J. (2006) 'Social patterning of individual health behaviours: The case of cigarette smoking', in M. Marmot and R. Wilkinson (eds.) *The social determinants of health*, Oxford: Oxford University Press

Karanikolos, M., Mladovsky, P., Cylus, J., Thomson, S., Basu, S., Stuckler, D., et al. (2013) Financial crisis, austerity, and health in Europe. *The Lancet*, 381 (9874): 1323–1331

Katikireddi, S. V., Niedzwiedz, C. L., and Popham, F. (2012) Trends in population mental health before and after the 2008 recession: a repeat cross-sectional analysis of the 1991–2010 Health Surveys of England. *BMJ*, 2(5)

Khaw, K., Wareham, N., Bingham, S., Welch, A., Luben, R., and Day, N. (2008) Combined impact of health behaviours and mortality in men and women: The EPIC-Norfolk prospective population study, *Plos Medicine*, 5(3): 39–47

Kondo, N., Subramanian, S., Kawachi, I., Takeda, Y. and Yamagata, Z. (2008) Economic recession and health inequalities in Japan: analysis with a national sample, 1986–2001. *Journal of Epidemiology and Community Health*, 62: 869–875

Krieger N. (2003) 'Theories for social epidemiology in the twenty-first century: an ecosocial perspective', in: R. Hofrichter (ed) Health and social justice: Politics, ideology, and inequity in the distribution of disease – A public health reader. San Francisco: Jossey-Bass, pp. 428–450

Krieger, N., et al. (2008) The fall and rise of US inequities in premature mortality: 1960–2002. *Plos Medicine.* 5(2): 227–241

Lahelma, E., Kivelä, K., Roos, E., Tuominen, T., Dahl, E., Diderichsen, F. and Yngwe, M. Å. (2002) Analysing changes of health inequalities in the Nordic welfare states. *Social Science and Medicine*, 55(4): 609–625

Levell, P. and Oldfield, Z. (2011) The spending patterns and inflation experience of low-income households over the past decade, in IFS Commentary C119, Institute of Fiscal Studies: London

Litt, J., Tran, N., and Burke, T. (2002) Examining urban brownfields through the public health 'macroscope', *Environmental Health Perspectives*, 110(2): 183–193

Lundberg, O., Diderichsen, F., and Yngwe, M. Å. (2001) Changing health inequalities in a changing society? Sweden in the mid-1980s and mid-1990s. *Scandinavian Journal of Public Health*, 29: 31–39

Macintyre, S. (2007) Deprivation amplification revisited; or, is it always true that poorer places have poorer access to resources for healthy diets and physical activity? *International Journal of Behavioral Nutrition and Physical Activity*, 4(32): 1–7

Macintyre, S., A. Ellaway, and S. Cummins (2002) Place effects on health: How can we conceptualise, operationalise and measure them? *Social Science & Medicine.* 55(1): 125–139

MacLeavy, J. (2011) A 'new politics' of austerity, workfare and gender? The UK coalition government's welfare reform proposals. *Cambridge Journal of Regions Economy and Society.* 4(3): 355–367

Maas, J., Verheij, R., de Vries, S., Spreeuwenberg, P., and Groenewegen, P. (2005) Green space, urbanity, and health: how strong is the relation? *European Journal of Public Health*, 60(7): 587–592

Manderbacka, K., Lahelma, E., and Rahkonen, O. (2001) Structural changes and social inequalities in health in Finland, 1986–1994. *Scandinavian Journal of Public Health*, 29: 41–54

Markowitz, G., and Rosner, D. (2003) Deceit and denial: The deadly politics of industrial pollution, New York: University of California Press

Marmot, M. (chair) (2010) Fair Society Health Lives: The Marmot Review. London: University College

M'Gonigle GCM. (1936) Poverty and public health. London, Victor Gollantz

Moeller, H. (2013) Rising unemployment and increasing spatial health inequalities in England: further extension of the North-South divide. *Journal of Public Health*. 35(2): 313–321

Niedzwiedz, C. L. Mitchell, R. J. Shortt, N. K. and Pearce, J. R. (2016) Social protection spending and inequalities in depressive symptoms across Europe. *Social Psychiatry and Psychiatric Epidemiology*, pp. 1–10

Novo, M., Hammerstrom, A. and Janlert, U. (2000) Smoking habits – a question of trend and unemployment? A comparison of young men and women between boom and recession. *Public Health*, 114: 460–463

Novo, M., Hammerstrom, A. and Janlert, U. (2001) Do high levels of unemployment influence the health of those who are not unemployed? A gendered comparison of young men and women during boom and recession. *Social Science and Medicine*, 53: 293–303

ONS – Office for National Statistics (2014) Suicides in the United Kingdom: 2012 Registrations

ONS (2015) Inequality in healthy life expectancy at birth by national deciles of area deprivation: England, 2011 to 2013.

Pearce, J. (2013) Financial crisis, austerity policies, and geographical inequalities in health. Introduction/Commentary. *Environment and Planning A*, 45(9): 2030–2045

Pearce, J. and Dorling, D. (2006) Increasing geographical inequalities in health in New Zealand, 1980–2001. *International Journal of Epidemiology*. 35(3): 597–603

Pearce, J., et al. (2006) Geographical inequalities in health in New Zealand, 1980–2001: the gap widens. *Australian and New Zealand. Journal of Public Health*. 30(5): 461–466

Pearce, J., Blakely, T., Witten, K., and Bartie, P. (2007) Neighborhood deprivation and access to fast-food retailing – A national study, *American Journal of Preventive Medicine*, 32(5): 375–382

Pearce, J., Richardson, E., Mitchell, R., and Shortt, N. (2010) Environmental justice and health: the implications of the socio-spatial distribution of multiple environmental deprivation for health inequalities in the United Kingdom, *Transactions of the Institute of British Geographers*, 35(4): 522–539

Petersen, C. B., Mortensen, L. H., Morgen, C. S., Madsen, M., Schnor, O., Arntzen, A., Gissler, M., Cnattingius, S. and Nybo Andersen., A. (2009) Socio-economic inequality in preterm birth: a comparative study of the Nordic countries from 1981 to 2000. *Paediatric and Perinatal Epidemiology* 23(1): 66–75

PHE (Public Health England) (2017) Public Health Outcome Framework.

Priestley, J. B. (1934) English Journey. Heinemann/Gollancz, London.

Putnam, R. (1993) Making democracy work: Civic traditions in modern Italy, Princeton: Princeton University Press

Reeves, A., Basu, S., McKee, M., Marmot, M., and Stuckler, D. (2013) Austere or not? UK coalition government budgets and health inequalities. *Journal of the Royal Society of Medicine*, 106(11): 432–436, doi: 10.1177/0141076813501101

Ruhm, C. J. (1995) Economic conditions and alcohol problems. *Journal of Health Economics*, 14, 583–603

Ruhm, C. J. (2000) Are recessions good for your health? *Quarterly Journal of Economics*, 617–50

Schrecker, T., and Bambra., C. (2015) How politics makes us sick: Neoliberal epidemics, London: Palgrave Macmillan

Scott-Samuel, A., Bambra, C., Collins, C., Hunter, D., McCartney, G., and Smith, K. (2014) The impact of Thatcherism on health and well-being in Britain, *International Journal of Health Services*, 44(1): 53–71

Shaw, C., et al. (2005) Do social and economic reforms change socioeconomic inequalities in child mortality? A case study: New Zealand 1981–1999. *Journal of Epidemiology and Community Health.* 59(8): 638–644

Skalická, V., Lenthe, F., Bambra, C., Krokstad, S., and Mackenbach J. (2009) Material, psychosocial, behavioural and biomedical factors in the explanation of socio-economic inequalities in mortality: evidence from the HUNT study. *International Journal of Epidemiology*, 38: 1272–1284

Spence, R. (2014) Antidepressant prescribing:, Trends in the prescribing of antidepressants in primary care. The Health Foundation, Nuffield Trust

Stuckler, D. and Basu, S. (2013) The body economic: Why austerity kills, London: Allen Lane

Stuckler, D., Basu, S., Suhrcke, M., Coutts, A. and McKee, M. (2009) The public health effect of economic crises and alternative policy responses in Europe: an empirical analysis. *Lancet*, 374: 315–23

Tapia Granados, J. A. (2005) Increasing mortality during the expansions of the US economy, 1900–1996. *International Journal of Epidemiology*, 34: 1194–1202.

Thomas, B., Dorling, D. and Smith, G. D. (2010) Inequalities in premature mortality in Britain: observational study from 1921 to 2007. *British Medical Journal*, 341

Thompson, L., Pearce, J., and Barnett, R. (2007) Moralising geographies: stigma, smoking islands and responsible subjects, *Area*, 39(4): 508–17

Trussell Trust (2013) Biggest ever increase in UK foodbank use: 170% rise in numbers turning to foodbanks in last 12 months. https://trusselltrust.org/wp-content/uploads/sites/2/2015/06/BIGGEST-EVER-INCREASE-IN-UK-FOODBANK-USE.pdf

Valkonen, T., Martikainen, P., Jalovaara, M., Koskinen, S., Martelin, T. and Makela, P. (2000) Changes in socioeconomic inequalities in mortality during an economic boom and recession among middle-aged men and women in Finland. *European Journal of Public Health*, 10: 274–80

Vizard, P. and Obolenskaya, P. (2015) The coalition's record on health: Policy, spending and outcomes 2010–2015. Social Policy in a Cold Climate Working Paper, 16

Walton, H., Dajnak, D., Beevers, S., Williams, M., Watkiss, P., and Hunt, A. (2015) Understanding the health impacts of air pollution in London, London: Kings College

Whitehead, M., Burström, B. and Diderichsen, F. (2000) Social policies and the pathways to inequalities in health: a comparative analysis of lone mothers in Britain and Sweden. *Social Science and Medicine*, 50(2): 255–270

Whitehead, M. (chair), Bambra C., Barr B., Bowles J., Caulfield R., Doran T., Harrison D., Lynch A., Pleasant S., and Weldon, J. (2014) Due North: Report of the inquiry on health equity for the North University of Liverpool and Centre for Local Economic Strategies, Liverpool and Manchester (www.cles.org.uk/publications/due-north-report-of-the-inquiry-on-health-equity-for-the-north/)

WHO – World Health Organization (2008) Commission on the Social Determinants of Health: Closing the gap in a generation, World Health Organization: Geneva

Zavras, D., Tsiantou, V., Pavi, E., Mylona, K., and Kyriopoulos, J. (2013) Impact of economic crisis and other demographic and socio-economic factors on self-rated health in Greece. *The European Journal of Public Health*, 23(2): 206–210

TWO

Austerity Then and Now

Mike Langthorne

Introduction

This chapter uses extensive archival research, to examine the political, economic and social determinants of health and health inequalities during the 1930s within the historical perspective of Stockton-on-Tees. This was the period of the Great Depression – another time in which severe economic downturn as a result of collapsing financial markets was met with austerity by the UK government and the poor were blamed for their own diminished circumstances. This chapter outlines the effects of government spending cutbacks on unemployment, housing provision and healthcare in 1930s Stockton-on-Tees, charting the detrimental consequences for health and health inequalities between neighbourhoods and social classes. It also highlights the pioneering work of Dr George M'Gonigle, medical officer of health for Stockton Borough from 1924–39. The parallels, consistencies, continuities and discontinuities between 1930s Stockton and Stockton today are also examined: austerity then and now. It thereby engages with contemporary debates about health and austerity as well as a long-running debate within historical research about the effects of the Great Depression on health and social inequalities.

The 1930s provide a benchmark against which unemployment and its effects on communities are measured. 'The Depression', and the depression which it brought both economically, socially and psychologically, have left a lasting impression on the collective memory. Phrases such as 'a return to the conditions of the thirties' are often used in the media and politics, but what does that mean and is such an analogy justified? This chapter will examine the themes of unemployment, housing, healthcare and the health of Stockton during this period of austerity. The austerity imposed in response to the 2007/08 recession echoes to some extent the austerity experienced in the 1930s. Both periods involve a reduction of state spending particularly in welfare and public services. As such, this provides an opportunity to reflect on the effects of austerity on health inequality across the two eras. Comparing the political and social effects on Stockton in the 1930s with those experienced currently – austerity then and now – will indicate whether or not the results are consistent between these two periods.

Background to the 1930s

A slow economic recovery following the First World War had become impeded by Britain rejoining the gold standard at the end of 1925 at an exchange rate which made British exports expensive to the world market. The gold standard is a monetary system where the value of a country's currency is directly linked to the value of gold. A country that uses the gold standard sets a fixed price for gold and buys and sells gold at that price. In the case of Britain, this exchange rate 'almost certainly overvalued the pound in relation to other currencies' (McKibbin, 1975, p. 110), not least the US, German, French and Belgian currencies (Skidelsky, 1998), leading to the export difficulties. The subsequent Wall Street Crash in 1929, whereby share values in the US plummeted rapidly and the resultant global financial crisis followed, further exacerbated an already difficult situation. Demand for British manufactured goods, coal, agricultural produce and shipping collapsed (Williamson, 1992). National income fell while costs of supporting unemployment rose due to the higher numbers of those claiming benefits. The incumbent minority Labour government, headed by Ramsay MacDonald, disintegrated over disagreements regarding imposition of austerity measures in response to the recession: more specifically the dispute revolved around an unwillingness to implement cuts to public sector wages and public spending, including reductions in benefits and increases to insurance contributions which had been recommended by the Royal Commission on Unemployment Insurance in June 1931 (Macmillan, 1966; McKibbin, 1975). Economist John Maynard Keynes advocated government spending to invest in the economy, which would sustain businesses and employment. He believed that cuts at this point would be 'self-defeating' and would 'inadvertently prolong' the recession (Burton, 2016, p. 13). However, fearing a budget deficit, the recommendations of the royal commission advocated increased taxes on the rich to recoup £24 million and economies totalling £96 million, including £64 million via a reduction in unemployment assistance (Taylor, 1965). An interim coalition 'national government' was formed, and a general election soon followed which resulted in a Conservative-dominated national government, although MacDonald remained as prime minister. Public sector wages were cut – by 25% in some sections of the Royal Navy – unemployment benefits were reduced by 10% alongside increased national insurance contributions (Needham, 2013), and taxes increased. However, recovery did not begin until Britain again withdrew from the gold standard in September 1931, devaluing the pound and stimulating exports. Unemployment began to decline through the middle of the decade, although improvements were mainly experienced in the south of the country.

Teesside's, and particularly Stockton's, economy relied heavily on iron and steel, shipbuilding and heavy engineering, much of the latter dependent on marine engineering and bridge building (Beynon et al., 1994). Indeed, by 1914 it was an important centre of industry, and Teesside was one of the world's leading shipbuilding areas. However, nationally 36 shipyards had closed by the end of the decade (Perry, 2000, p. 54), and output had fallen by 85% by 1933 due largely to the economic slump caused by the Wall Street Crash and the accompanying fall in exports on which the area relied. A sharp rise in unemployment followed, suffered disproportionately by the major industrial areas such as the North East of England.

Unemployment

A marked increase in unemployment occurred nationally from 1929 to 1932, as illustrated in Figure 2.1. For example, by 1934 while the rate for unemployment was 16.7% the rate for long-term unemployment nationally was 29.7%, and was as high as 51.4% in the most depressed areas (Denman and McDonald, 1996, pp. 5–11; Perry, 2000, p. 47).

The unemployed had three potential sources of financial assistance – unemployment benefit for those who had accrued enough unemployment insurance; government-funded transitional benefit for those who had not accrued enough insurance, or who had exhausted their unemployment benefit; out-relief (also called outdoor relief or public assistance) for the most destitute who had no entitlement to insurance-funded unemployment benefit. Levels of benefits varied and fluctuated throughout the decade.

By November 1930, County Durham, which at this time included Stockton, had the worst unemployment rate in the country at 29.6% of the working population (*Darlington & Stockton Times*, 1930a, p. 14). The Bishop of Durham, Hensley Henson, commented on the effects of unemployment. He acknowledged that some unemployed people accepted life on the dole easily, but held that the majority 'bitterly

Figure 2.1: UK unemployment 1929–39, yearly average

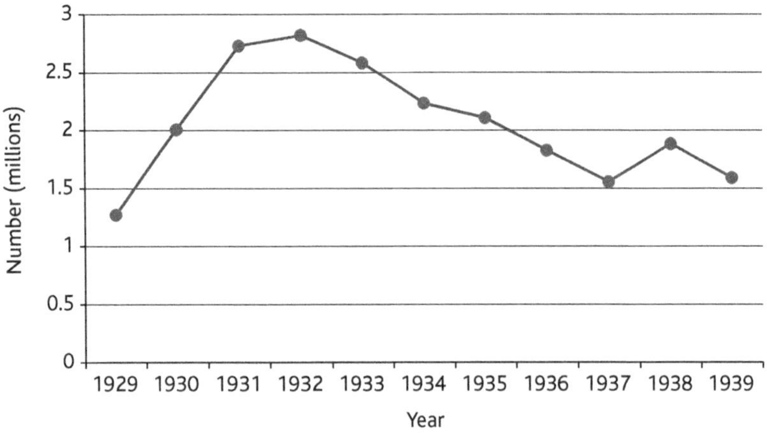

Source: Created using data from Denman and McDonald 1996, pp. 5–11

resented their misfortune'. The major consequences of unemployment that he observed were the low morale and loss of self-respect of workmen due to idleness (*Darlington & Stockton Times*, 1930b, p. 13). Conditions had not markedly improved by 1934 when a report by the government's special investigator, Conservative MP Captain D. Euan Wallace, stated that in County Durham '... it has been impossible to avoid a strong general impression that the area as a whole is losing hope' (Ministry of Labour, 1934, p. 74). He went on to say that

> Prolonged unemployment is destroying the confidence and self-respect of a large part of the population. Their fitness for work is being steadily lost and the anxiety of living always upon a bare minimum without any margin of resources... is slowly sapping their nervous strength and their powers of resistance. (*Darlington & Stockton Times*, 1934a, p. 3; Ministry of Labour, 1934, p. 76)

National and regional politics of unemployment

A struggling export market alongside failing businesses meant that the national economy was faltering and income to the Treasury was suffering. The rise in unemployment further depleted government funds. The unemployment insurance scheme was paying out more in benefits than it was taking in contributions, and therefore had to be subsidised from central government.

In July 1931 the Committee on National Expenditure – named the 'May Committee' after its chairman – predicted, incorrectly, a budget deficit of £120 million for 1931/32. This figure was used to justify the imposition of austerity which followed. Targeting savings of £96 million the Conservative-dominated national government cut unemployment benefits by 10%. Furthermore, qualification for transitional benefit was means-tested by the Public Assistance Committee (PAC) of Durham County Council (Taylor, 1965; Garside, 1990, pp. 59–60).

Every category of benefits suffered the 10% reduction apart from the amount for dependent children (see Table 2.1).

The 10% cut in unemployment benefit was not restored until July 1934. Additionally, means testing for transitional benefits (the 'dole') became more stringent. Prior to 1931 any means testing had examined the economic status of an individual. From 1931 the means test instead determined whether a household as a whole had sufficient income to disqualify them for assistance. Cases could be harshly dealt with:

> a young married man paid £1 per week rent and rates. His only income was 10s per week which he received for renting out 2 rooms. The PAC decided he did not need assistance and reduced his benefit from 23s 3d to nil. (*Darlington & Stockton Times*, 1932, p. 3)

Table 2.1: Unemployment Benefit before and after the cuts

	Old payment	New payment
Man over 21	17s 0d[a]	15s 3d
Woman over 21	15s 0d	13s 6d
Dependent child	2s 0d	2s 0d
Young man 18–21	14s 0d	12s 6d
Young woman 18–21	12s 0d	10s 9d
Boy aged 17	9s 0d	8s 0d
Girl aged 17	7s 6d	6s 9d
Boy aged 16	6s 0d	5s 6d
Girl aged 16	5s 0d	4s 6d

Note: [a] s = shilling; d = pence. During the 1930s in the UK the units of currency were pounds (£), shillings and pence (or pennies). A pound equalled 20 shillings, and a shilling equalled 12 pence. A shilling equates to approximately £3.10 in today's money.

Source: County Council of Durham 1933, p. 48; *Darlington & Stockton Times* 1931c, p. 5

Unemployment in Stockton

Stockton suffered a sharp rise in unemployment following the onset of the Depression in 1929 (Figure 2.2).

In 1931 Neville Chamberlain, UK Chancellor of the Exchequer, wrote to local authorities urgently advocating economy in municipal spending. He stated that local authorities should decide themselves how best to reduce the drain on their economic resources, either through cuts or by raising rates. A number of schemes in Stockton that would have provided training or employment were adversely affected. Stockton Corporation proposed seven infrastructure projects as part of a programme of unemployment relief works. Funding for such schemes relied on the support of a 75% grant from the government's Unemployment Grants Committee (Markets and Properties Committee, 1931). The 'May Committee' report recommended that the Unemployment Grants Committee should reduce expenditure, reflecting the adoption of austerity. Consequently, in December 1931 the Committee decided to accept no further applications for grant aid. A request from Stockton Council to the government that they restore the grants for approved local unemployment schemes was rejected on the grounds of expense to both the state and to local authorities, and the poor provision of real employment (*Darlington & Stockton Times*, 1933a, p. 3; Parliamentary, Finance and General Purposes Committee, 1933a).

Figure 2.2: Unemployment in Stockton, 1929–38

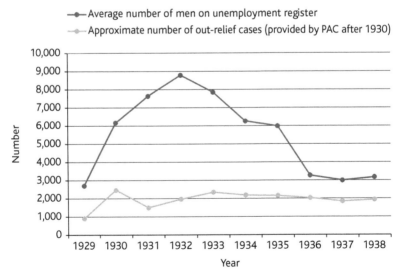

Source: Based on M'Gonigle 1929–32, 1933a, 1934, 1935a, 1936–38

Stigma and support

Sympathy for the unemployed existed, but was not universal. The local newspaper attached a stigma particularly to those on the 'dole' as being scroungers seeking to exploit the benefit system (*Darlington & Stockton Times*, 1935a, p. 10). Comment was made that, although the unemployed may have resented 'what seem to be the inquisitional methods' of the PAC in applying the means test, it was necessary as there had been so many cases of deception (*Darlington & Stockton Times*, 1931a, p. 9). There was a complaint that, to circumvent the rule that assessed income for the household rather than the individual, claimants had left home to move into lodgings, thereby having no other income available for support from family members and therefore qualifying for transitional benefit. This was regarded as a 'trick' (*Darlington & Stockton Times*, 1931b, p. 8).

Despite some vilification of the unemployed, charities and churches made efforts to ameliorate their suffering. Stockton and Thornaby District Women's Association (1935) donated clothing and blankets. The Mayor's Clothing Bureau, alongside the Personal Service League, had distributed 40,000 garments by 1935 (*Darlington & Stockton Times*, 1935b, p. 3). Affordability of a nutritious diet was a major problem for those on low incomes. In 1932, 250 allotments were provided for the use of the unemployed by the Mayor's Committee for the Help of the Unemployed, with the assistance of Durham County Education Committee (*Darlington & Stockton Times*, 1931d, p. 10; M'Gonigle, 1935a). Food produced from these allotments provided a valuable addition to the diet of the unemployed families. Men working on the allotments confirmed that working on the allotments had also greatly alleviated their depression (*Darlington & Stockton Times*, 1933b, p. 7). The Salvation Army were also a source of free food: 'If the band was playing round the streets when I was young I always used to follow it and get a basin of soup ... I'd join anything for a bite to eat, I'll tell you that' (Nicholas, 1986, p. 182).

The Mayor's Committee also provided boot-repair shops and, with the support of local churches, arranged meetings and concerts, provided rest rooms and organised recreational activities and sports (Stockton Baptist Tabernacle, March 1927 to September 1944; Stockton Unitarian Church, October 1927 to September 1933; Cemeteries and Parks Committee, 1931; Yarm Road Congregational Church, 1935).

Unemployed workers also organised themselves to take action. Both the National Unemployed Workers' Movement (NUWM) and the Stockton and Thornaby Unemployed Workers Association were active in Stockton. Predominantly these organisations lobbied the local council for improved benefits, lower rents, food and employment schemes (Town Council, 1931a; Parliamentary, Finance and General Purposes Committee, 1931b). The NUWM organised hunger marches and demonstrations, and provided legal support for claimants to challenge harsh benefits rulings (Croucher, 1987, p. 114). The NUWM also carried out local charitable work:

> ... we used to run jumble sales but ... it was hard to get old clothes. Also we joined together to help somebody who was really poor and having a baby, say, we'd have a street collection round the doors, even if they could just give you a piece of bread. (Watson, 2014, p. 108)

Housing: unhealthy areas

The town of Stockton grew from the banks of the River Tees, and expanded over time to encompass outlying villages within its suburbs. The older areas closest to the centre of town and to the riverbank included some of the most dilapidated and unhealthy housing, as Figure 2.4 illustrates. Outlying areas such as Hartburn ward benefited from having more modern, less densely packed housing. By the 1930s

Figure 2.3: Constables Yard, Stockton, circa 1925

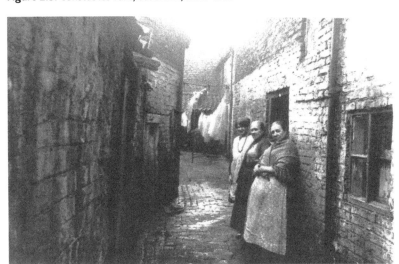

Source: Stockton Archives, courtesy of Stockton Libraries and Heritage Service, Stockton Borough Council

Figure 2.4: 1930s Stockton – approximate locations of old housing (King Street; Queen Street; Bay Street) and new housing (Manor House Terrace; Brisbane Grove)

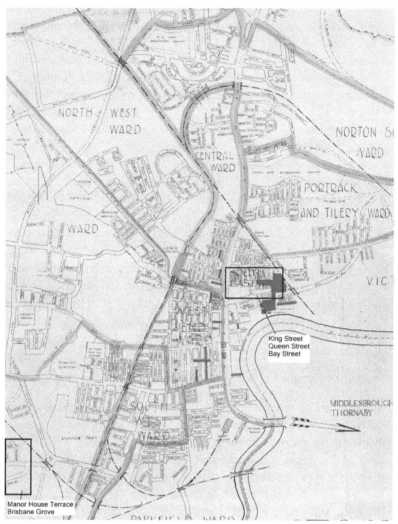

Base map reproduced by permission of Durham County Record Office (Durham County Record Office CC/X 185/4/64/4)

Source: M'Gonigle 1934; Housing Committee 1933

these differences in housing quality were reflected in the social status of the occupiers. The Hartburn area attracted predominantly – though not entirely – professionals, artisans and office workers. Conversely, the older areas consisted more of the skilled or unskilled industrial workers. It is probable that these areas of working-class residents had a higher proportion of unemployed, since 'unskilled manual workers were more likely to be unemployed … than clerical workers' (McKibbin, 1998, p. 114).

Much of the town's original housing had been demolished by the 1930s, but old housing still existed, for example King Street and its near neighbour Queen Street. By the 1930s, King Street consisted of a mix of the professions alongside manual skilled and unskilled trades. Queen Street conversely was largely an area of industrial and manual occupations. The nearby Bay Street bordered the slum clearance areas identified in the 1930s. This street also housed almost exclusively those in manual trades. In contrast, Manor House Terrace in suburban Hartburn was a much 'younger' area. By the 1930s this was a predominantly 'middle-class' area, with fewer manual workers and more professionals and businessmen. Also in Hartburn, Brisbane Grove first appeared in directories in 1930–31. Consisting of much lower density semi-detached houses, this was predominantly an area of professionals and artisans, with a small number of manual tradesmen (*Ward's Directory*, 1885, 1896, 1904, 1914, 1924, 1930, 1934; Ordnance Survey, 2017). The inequality of economic status of these areas, signified by the types of housing and the occupational classes, is reflected in the inequality of health suffered by these areas. Figure 2.4 indicates the locations of these areas. Zones identified for slum clearance are highlighted in dark grey.

Housing conditions

Most housing was adequate, but this was not universally true. Individual residences commonly experienced multiple problems, as illustrated by a single inspection of 21 Thompson Street: 'ground damp in front living room; excessive dampness in front bedroom; defective rear eves gutter; defective water closet door frame; defective floor boards in back bedroom; defective back bedroom window frame' (Health Committee, 1932).

Medical officer reports suggest that vermin infestation worsened, from 33 houses in 1930 to 132 houses in 1937 (M'Gonigle, 1930-1932, 1933a, 1934, 1935a and b, 1936-1938). In 1935, bug infestation of slum housing was conservatively estimated at 60–70% (M'Gonigle, 1935b).

Slum clearance

Slum housing existed in many areas of the country. A slum neighbourhood was an area where the:

narrowness, closeness and bad management, or the bad condition of the streets and houses or groups of houses within such an area, or the want of light, air, ventilation and proper conveniences and other sanitary defects, or one or more of such causes are dangerous or injurious to the health of the inhabitants of the buildings in the said area, or of the neighbouring buildings. (Allan, 1890, p. 4)

In 1930 Dr George M'Gonigle, medical officer of health (MOH) for Stockton, highlighted several areas as having major housing problems, totalling approximately 250 houses (M'Gonigle, 1930, pp. 39–41). A similar survey in 1931 was not acted on due to the need for the local authority to economise. In September 1931 the Ministry of Health called for reductions in local expenditure. The government wished to 'make large reductions in the national expenditure, some of which are such as to involve heavy sacrifices by the community' (M'Gonigle, 1933b, p. 17). In 1933, a five-year action plan on slum clearance began. As part of the austerity measures, the subsidy for general house building was abolished under the 1933 Housing (Financial Provisions) Act, but subsidies remained for housing to replace slum clearance (Yelling, 1988 pp. 282–6; Lund, 2011, p. 50). Surveys in Stockton resulted in five areas recommended for demolition totalling 941 houses, to be replaced with 1,046 new houses. These schemes were to be completed by 1938. Following subsequent public enquiries by the Ministry of Health, 578 houses were eventually demolished, with others being instead reconditioned. Seven hundred families were rehoused. By September 1937 all but 30 individual houses had been dealt with (Housing Committee, 1937).

Overcrowding and the link with rent

Living in close, cramped conditions accelerated the spread of communicable disease. Alongside this, the psychological stresses of overcrowding could exacerbate high blood pressure – a major cause of heart disease, which was the biggest killer of adults in Stockton during the decade (M'Gonigle, 1929-1932, 1933a, 1934, 1935a, 1936-1938; NHS, 2014, 2017a). Many local authorities in County Durham did not want housing with low rateable value as they could not recoup the cost of new housing from rates, and this then placed the burden on other rate-payers. If authorities kept rents low, then rates would have to increase to compensate for this. The burden would largely fall on those living in low-rate houses. If they set rents at the maximum in order to minimise rate rises, then this would reduce often already low family budgets. To keep rents down, some local authorities were building working-class housing which was below the recognised national standard (Bottomley and M'Gonigle, 1934, pp. 3–8).

Overcrowding in Stockton

Overcrowding could be assessed by either floor area or number of rooms. The permitted number of persons would be whichever produced the lower figure. A 1935 survey reported a total of 665 houses in the borough were overcrowded, 4–5% of total housing stock, or 6% of the total population of approximately 67,000 (M'Gonigle, 1935a, pp. 22–3). As Figure 2.5 illustrates, South East and Victoria wards suffered most, and these wards also suffered significantly from slum housing. These areas reflected some of the worst mortality figures.

Rents for council housing varied greatly depending on location and size of house – from 2s 6d per week for a single bedroom with kitchen to 12s 6d for the largest houses (M'Gonigle, 1929, p. 26; Housing Committee, 1936b). M'Gonigle commented that most lower-rent houses tended to be two-bedroom dwellings – unsuitable for families, but nevertheless rented by low-income families as they could not afford higher rents. The Housing Committee acknowledged that an unemployed family applying for a house may have had to wait longer than an employed family, as the date on which they could obtain a house 'would depend on the amount of income pending the applicant obtaining employment'. In other words, they may have to wait until a house became available at a rent they could afford, dependent on their level of benefits (Housing Committee, 1932), a situation not helped by the benefit cuts.

Similar fluctuations in rent existed in the private sector, partly influenced by the regulations on 'controlled' and 'decontrolled' housing.[1] For example, in 1939 in the Calf Fallow Lane area controlled rents were between 6s 3d and 7s 5d, while uncontrolled rents ranged from 7s 5d to 7s 11d (Housing Committee, 1939). Private landlords acknowledged that profiteering existed. As a meeting of the Northumberland and Durham Property Owners' and Ratepayers' Association reported, strong demand for housing had enabled landlords to over-charge on properties with, for example, houses worth 12s per

---

[1] Controlled housing had restrictions placed on the amount of rent which could be charged; decontrolled housing had no restrictions (Heath, 2013).

Figure 2.5: Overcrowding by ward, private housing only, 1935

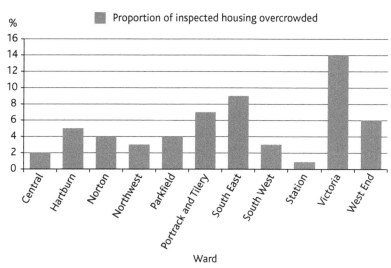

Source: Housing Committee 1936a

week being rented instead for between 15s to 25s per week (*Darlington & Stockton Times*, 1935c, p. 19).

M'Gonigle reported an acute shortage of houses, with two families often occupying houses intended only for one: 'much of the overcrowding ... is due to inability to pay the rents. ... Many families are compelled, on account of reduced income owing to unemployment, to share their houses with other families' (M'Gonigle, 1930, p. 36).

Families rehoused as a result of slum-clearance or to eradicate overcrowding could find that their rent increased in the new housing. M'Gonigle analysed two neighbourhoods of Stockton, one a low-rent area of slum housing, and one a high-rent area of new housing populated by families moved from recently cleared slums. Contrary to assumptions, those living in the new housing suffered more ill-health than those who remained in the slums. M'Gonigle argued that the higher rents paid in the new housing reduced the available income to spend on food. This resulted in a poorer, less nutritious diet – the catalyst for deteriorating health (M'Gonigle and Kirby, 1936).

Applications for council housing were consistently high from those living in overcrowded conditions. 'Not a few of the applications are on medical grounds from people who are recommended by their doctors to move to the more salubrious environment of the Council Estates' (M'Gonigle, 1932, p. 23). However, the borough council's funding constraints for house building influenced both overcrowding and associated health impacts: '…the only reason for the persistence of bad environmental conditions such as insanitary and overcrowded houses is financial' (M'Gonigle, 1934, p. 6).

The council called for the government to reinstate the subsidy for general house building – previously withdrawn in 1933 – to enable low-rent houses to be built (Housing Committee, 1934). In 1937 the Ministry of Health agreed to subsidise houses required for the abatement of overcrowding. This was offered due to the council's financial difficulty in funding new housing (Town Council, 1937). Conditions further improved when the Exchequer also agreed to subsidise new houses provided for slum clearance (Housing Committee, 1938).

Health and healthcare

Healthcare services

Access to healthcare was obviously an important determinant of health. However, access could be precarious for those on low incomes. In a time prior to the NHS, healthcare often had to be paid for. This could be difficult, if not impossible, for the poor. Families could choose not to pay for health insurance, but then risked ill health and being means tested in order to receive free care – a situation which many feared since access to such care was not guaranteed. M'Gonigle entreated the agencies involved in the provision and awarding of benefits to be sympathetic to family needs:

> … services such as those of … unemployment insurance, public assistance and the unemployment assistance board can by a liberal and generous interpretation of their powers raise the nutritional status of certain parts of the population and so raise the powers to resist disease. (M'Gonigle, 1934, p. 7)

Access to an adequate diet benefited the physical and mental wellbeing of a family, but also, in the opinion of John Boyd Orr of the Rowett Institute, made financial sense as well: 'It is probable that … the cost of bringing a diet adequate for health within the reach of the poorest would be less than the cost of treating disease which by this means would be prevented' (Orr, 1936).

The main clinical health services are located on the following map (Figure 2.6). This map concentrates on the identified slum clearance areas of Stockton. Slum residence tends to be an enforced economic

Figure 2.6: Stockton, 1936 – slum clearance areas; doctors; midwives; health care facilities

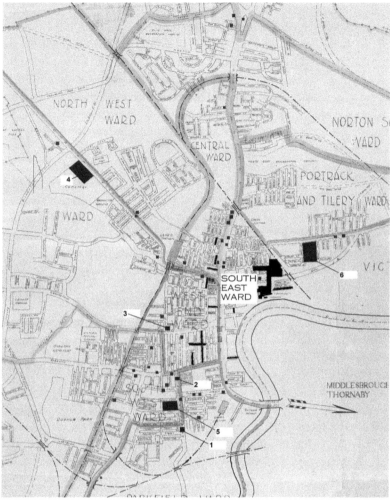

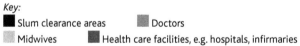

Key:

■ Slum clearance areas   ■ Doctors
■ Midwives   ■ Health care facilities, e.g. hospitals, infirmaries

The numbers correspond to the following health care facilities:
1 Durham County Council Tuberculosis Dispensary
2 Robson Maternity Home
3 Stockton Dispensary
4 Stockton Fever Hospital/Isolation Hospital
5 Stockton and Thornaby Hospital (voluntary)
6 Poor Law Infirmary (Public Assistance Institution – former workhouse)

Base map reproduced by permission of Durham County Record Office (Durham County Record Office CC/X 185/4/64/4)

Sources: Ward's Directory 1928, 1930, 1932, 1934, 1938; Kelly's Directory 1934, 1938; M'Gonigle 1934

necessity rather than a personal choice. These areas therefore represent some of the poorest areas of the borough.

Poor areas tend to have poor health. Thus they need good healthcare, but conversely tend to suffer poor healthcare as well. This is the essence of the 'Inverse Care Law' which is most prominent 'where medical care is most exposed to market forces' (Hart, 1971, p. 405). The proximity of health services to the poorest areas indicates that this 'law' did not operate within Stockton. Services, however, had to be paid for. National health insurance funded doctors for those in insured occupations. An unemployed person could also voluntarily contribute to this scheme at a rate, in 1937, of 1s 8d per week (Parliament. House of Commons, 1931, 1936; *Darlington & Stockton Times*, 1935d, p. 17; *Darlington & Stockton Times*, 1937c, p. 18). However, insurance committees recognised that the provision of medical assistance from insurance was limited, and that 'a long and severe illness means almost disaster to a worker' (*Darlington & Stockton Times*, 1930c, p. 5). The poorest who had neither national nor private insurance depended on the PAC to determine whether they qualified for assistance. The most impoverished could access a doctor for free, paid for by the PAC. This, however, brought a stigma of destitution and 'scrounging'[2] from the state.

Stockton was served by both municipal and private hospitals. Charging varied depending on the institution. National insurance did not cover hospital treatment and so additional private insurance had to be funded, or patients had otherwise to rely on the availability of free treatment at the poor law infirmary. Treatment at the Isolation Hospital (for infectious diseases), for example, cost 4s 10d in 1935. Perhaps reflecting the extent of unemployment and associated poor diet, by 1933 this hospital had a ward dedicated solely to the treatment of malnutrition. The Robson Maternity Home charged 35s for a 12–15 day stay. Preference of admission was given to those whose home surroundings were such as to be unsuitable for a confinement (M'Gonigle, 1929, p. 61). It seems reasonable to assume that pregnant women from the overcrowded slum areas of Stockton might qualify. Additionally, 'No person is precluded from taking advantage of the Home by reason of poverty, the amount of fees paid being regulated by the income of the family' (M'Gonigle, 1929, p. 61).

The 1936 MOH report states that fees were remitted altogether where necessary. In 1931 M'Gonigle stated that the home was almost

---

[2] A scrounger – work-shy and claiming benefits by choice rather than obtain work, or someone in work but also fraudulently claiming benefit (Deacon, 1976; Welshman, 2013, pp. 35 and 56).

overwhelmed with clients. A plan to extend facilities had been postponed due to financial constraints. By 1932 requests for admission were being turned away. M'Gonigle intimates that this was due to the cancellation/postponement of the building of the extensions to the accommodation. This situation occurred again in 1934, until the accommodation was eventually extended in 1935.

The poor law infirmary was located in the former workhouse and was administered by the PAC. This hospital provided care for the most destitute who could not afford to pay for treatment. The hospital struggled to cope with the increasing admissions, exacerbated by a difficulty in recruiting sufficient nursing staff. Shortage of beds for female inmates was an ongoing problem. The facility operated, at times, at 100% capacity with no possibility of admitting new patients (Council of the County Palatine of Durham, 1938, p. 27; *Darlington & Stockton Times*, 1938c, p. 3).

Stockton and Thornaby Surgical Hospital treated patients 'having sustained injuries, or suffering from diseases, not infectious or contagious, requiring surgical or medical treatment' (Stockton and Thornaby Hospital, 1926, p. 4). The hospital included 140 beds – a ratio of 1 bed for every 480 residents (M'Gonigle, 1930, p. 14). Patients would be treated 'on such terms as may from time to time be agreed upon' (Stockton and Thornaby Hospital, 1926, p. 4). The poorest may therefore have been charged on sympathetic terms. No scales of subscriptions are provided, but in the early 1940s subscriptions to hospital contributory schemes ranged between 2d – 6d per week (British Hospitals Association, 1943, p. 11). Subscribers could use the services on a pro rata basis: once per year as an in-patient for every £3 3s 0d subscribed; once per year as an out-patient for every 10s 6d subscribed (Stockton and Thornaby Hospital, 1930, p. 28).

Patients were admitted via a 'recommendation', which appears to have operated essentially as a voucher system since a recommendation was valid 'for 1 year from the date of issue' (Stockton and Thornaby Hospital, 1926, p. 6). Some unemployed continued to pay insurance subscriptions for hospital costs. This could be a potentially significant financial burden. For those without such insurance, the prospect of paying from their own meagre resources may have been prohibitive. The hospital encouraged subscribers to assist those unable to fund their own treatment: 'The Secretary will much appreciate the receipt of Recommendations from Subscribers not in a position to use them for the use of deserving cases' (Stockton and Thornaby Hospital, 1930, inside front cover).

The term 'deserving' may be revealing. Benefit claimants accused of choosing to live on benefits rather than find work, who 'scrounged', were seen as 'undeserving'. Those considered to be 'genuinely seeking work' were regarded as 'deserving' (Thane, 1996, pp. 64–5; Welshman, 2013, p. 8). Potentially, however, in this context 'deserving' patients were merely those unable to fund their own care. In either case, this would have been a precarious method for the unemployed to rely on.

Stockton was well served by welfare clinics and centres, but the service was under stress. A proposed new centre in the North West ward was turned down in 1931 due to the need for economy (*Darlington & Stockton Times*, 1931e, p. 3). In 1932 M'Gonigle commented: 'Finance, unfortunately, remains the dominant factor … It dictates and moulds policy, limits staffs and prevents the application of modern knowledge' (M'Gonigle, 1932, p. 11), although in fairness a new clinic was opened the same year, and another in 1938 (M'Gonigle, 1932, 1938). Maternity and child welfare centres provided milk and food to mothers. In 1935 M'Gonigle asserted that poorly fed mothers could not produce the breast milk required to sustain the health of infants. Providing a good daily meal to the mother would benefit both her and her baby's health. This service was provided free, or at cost or reduced price (M'Gonigle, 1937, p. 40).

Health

Particularly from 1932 onwards, the MOH reports comment on the detrimental health effects of low income concomitant with unemployment. M'Gonigle considered that the lower purchasing power of the unemployed had resulted in an inability to buy sufficient quantity and/or quality of food alongside other costs (M'Gonigle, 1932). Local clergy also worried that the allowances granted under the means test were inadequate even for a family's basic needs (Parliamentary, Finance and General Purposes Committee, 1933b). This was particularly pertinent between 1931–34 when benefits were cut, but continued to be a problem once benefit levels had been reinstated. Priorities had to be decided, with diet often being the easiest area to economise. The poorest areas of Stockton appear to have suffered disproportionately high infant and overall mortality. Infant mortality in particular was influenced by poor diet, with causes of death linked to malnutrition, such as premature birth or marasmus,[3] consistently ranking as major causes of death.

---

[3] Marasmus – wasting of muscle tissue and fat which the body breaks down to create energy. A result of acute malnutrition (UNICEF n.d.).

The difficulty of eating healthily on low incomes was an ongoing controversy among researchers, the media and the government. In response, in 1933 the British Medical Association formed a 'Committee on Nutrition' – which included M'Gonigle. The committee argued that the suggested standard daily requirement of 3,000 calories (2,700 after allowing for wastage) was only adequate for a man who was largely sedentary, and not engaged in regular physical activity.[4] The committee adopted 3,400 calories *as purchased* as their standard requirement for an average man with moderate physical exertion. Example diets for various family units were also devised (British Medical Association, 1933). The government criticised the production of the report as being socialistically motivated (Mayhew, 1988). Calculations of the costs of suitable diets, alongside other outgoings such as rent and fuel, showed that some of the poorest on benefits could not afford even the minimum recommended diet.

As illustrated in Figure 2.7, the overall mortality rate for Stockton indicated a generally improving trend, perhaps contradicting an assumption that the 1930s brought universally adverse health effects for the depressed areas.

However, mortality statistics for each ward show that not all wards displayed the same positive results, and some wards suffered higher mortality rates than the national figures.

Apart from 1929, heart disease was consistently the biggest cause of adult mortality in the borough, with cancer or pneumonia predominantly recorded as the second biggest killer (M'Gonigle, 1930-1932, 1933a, 1934, 1935a, 1936–1938). After 1935, however, causes of death were recorded as groups of principal and associated causes, and figures are therefore more difficult to compare. Occurrences of cancer and particularly heart disease rose significantly from 1932 (M'Gonigle, 1930–1932, 1933a, 1934, 1935a, 1936–1938). Modern medical science suggests that the stress associated with unemployment could have contributed to the high incidence of both diseases.[5] Respiratory diseases like pneumonia can be linked to poor housing conditions, such as inadequate ventilation, damp and airborne mould spores (WHO, 2010; NHS, 2015).

---

[4] Modern recommendations are approximately 2,500 calories per day for a man and approximately 2000 calories for a woman, varying depending on age and level of physical activity (NHS Choices, 2016)

[5] Depression and anxiety have been linked to an increased risk of death from cancer (NHS, 2017b); chronic psychological stress is believed to cause inflammation of the blood vessels, which may in turn lead to heart damage (NHS, 2014, 2017a)

Figure 2.7: Overall death rate, 1929–39 (per 1,000 population)

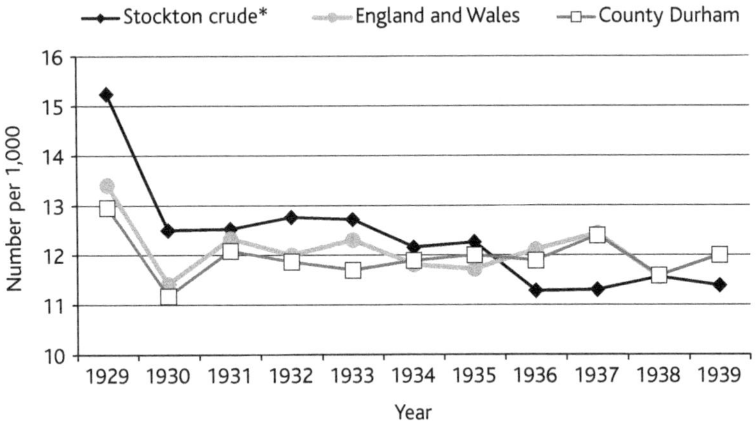

Note: * 'Adjusted' figures are those to which an 'Areal Comparability Factor' has been applied. The crude figures are multiplied by this factor so that local figures are comparable with national figures taking into account local age and sex demographics (Report of the Medical Officer of Health for Hayes, 1940, p. 4). Crude figures have been used for the graph as the figures provided for County Durham were not adjusted.

Source: M'Gonigle, 1930–1932, 1933a, 1934, 1935a, 1936–1938; Council of the County Palatine of Durham, 1930–1940; Health Committee 1938a, 1938b, 1939a–1939g

Infant mortality refers to death within the first year of birth and is a particularly sensitive indicator of an area's health. As Figure 2.8 shows, death rates were higher than the average for England and Wales until the mid-1930s when Stockton began to reflect an improving picture, although there was a substantial increase in 1937.

These trends signify an improving picture at national, regional and local levels. Infant mortality rate nationally had been improving since 1900. However, as Mitchell (1985, p. 107) has identified, improvement slowed dramatically during the 1930s:

> From 1900–1910 the rate fell by 44[6]
> From 1910–1920 the rate fell by 26
> From 1920–1930 the rate fell by 20
> From 1930–1940 the rate fell by 4
> From 1940–1950 the rate fell by 26

Mitchell contends that this poor rate of decline suggests a link between the economic difficulties and infant mortality. Young infants would, she states, have been most susceptible to the poor nutrition of

---

[6] Deaths per 1,000 live births.

Figure 2.8: Infant mortality rate, 1929–38 (per 1,000 births)

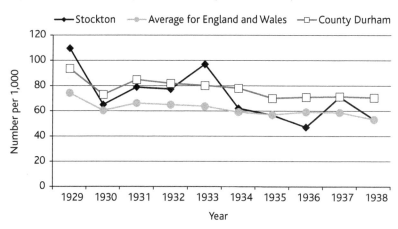

Source: M'Gonigle, 1930–1932, 1933a, 1934, 1935a, 1936–1938; Council of the County Palatine of Durham, 1939, p. 16; 1940, p.14

their mothers. Except in 1929, the biggest causes of infant mortality were premature birth, pneumonia, and the combined symptoms of atrophy, debility and marasmus – physical effects associated with malnutrition.[7]

Ward-level analysis: localised health inequalities highlighted

In 1936, for the only time in the decade, overall death rates by ward were reported (Figure 2.9).

The slum clearance areas were located in the Central, South East and West End wards. Additionally, an improvement area called the 'Victoria Ward area' included the demolition of 300 houses unfit for human habitation (M'Gonigle, 1933a, p. 18), although no description is provided to enable the marking of this area on the map. These wards recorded the highest death rates in the above data. This indicates a correlation between the poorest areas and the highest mortality rates.

In 1935 ward-based data on infant deaths, stillbirths and neonatal deaths was also produced. Infant death rates are summarised in Figure 2.10

---

[7] Atrophy – wasting away of body tissues or organs; debility – loss of muscle function, which can include heart muscle (OED, 2017a, 2017b); for the definition of marasmus see note 3.

Figure 2.9: Overall death rate by ward, 1936

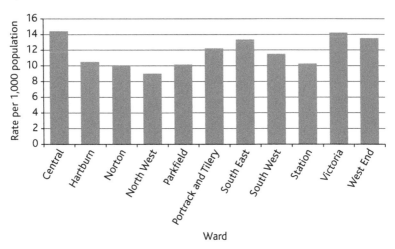

Source: M'Gonigle 1936, p. 11

Figure 2.10: Infant mortality by ward, 1935

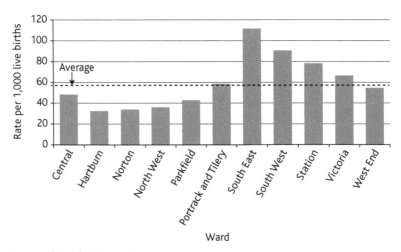

Source: M'Gonigle 1935, p. 54

Combining infant mortality and stillbirth figures, illustrated in Figure 2.11, five wards suffered above average rates. South East, Station and Victoria wards all reflect poor mortality rates in both graphs. South East ward and Victoria ward suffered from significant slum areas and the worst overcrowding.

Figure 2.11: Combined infant mortality and stillbirth rates, 1935

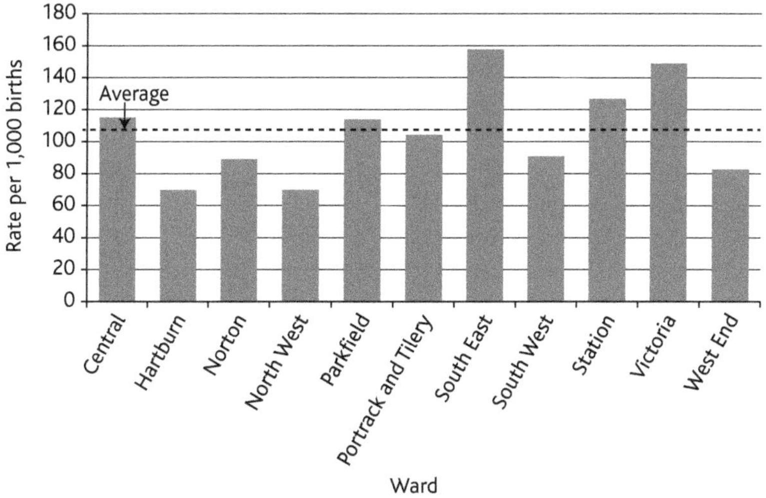

Source: M'Gonigle 1935, p. 54

Medical officer of health observations

A major killer of infants was developmental defect, for example imperfectly developed cranium or congenital heart defect. Although such defects were not well understood, M'Gonigle speculated that a deficient maternal diet had adverse effects on the anatomical development of the foetus (M'Gonigle, 1930, p. 71).[8] He also suspected dietary deficiencies influenced cases of premature birth[9] – the biggest cause of infant mortality. By 1931 he believed that the unemployed were suffering malnutrition, and that malnourished children were dying of diseases that would be resisted in well-nourished children. The impact of poor diet continued into 1936, when M'Gonigle stated:

> The importance of good nutrition cannot be over-emphasised ... inadequate purchasing power due to unemployment ... is reflected in the quality of the food supplied to children ... the protective foods are expensive and families with low income levels cannot afford to

---

[8] Recent research also suggests a link (for example, Belkacemi et al., 2010; Ford and Long, 2011).

[9] This is also suggested by recent studies (for example, Abu-Saad and Fraser, 2010; Bloomfield, 2011).

purchase adequate quantities … [this] explains why so many children of the poor are sub-normally nourished. (*Darlington & Stockton Times*, 1936, p. 3)

The assertion that poverty was a crucial contributor to poor diet, and that low benefit levels could create poverty, brought M'Gonigle and the medical profession into conflict with the government. Results discussed in this chapter support M'Gonigle's belief in the association between poverty and morbidity/mortality – and thus between government policy and morbidity/mortality. The suggestion of this link was problematic for a government intent on imposing austere policies. Chief medical officer George Newman, after initial hostility, did however illustrate sympathy for the existence of a link: 'There has been a rise in the maternal mortality rate, and there is evidence of malnutrition in young men and women who are unemployed … People cannot buy good food unless they can afford it' (*Darlington & Stockton Times*, 1934b, p. 8).

Although it is unclear that it resulted from this argument, it may be significant that when the 10% cut in benefits was restored in 1934, the benefit allowed for a child was increased by 50%.

Stockton in the Recession: comparing the 1930s with today

In some respects, the political and social responses to economic downturn in the recession stimulated by the banking collapse of 2007/08 echo those of the 1930s. Currently, foodbanks proliferate, mirroring the difficulties of financing a healthy diet. Those who use them are targeted as 'undeserving', as people who abuse the system, similar to the 'scroungers' of the 1930s (Garthwaite, 2016). As in the 1930s, benefits have been targeted as a means of reducing government spending, and have become more difficult to access. Harsh means testing for benefits has been imposed, causing severe difficulties for some claimants (BBC, 2017a). In June 2017 the government's proposals to cap certain benefits were overruled by the High Court due to the 'real misery' which this would impose for 'no good purpose' (BBC, 2017b). The government and elements of the media stigmatise the unemployed as workshy, for example the Channel 4 television programme 'Benefits Street', or newspapers such as the *Daily Mail* (Ramesh, 2013; Toynbee and Walker, 2015). Also paralleling the 1930s, harsh sanctioning of claimants for missing appointments with benefits officials has led to loss of benefits:

A man was sanctioned for being two minutes late, even though he had turned up 15 minutes early but wasn't allowed to go upstairs to see his advisor until the security guard said so;

A woman who went on a health and social care course the jobcentre sent her on was sanctioned for not going to her jobcentre appointment, even though she was on the course the jobcentre had sent her on. (Garthwaite, 2016, p. 84)

Mitchell (1985) identified a significant slow-down in improvement in infant mortality rates during the 1930s, suggesting that this was linked to the malnutrition experienced due to economic difficulties. Michael Marmot, director of the Institute of Health Equity at University College London and a health adviser to both the UK government and the World Health Organization, has identified a similar slow-down in improvements to life expectancy in England since 2010. Marmot believed it was 'entirely possible' that this was due to austerity and cuts to health and social care spending (Coghlan, 2017; Triggle, 2017).

Austerity, income and malnutrition

Benefits changes have particularly affected working-age families and their children (Toynbee and Walker, 2015, p. 109). The 2012 Welfare Reform Act capped levels of entitlement and lengthened the period between becoming unemployed and becoming eligible for benefits. The recent roll-out of universal credit includes a wait of six weeks before benefits commence (Millar and Bennett, 2016; Rampen, 2016). Sanctioning of claimants can stop benefit payments for weeks or months (even years in extreme cases), and even discretionary hardship payments for the neediest cannot be claimed for two weeks. Changes to benefit levels and the complete halt on payments for those who are sanctioned have created poverty for those affected. The reduction in income, combined with the difficulty of paying for fuel or food – the 'heat or eat' quandary – has resulted in rising malnutrition, echoing the 1930s. This has stimulated a rise in the use of foodbanks across the country, including within Stockton (Garthwaite, 2016). Echoing the accusation in the 1930s that the British Medical Association's report on minimum diets was politically motivated, a similar accusation has been raised against the Trussell Trust, a major provider of foodbanks. As Toynbee and Walker (2015, p. 108) suggest, it is as if the Trust were 'deliberately giving people food … to shame the government'. The link between benefits, low income and malnutrition indicates that in some respects we have returned to the conditions of the 1930s. This link is contested by the government, echoing the political response in the 1930s.

Stockton-on-Tees

In the following maps, the circled area on the 1930s map (Figure 2.12) highlights the slum clearance areas. The modern map of Stockton

Figure 2.12: Stockton 1930s – 'slum' wards (circled area)

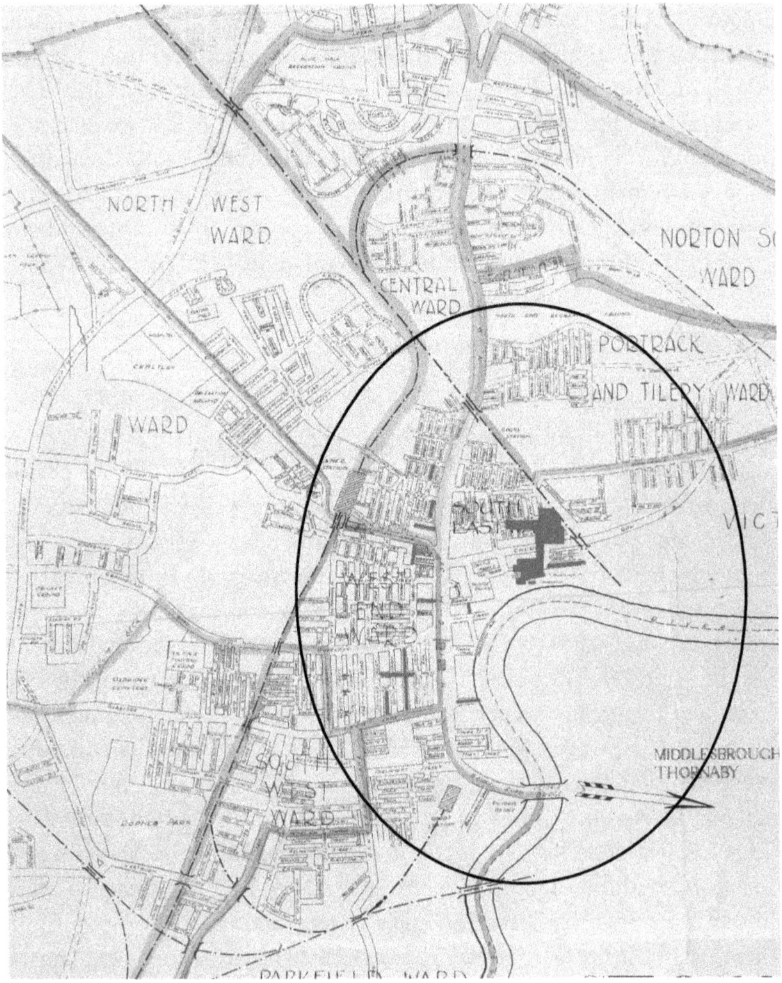

Base map reproduced by permission of Durham County Record Office (Durham County Record Office CC/X 185/4/64/4)

Source: M'Gonigle, 1934; Housing Committee, 1933

(Figure 2.13) shows the most and least deprived areas. The circled area on this map shows the approximate position of the circled slum areas on the 1930s map. Substantially the slum wards from the 1930s have been incorporated into the new ward of 'Stockton Town Centre'. Thus, the slum areas from the 1930s are still among the most deprived areas of Stockton now. There does not appear to have been any 'social mobility of place'.

Unemployment

Mirroring the 1930s, unemployment in Stockton rose from 2008 to a peak from October 2011 to September 2012 before generally declining from 2012 to 2017. Unemployment rates regionally, nationally and

Figure 2.13: Stockton-on-Tees, 2015, with 1930s 'slum' areas circled

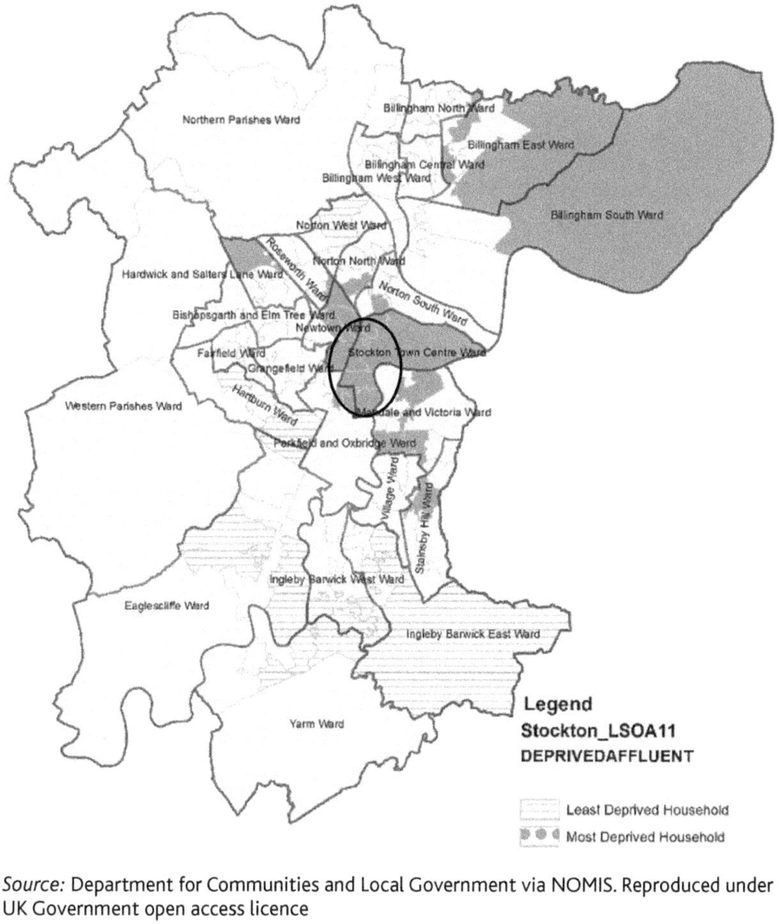

Source: Department for Communities and Local Government via NOMIS. Reproduced under UK Government open access licence

in Stockton were not as significant as during the 1930s. The national rate peaked at 8.1% and fell to a low of 4.7% between 2008 and 2017 (Figure 2.14). Stockton compared unfavourably with the national rates, peaking at 11.1% and reaching a low of 6.4%.

It should be noted that unemployment had begun to climb from 2006, prior to the recession. Additionally, the population of Stockton is larger than that of the 1930s.

Figure 2.14: Unemployment in Stockton, 2008–17

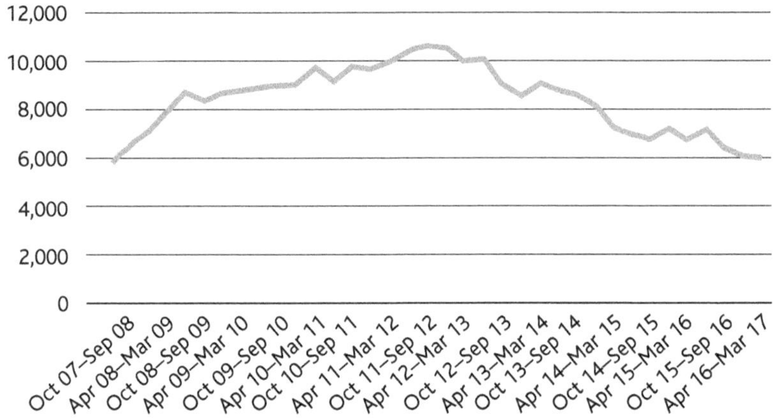

Source: Created using data from ONS, 2017

Ward-level comparison

Included earlier was an overview of the socioeconomic makeup of the poorer South East ward, and the more affluent Hartburn ward, in the 1930s. Hartburn ward now has a larger geographical area and South East ward has been subsumed into Town Centre ward, but these contemporary wards can still be used to provide a comparison in modern-day Stockton. A profile of Town Centre ward (Stockton-on-Tees Borough Council, 2015a) reported high levels of claimants for unemployment benefit, and above average levels of poor health. The ward was the most deprived in the borough. Almost 11% of working-age residents claimed job seeker's allowance benefits, and over 4% had been unemployed for more than a year. Over 44% of households were thought to be struggling to cope on their incomes. Socially rented housing accounted for 53% of households, and 37% of all households could not afford to heat their homes adequately. Almost half of children up to 15 years old lived in households claiming benefits. Life expectancy was the lowest in the borough – 67.7 years for men, 74.8 for women. The averages for the borough were 77.8 and 81.9 respectively. Almost 27% of people had long-term health problems, and almost 11% of births were of low birth weight. This evidence supports Gregory's (2009) contention that areas that have historically suffered deprivation will tend to experience similar effects in the future.

In comparison, a Hartburn Ward profile (Stockton-on-Tees Borough Council, 2015b), reported that most residents were either working or retired. Incomes were sufficient to live comfortably, mostly in owner-occupied semi-detached housing. Health was generally good. Hartburn was the third least deprived ward in the borough, ranking it 23 wards higher than Town Centre ward. Eleven per cent of children lived in 'income deprived' households – the average for the borough was 22%. Only 1.5% of working-age residents claimed job seeker's allowance, and just 0.3% had been long-term unemployed. Just under 18% of households were struggling to cope on their incomes, but 22% could not afford to heat their homes properly. Life expectancy was higher than average for the borough, at 80.9 years for men and 88.1 years for women. Approximately 19% of people had long-term health problems, and just 4.4% of births were of low birth weight.

In every item discussed above life appears to have been better in Hartburn ward than in Town Centre ward. There is an apparent correlation between low incomes – influenced by benefits, and the quality of housing and poor health in Town Centre Ward. It may be expected that quality of life and health was adversely affected by the welfare changes discussed by Garthwaite (2016) above. This was not the experience in Hartburn ward, where better incomes were less affected by the austerity-hit benefits system and reflected in better quality housing and better health.

Housing

Using occupancy data from the 2011 census, the Strategic Housing Market Assessment (Stockton-on-Tees Borough Council 2016) calculated that overcrowding in Stockton stood at 3,580 households. However, adopting a more stringent 'bedroom standard' advocated by the secretary of state, it was estimated that Stockton had 1,253 overcrowded households in 2014. Stockton was by then a much larger geographical area than in the 1930s. From a total housing stock of 82,200 in 2011 this equates to an approximate overcrowding rate of 1.5% – better than the rate observed in 1935. However, if the original 'census occupancy rate' method was used then overcrowding increased to 4.5% – similar to the 1935 rate. No breakdown of overcrowding by ward is provided, and ward-level rates may have been higher in some cases.

The term 'slum' has been replaced by the term 'non-decent' housing. The criteria for 'decent' housing are that the house must:

- be above the legal minimum standard for housing (currently the Housing Health and Safety Rating System, HHSRS); and
- be in a reasonable state of repair; and
- have reasonably modern facilities (such as kitchens and bathrooms) and services; and
- provide a reasonable degree of thermal comfort (effective insulation and efficient heating). (Stockton-on-Tees Borough Council, 2016, p. 41)

No figures on non-decent housing for Stockton were provided. However, the national trend is that while social housing is likely to comply with the standard for decent housing, approximately 33% of private rented housing did not. This trend tended to exist at a local level.

House building in Stockton fell sharply after 2007, although rates for following years were close to the national average. Nevertheless, echoing the 1930s, some overcrowding was due to a shortage of affordable housing, and some families were 'forced to live together due to affordability difficulties' (Stockton Borough Council, 2016, p. 105). Data from the Department of Work and Pensions reported that, in Stockton, the numbers claiming housing benefit had risen – from 14,100 in 2008–09 to 16,600 in 2014–15. The vast majority of this increase occurred in private rented housing. Again, these figures are for Stockton overall, and there is no breakdown by ward.

In the 1930s the government provided subsidies for house building to replace slum properties and abate overcrowding. In the current period the government had introduced initiatives to encourage house building, for example:

- Affordable Homes Programme – the 2015–18 programme intended to provide 43,821 new affordable homes across England;
- Care and Support Specialised Housing Fund – to accelerate the provision of housing for older and disabled people;
- Community Right to Build – to include some affordable housing provision.

However, the report identified a number of government policies which were depressing the house building market. These included welfare reform, with landlords and house builders concerned that changes to benefits could adversely affect their revenue; reductions in grants, which were discouraging developers – an echo of the reduction in general house building subsidies in the 1930s; and cuts in social housing rents, which reduces available income to support local authority house building.

Mortality and morbidity

In 2016 it was reported that male life expectancy was 16.6 years higher in the most affluent areas of Stockton than in the least affluent. A similar inequality in female life expectancy indicated a gap of 12.2 years between the most and least affluent areas (Public Health England, 2016). Town Centre ward, identified as the most deprived in the borough, suffered the highest five-year average standardised mortality rate at more than three and a half times the national average for males between 0 and 64, and two and a half times the national average for females of similar age. The more affluent Northern Parishes ward, for example, suffered a mortality rate that was significantly below the national average for both genders (Elias, 2015).

Recent research suggests that austerity is responsible for similar inequality on a national level. Malnutrition has increased across much of England, but more so in the less affluent north than in the more affluent south. Mortality rates among lower socioeconomic status women have improved in the south, but have worsened in the north. Similarly, rates of morbidity and mortality overall are higher in the north than the south, a gap which has widened as unemployment has increased (Bambra and Garthwaite, 2015). The strain of unemployment and poverty is a catalyst for mental health problems, and government cuts to mental health services further aggravate this situation (Mattheys, 2015). Inequality in mental health between the most and least affluent areas is evident in Stockton, with the poorest areas being at greater risk than the prosperous (Mattheys et al., 2016).

Conclusion

Austere policies during the 1930s saw cuts to benefits and housing subsidies. Stockton suffered from unemployment, and those relying on benefits suffered from the cuts imposed. This often manifested in a poor diet and subsequent health detriment, although the government contested the idea that their policies contributed to poverty. Alongside the malnutrition which M'Gonigle observed, slum and overcrowded housing further exacerbated conditions for some of the poorest. The combination of bad housing and ill-nourishment was reflected in the worst mortality statistics being observed in the poorest wards. This suggests that an association existed between poverty and ill health, and furthermore, between government austerity and ill health – that austerity caused or exacerbated reductions in household income via benefit cuts; that reduced incomes caused or contributed to poverty; that poverty caused or contributed to poor diet due to the need to economise on food expenditure; and in consequence, poor diet led to malnutrition and malnutrition caused or contributed to mortality.

Webster's *Healthy or Hungry Thirties?* (1982) discussed the debate about whether the 1930s were as bad as had previously been considered: whether, in fact, the positive state of health in the country promoted by the government and other commentators was accurate, or was unduly optimistic or intentionally inaccurate. The conclusion presented by Webster is that the data used by the government to illustrate an improving picture was unreliable or misleading. Taken as a national average health could, from some points of view at least, have been regarded as improving. However, a closer examination of the evidence illustrated diverse regional and local results, with the depressed areas suffering significantly worse health than more affluent areas. Framing this chapter in the context of this debate, Stockton in the 1930s reflects a microcosm of the rest of the country. General trends in mortality in Stockton were indeed downward, but ward-level statistics illustrate that poorer wards suffered higher rates than the average for the town as a whole. Thus, although Stockton could be regarded as having improving health overall, the improvement was unequally distributed and poorer areas reflected higher mortality rates. The localised, ward-level picture of health therefore looks quite different, and less positive, than the overall image. With malnutrition a significant problem in the borough, some of the poorest in Stockton appear to have been more hungry than healthy.

Overall, Stockton seems to have fared better during the austerity following the 2007/08 recession than during the 1930s. Unemployment is not as bad, but the rise in foodbank use is a worrying trend and this, alongside inequalities in mortality between poor and affluent areas, perhaps indicates that elements of Stockton remain hungry and unhealthy. Housing is still a problem, although less so than in the 1930s. Overcrowding still exists, and it is estimated that a third of private rented housing is unsuitable. While house building programmes exist, however, government policies have in some respects discouraged developers. The major difference in healthcare is probably, for most people, the NHS (National Health Service), which provides, at least in theory, an equal right of access to care for all. Benefit cuts have not brought the apprehension over costs that existed during the 1930s. There is no trepidation regarding ability to pay, or worries about whether people qualify for free or subsidised health treatment, both of which were a cause of anxiety for the poor during the 1930s. No stigma is attached to receiving this care, unlike, for instance, the stigma associated with the use of the poor law infirmary in the 1930s. This has not, however, eradicated health inequality. It would appear, then, that the improvements in clinical healthcare accessibility have not been able to overcome the detrimental effects of the social determinants of health. Poorer areas tend to experience higher unemployment and thus suffer more from cuts to benefits, and worse health statistics are still reflected in areas of poorer housing, low incomes and higher unemployment, as experienced in Town Centre ward for example. Stockton's most deprived areas have suffered disproportionately when compared to more affluent areas and appear to be anchored in this position. It would appear that they may have remained anchored since at least the 1930s, and suffered from both historical and contemporary austerity.

Acknowledgements

I would like to offer my thanks and appreciation to my supervisors for their guidance in the initial stages: Dr Gordon Macleod of Durham University Geography Department, Dr Matt Perry of Newcastle University School of History, Classics and Archaeology, Dr Andrzej Olechnowicz of Durham University History Department and Professor Clare Bambra of Newcastle University Institute of Health and Society.

References

Abu-Saad, K. and Fraser, D. (2010) Maternal Nutrition and Birth Outcomes. *Epidemiologic Reviews*, 32, 5–25.

Allan, C. E. (1890) The Housing of the Working Classes Act, 1890, annotated, with appendices containing the Incorporated Statutory Provisions, the Working Classes Dwellings Act, 1890, the Standing Orders of Parliament related to Provisional Orders, and the Circulars, Memoranda and Orders of the Local Government Board under the Act. London: Knight and Co.

Bambra, C. and Garthwaite, K. (2015) Austerity, welfare reform and the English health divide. *Area*, 47(3), 341–343.

BBC (2017a) Concentrix tax credit cases to be reviewed, government says. www.bbc.co.uk/news/business-38873311

BBC (2017b) Single parents win benefits cap High Court challenge. www.bbc.co.uk/news/business-40367686

Belkacemi, L., Nelson, D. M., Desai, M. and Ross, M. G. (2010) Maternal undernutrition influences placental-fetal development. *Biology of Reproduction*, 83(3), 325–331.

Beynon, H., Hudson, R. and Sadler, D. (1994) *A Place Called Teesside: A Locality in a Global Economy*. Edinburgh: Edinburgh University Press.

Bloomfield, F. H. (2011) How Is Maternal Nutrition Related to Preterm Birth? *Annual Review of Nutrition*, 31, 235–261.

Bottomley, H. and M'Gonigle, G. C. M. (1934) *Overcrowding in County Durham*. Darlington: North of England Newspaper Co. Ltd. PP/ GMG/E/7. Wellcome Library, London.

British Hospitals Association, The (1943) *800 Years of Service: The Story of Britain's Voluntary Hospitals*. The British Hospitals Association: London.

British Medical Association (1933) Report of Committee on Nutrition. *British Medical Journal Supplement*, 2 (3803), November.

Burton, M. (2016) *The Politics of Austerity*. London: Palgrave Macmillan.

Cemeteries and Parks Committee (1931) 'Recreation for the Unemployed'. *Minutes of Cemeteries and Parks Committee meeting 7 December 1931*, Borough of Stockton, Stockton.

Coghlan, A. (2017) 'Rising life expectancy in England has slowed since recession'. *New Scientist*, 18 July. www.newscientist.com/ article/2140907-rising-life-expectancy-in-england-has-slowed-since-recession/

Council of the County Palatine of Durham (1930) *Annual Report of the Medical Officer of Health, and Other Records For The Year 1929*. Durham: Durham County Council.

Council of the County Palatine of Durham (1931) *Annual Report of the Medical Officer of Health, and Other Records For The Year 1930*. Durham: Durham County Council.

Council of the County Palatine of Durham (1932) *Annual Report of the Medical Officer of Health, and Other Records For The Year 1931*. Durham: Durham County Council.

Council of the County Palatine of Durham (1933) *Annual Report of the Medical Officer of Health, and Other Records For The Year 1932*. Durham: Durham County Council.

Council of the County Palatine of Durham (1934) *Annual Report of the Medical Officer of Health, and Other Records For The Year 1933*. Durham: Durham County Council.

Council of the County Palatine of Durham (1935) *Annual Report of the Medical Officer of Health, and Other Records For The Year 1934.* Durham: Durham County Council.

Council of the County Palatine of Durham (1936) *Annual Report of the Medical Officer of Health, and Other Records For The Year 1935.* Durham: Durham County Council.

Council of the County Palatine of Durham (1937) *Annual Report of the Medical Officer of Health, and Other Records For The Year 1936.* Durham: Durham County Council.

Council of the County Palatine of Durham (1938) *Annual Report of the Medical Officer of Health, and Other Records For The Year 1937.* Durham: Durham County Council.

Council of the County Palatine of Durham (1939) *Annual Report of the Medical Officer of Health, and Other Records For The Year 1938.* Durham: Durham County Council.

Council of the County Palatine of Durham (1940) *Annual Report of the Medical Officer of Health, and Other Records For The Year 1939.* Durham: Durham County Council.

Croucher, R. (1987) *We Refuse to Starve in Silence.* London: Lawrence and Wishart.

Darlington & Stockton Times (1930a) 'Tragedy of Unemployment', 1 November, p. 14.

Darlington & Stockton Times (1930b) 'The Disaster of the Dole', 21 June, p. 13.

Darlington & Stockton Times (1930c) 'Medical Services', 11 October, p. 5.

Darlington & Stockton Times (1931a) 'Notes Of The Week', 5 December, p. 9.

Darlington & Stockton Times (1931b) 'A New "Dole" Trick', 19 December, p. 8.

Darlington & Stockton Times (1931c) 'Extra Burdens For Everybody', 12 September, p. 5.

Darlington & Stockton Times (1931d) 'Gardening for the Unemployed', 30 May, p. 10.

Darlington & Stockton Times (1931e) 'Stockton Town Council', 10 October, p. 3.

Darlington & Stockton Times (1932) 'The Means Test', 9 January, p. 3.

Darlington & Stockton Times (1933a) 'Ministry and Unemployment Schemes', 11 March, p. 3.

Darlington & Stockton Times (1933b) 'Stockton Unemployed', 14 October, p. 7.

Darlington & Stockton Times (1934a) '"Back To The Land" Move In Durham County', 10 November, p. 3.

Darlington & Stockton Times (1934b) 'The National Health', 22 September, p. 8.

Darlington & Stockton Times (1935a) 'More Workers', 13 July, p. 10.

Darlington & Stockton Times (1935b) 'Looking After Stockton's Unemployed', 30 November, p. 3.

Darlington & Stockton Times (1935c) 'Property Owners and Slum Clearance', 12 October, p. 19.

Darlington & Stockton Times (1935d) 'Information Bureau', 7 September, p. 17.

Darlington & Stockton Times (1936) 'The Work of Stockton's School Services', 27 June, p. 3.

Darlington & Stockton Times (1937) 'Information Bureau', 24 April, p. 18.

Darlington & Stockton Times (1938) 'Christmas Gifts', 8 January, p. 3.

Deacon, A. (1976) *In Search Of The Scrounger*. London: G. Bell & Sons.

Denman, J. and McDonald, P. (1996) Unemployment statistics from 1881 to the present day. *Labour Market Trends*, 104 (15–18), pp. 5–18.

Elias, P. (2015) *Standardised Mortality Rates for Tees Valley Wards*. Tees Valley Unlimited, February 2015. https://teesvalley-ca.gov.uk/wp-content/uploads/2016/03/1.-TVU-Mortality-by-Ward-to-Mid2013.pdf

Ford, S. P. and Long, N. M. (2011) Evidence for similar changes in offspring phenotype following either maternal undernutrition or overnutrition: potential impact on fetal epigenetic mechanisms. *Reproduction, fertility and development*, 24(1), 105–111.

Garside, W. R. (1990) *British Unemployment 1919–1939: A study in public policy*. Cambridge: Cambridge University Press.

Garthwaite, K. (2016) *Hunger Pains: Life inside foodbank Britain*. Bristol: Policy Press.

Gregory, I. N. (2009) Comparisons between geographies of mortality and deprivation from the 1900s and 2001: spatial analysis of census and mortality statistics. *British Medical Journal*, 339 (7722), 676–679.

Hart, J. T. (1971) The Inverse Care Law. *Lancet*, 297 (7696), 405–412.

Health Committee (1932) 'Nuisances – Public Health Acts'. *Minutes of Health Committee Meeting 11 November 1932*, Borough of Stockton, Stockton.

Health Committee (1938a) 'Medical Officer's Report'. *Minutes of Health Committee Meeting 14 November 1938*, Borough of Stockton, Stockton.

Health Committee (1938b) 'Medical Officer's Report'. *Minutes of Health Committee Meeting 12 December 1938*, Borough of Stockton, Stockton.

Health Committee (1939a) 'Medical Officer's Report'. *Minutes of Health Committee Meeting 9 January 1939*, Borough of Stockton, Stockton.

Health Committee (1939b) 'Medical Officer's Report'. *Minutes of Health Committee Meeting 6 February 1939*, Borough of Stockton, Stockton.

Health Committee (1939c) 'Medical Officer's Report'. *Minutes of Health Committee Meeting 6 March 1939*, Borough of Stockton, Stockton.

Health Committee (1939d) 'Medical Officer's Report'. *Minutes of Health Committee Meeting 3 April 1939*, Borough of Stockton, Stockton.

Health Committee (1939e) 'Medical Officer's Report'. *Minutes of Health Committee Meeting 8 May 1939*, Borough of Stockton, Stockton.

Health Committee (1939f) 'Deputy Medical Officer's Report'. *Minutes of Health Committee Meeting 12 June 1939*, Borough of Stockton, Stockton.

Health Committee (1939g) 'Deputy Medical Officer's Report'. *Minutes of Health Committee Meeting 10 July 1939*, Borough of Stockton, Stockton.

Heath, S. (2013) *The Historical Context of Rent Control in the Private Rented Sector*. http://researchbriefings.parliament.uk/ResearchBriefing/Summary/SN06747#fullreport

Housing Committee (1932) 'Allocation of Houses'. *Minutes of Housing Committee Meeting 11 March 1932*, Borough of Stockton, Stockton.

Housing Committee (1933) 'Housing Act, 1930 – Riverside Area'. *Minutes of Housing Committee Meeting 15 December 1933*, Borough of Stockton, Stockton.

Housing Committee (1934) 'Overcrowding'. *Minutes of Housing Committee Meeting 12 January 1934*, Borough of Stockton, Stockton.

Housing Committee (1936a) 'Overcrowding Survey'. *Minutes of Housing Committee Meeting 7 February 1936*, Borough of Stockton, Stockton.

Housing Committee (1936b) 'Erection of 214 Houses, 90 Houses and 76 Houses, Blue Hall Estate – erection of 66 Houses, Gilpin Brown Estate – Rents'. *Minutes of Housing Committee Meeting 21 September 1936*, Borough of Stockton, Stockton.

Housing Committee (1937) 'Slum Clearance – Five Years' Programme'. *Minutes of Housing Committee Meeting 12 November 1937*, Borough of Stockton, Stockton.

Housing Committee (1938) 'Housing (Financial Provisions) Act, 1938'. *Minutes of Housing Committee Meeting 16 May 1938*, Borough of Stockton, Stockton.

Housing Committee (1939) 'Calf Fallow Lane Houses – Rents'. *Minutes of Housing Committee Meeting 3 February 1939*, Borough of Stockton, Stockton.

Kelly's Directory (1934) *of Durham and Northumberland*. London: Kelly's Directories Limited.

Kelly's Directory (1938) *of Durham*. London: Kelly's Directories Limited.

Lund, B. (2011) *Understanding Housing Policy*. Bristol: Policy Press.

Macmillan, H. (1966) *The Winds of Change 1914–1939*. London: Macmillan.

Markets and Properties Committee (1931) 'New Baths and Wash-houses'. *Minutes of Markets and Properties Committee meeting 25 February 1931*, Borough of Stockton, Stockton.

Mattheys, K. (2015) The Coalition, austerity and mental health. *Disability & Society*, 30 (3), 475–478.

Mattheys, K., Bambra, C., Warren, J., Kasim, A. and Akhter, N. (2016) Inequalities in mental health and well-being in a time of austerity: Baseline findings from the Stockton-on-Tees cohort study. *SSM – Population Health*, 2, 350–359.

Mayhew, M. (1988) The 1930s Nutrition Controversy. *Journal of Contemporary History*, 23, 445–464.

McKibbin, R. (1975) The Economic Policy of the Second Labour Government. *Past and Present*, 68 (1), pp. 95–123.

McKibbin, R. (1998) *Classes and Cultures: England 1918–1951*. Oxford: Oxford University Press.

M'Gonigle, G. C. M. (1929) *Report of the Medical Officer of Health to the Town Council*. Stockton-on-Tees: Stockton-on-Tees Corporation.

M'Gonigle, G. C. M. (1930) *Report of the Medical Officer of Health to the Town Council*. Stockton-on-Tees: Stockton-on-Tees Corporation.

M'Gonigle, G. C. M. (1931) *Report of the Medical Officer of Health to the Town Council*. Stockton-on-Tees: Stockton-on-Tees Corporation.

M'Gonigle, G. C. M. (1932) *Report of the Medical Officer of Health to the Town Council*. Stockton-on-Tees: Stockton-on-Tees Corporation.

M'Gonigle, G. C. M. (1933a) *Report of the Medical Officer of Health to the Town Council*. Stockton-on-Tees: Stockton-on-Tees Corporation.

M'Gonigle, G. C. M. (1933b) Poverty, Nutrition and the Public Health. *Proceedings of the Royal Society of Medicine*, April 1933, pp. 677–687.

M'Gonigle, G. C. M. (1934) *Report of the Medical Officer of Health to the Town Council*. Stockton-on-Tees: Stockton-on-Tees Corporation.

M'Gonigle, G. C. M. (1935a) *Report of the Medical Officer of Health to the Town Council*. Stockton-on-Tees: Stockton-on-Tees Corporation.

M'Gonigle, G. C. M. (1935b) *Infestation of Houses by Bugs*. Report to the Chairman and Members of the Housing Committee, 7 February 1935, Borough of Stockton, Stockton. DC/ST 26/104, Teesside Archives, Middlesbrough.

M'Gonigle, G. C. M. (1936) *Report of the Medical Officer of Health to the Town Council*. Stockton-on-Tees: Stockton-on-Tees Corporation.

M'Gonigle, G. C. M. (1937) *Report of the Medical Officer of Health to the Town Council*. Stockton-on-Tees: Stockton-on-Tees Corporation.

M'Gonigle, G. C. M. (1938) *Report of the Medical Officer of Health to the Town Council*. Stockton-on-Tees: Stockton-on-Tees Corporation.

M'Gonigle, G. C. M. and Kirby, J. (1936) *Poverty and Public Health*. London: Victor Gollancz.

Millar, J. and Bennett, F. (2016) Giving back control? A contradiction at the heart of Universal Credit. http://eprints.lse.ac.uk/71478/1/blogs. lse.ac.uk-Giving%20back%20control%20A%20contradiction%20 at%20the%20heart%20of%20Universal%20Credit.pdf

Ministry of Labour (1934) *Ministry of Labour Reports of Investigations into the Industrial Conditions in Certain Depressed Areas*. London: His Majesty's Stationery Office.

Mitchell, M. (1985) The Effects of Unemployment on the Social Condition of Women and Children in the 1930s. *History Workshop Journal*, 19 (1), 105–127.

Needham, (2013) *Austerity Britain: It's de-ja-vu all over again*. www.cam. ac.uk/research/news/austerity-britain-its-d%C3%A9j%C3%A0-vu-all-over-again

NHS (National Health Service) (2014) *Stress 'causes damage to the heart,' study finds*. www.nhs.uk/news/2014/06June/Pages/Stress-causes-damage-to-the-heart.aspx

NHS (2015) *Can Damp and Mould Affect My Health?* www.nhs.uk/chq/ Pages/Can-damp-and-mould-affect-my-health.aspx?CategoryID=87

NHS (2017a) *A pattern of brain activity may link stress to heart attacks*. www.nhs.uk/news/2017/01January/Pages/A-pattern-of-brain-activity-may-link-stress-to-heart-attacks.aspx

NHS (2017b) *Anxiety and depression linked to increased cancer death risk*. www.nhs.uk/news/2017/01January/Pages/Anxiety-and-depression-linked-to-increased-cancer-death-risk.aspx

NHS Choices (2016) What should my daily intake of calories be? www.nhs.uk/chq/pages/1126.aspx?categoryid=51

Nicholas, K. (1986) *The social effects of unemployment in Teesside, 1919–1939*. Manchester: Manchester University Press.

OED (Oxford English Dictionary) (2017a) *Atrophy*. https://en.oxforddictionaries.com/definition/atrophy

OED (2017b) *Debility*. https://en.oxforddictionaries.com/definition/debility

ONS (Office for National Statistics) (2017) 'All people – Economically active – Unemployed (Model Based) Stockton-on-Tees'. www.nomisweb.co.uk/

Ordnance Survey (2017) *Digimap*. http://digimap.edina.ac.uk/roam/historic

Orr, J. B. (1936) 'Poverty and ill health', *Sunday Times*, 7 June, p. 9.

Parliament. House of Commons (1931) *National health insurance (prolongation of insurance)*. (Bill 11). London: His Majesty's Stationery Office.

Parliament. House of Commons (1936) *An act to consolidate the enactments relating to National Health Insurance*. (Bill 145). London: His Majesty's Stationery Office.

Parliamentary, Finance and General Purposes Committee (1931b) 'National Unemployed Workers Movement'. *Minutes of Parliamentary, Finance and General Purposes Committee meeting 22 September 1931*, Borough of Stockton, Stockton.

Parliamentary, Finance and General Purposes Committee (1933a) 'Unemployment Relief Works'. *Minutes of Parliamentary, Finance and General Purposes Committee meeting 23 February 1933*, Borough of Stockton, Stockton.

Parliamentary, Finance and General Purposes Committee (1933b) 'Means Test'. *Minutes of Parliamentary, Finance and General Purposes Committee meeting 22 September 1933*, Borough of Stockton, Stockton.

Perry, M. (2000) *Bread and Work: The Experience of Unemployment 1918–39*. London: Pluto Press.

Public Health England (2016) *Stockton on Tees Unitary Authority Health Profile 2016*. www.egenda.stockton.gov.uk/aksstockton/images/att29209.pdf

Ramesh, R. (2013) 'Is Britain a nation of lazy scroungers?', *The Guardian*, 24 April. www.theguardian.com/politics/reality-check/2013/apr/24/benefits

Rampen, J. (2016) 'Waiting for Universal Credit is unbelievably terrifiying – here's why'. www.mirror.co.uk/money/waiting-universal-credit-unbelievably-terrifying-7331079.

Report of the Medical Officer of Health for Hayes (1940) wellcomelibrary.org/moh/report/b19791409/6#?c=0&m=0&s=0&cv=6&z=0.0233%2C1.0118%2C0.9261%2C0.4334.

Skidelsky, R. (1998) The First 100 Years: A policy that crippled: The Gold Standard debate. *Financial Times*, 15 February www.skidelskyr.com/site/article/the-first-100-years-a-policy-that-crippled-the-gold-standard-debate/

Stockton and Thornaby District Women's Association (1935) *Minutes*. U/SWC/4, Teesside Archives, Middlesbrough.

Stockton and Thornaby Hospital (1926) *Statutes and Rules*. H/ST 7/2, Teesside Archives, Middlesbrough.

Stockton and Thornaby Hospital (1930) *54th Annual Report*. H/ST 4/10, Teesside Archives, Middlesbrough.

Stockton Baptist Tabernacle (March 1927 to September 1944) *Minutes*. R/B/S/1/5, Teesside Archives, Middlesbrough.

Stockton-on-Tees Borough Council (2015a) *Stockton Town Centre Ward Profile 2015*. Stockton: Stockton-on-Tees Borough Council.

Stockton-on-Tees Borough Council (2015b) *Hartburn Ward Profile 2015*. Stockton: Stockton-on-Tees Borough Council.

Stockton-on-Tees Borough Council (2016) *Strategic Housing Market Assessment 2016*. Swansea: Opinion Research Services. www.stockton.gov.uk/media/7717/strategic-housing-market-assessment-2016-part-1.pdf

Stockton Unitarian Church. (October 1927 to September 1933) *Minutes*. R/UN/S/1/3, Teesside Archives, Middlesbrough.

Taylor, A. J. P. (1965) *English History 1914–45*. Oxford: Clarendon Press.

Thane, P. (1996) *Foundations of the Welfare State*. Harlow: Addison Wesley Longman.

Town Council (1931a) 'Deputations'. *Minutes of Town Council meeting 7 October 1931*, Borough of Stockton, Stockton.

Town Council (1937) 'Housing Committee'. *Minutes of Town Council meeting 18 February 1937*, Borough of Stockton, Stockton.

Toynbee, P. and Walker, D. (2015) *Cameron's Coup*. London: Guardian Books.

Triggle, N. (2017) 'Life expectancy rises 'grinding to halt' in England'. *BBC News*, 18 July. www.bbc.co.uk/news/health-40608256

UNICEF (n.d.) *Acute Malnutrition: Marasmus (or Wasting)*. www.unicef.org/nutrition/training/2.3/4.html

Ward's Directory (1885) *of Redcar and Coatham, Middlesbrough, Stockton and Thornaby* 1885. Newcastle: R. Ward & Sons.

Ward's Directory (1896) *of Redcar and Coatham, Middlesbrough, Stockton and Thornaby* 1896–1897. Newcastle: R. Ward & Sons.

Ward's Directory (1904) *of Redcar and Coatham, Middlesbrough, Stockton and Thornaby* 1904–1905. Newcastle: R. Ward & Sons.

Ward's Directory (1914) *of Redcar and Coatham, Middlesbrough, Stockton and Thornaby* 1914–1915. Newcastle: R. Ward & Sons.

Ward's Directory (1924) *of Redcar and Coatham, Middlesbrough, Stockton and Thornaby* 1924–1925. Newcastle: R. Ward & Sons.

Ward's Directory (1928) *of Redcar and Coatham, Middlesbrough, Stockton and Thornaby* 1928–1929. Newcastle: R. Ward & Sons.

Ward's Directory (1930) *of Redcar and Coatham, Middlesbrough, Stockton and Thornaby* 1930–1931. Newcastle: R. Ward & Sons.

Ward's Directory (1932) *of Redcar and Coatham, Middlesbrough, Stockton and Thornaby* 1932–1933. Newcastle: R. Ward & Sons.

Ward's Directory (1934) *of Redcar and Coatham, Middlesbrough, Stockton and Thornaby* 1934–1935. Newcastle: R. Ward & Sons.

Ward's Directory (1938) *of Redcar and Coatham, Middlesbrough, Stockton and Thornaby* 1938–1939. Newcastle: R. Ward & Sons.

Watson, D. (2014) *No Justice Without A Struggle: The National Unemployed Workers' Movement in the North East of England 1920–1940.* London: Merlin Press.

Webster, C. (1982) Healthy or Hungry Thirties?, *History Workshop Journal*, 13 (1), 110–129.

Welshman, J. (2013) *Underclass.* London: Bloomsbury.

WHO (World Health Organization) (2010) International Workshop on Housing, Health and Climate Change. www.who.int/hia/house_report.pdf?ua=1

Williamson, p. (1992) *National crisis and National government.* Cambridge: Cambridge University Press.

Yarm Road Congregational Church (1935) *Church Minutes.* R/UR/S/3/4, Teesside Archives, Middlesbrough.

Yelling, J. A. (1988) The Origins of British Redevelopment Areas. *Planning Perspectives*, 3 (3), pp. 282–296.

THREE

Placing Health in Austerity

Ramjee Bhandari

Background

It is well acknowledged that place can create inequalities in health but there is a debate within geographical research as to whether the health and wellbeing of an individual is determined by their own attributes (the compositional theory) and/or the environmental attributes of the area where the person lives (contextual approach). More recently, it has been argued that these determinants interact with each other, signifying that they are 'mutually reinforcing' (relational). This chapter outlines this key debate and engages with it by using data from a longitudinal household survey conducted in the most and least deprived neighbourhoods of Stockton-on-Tees. It examines the explanatory role of compositional and contextual factors and their interaction. The survey results indicate that there is a significant gap in general and physical health in Stockton-on-Tees and compositional-level material factors, contextual factors and their interaction appear to be the major explanations of the health gap. The findings are discussed in relation to geographical theories of health inequalities and the political and economic context of austerity. It further highlights the importance of the 'relational approach' in understanding geographical inequalities in health.

Stockton-on-Tees has the highest health inequalities in England. Life expectancy at birth reveals a gap between the most and least deprived neighbourhoods of 17.3 years for men and 11.4 years for women (Public Health England, 2015). This is similar to differences in life expectancy between the US and Ghana or the UK and India (WHO, 2016). Life expectancy, though, is only a headline indicator, signifying the need to explore the extent and determinants of other aspects of health inequalities in that area (Bambra, 2016). A complex relationship exists between place, the people who live there and health. Complex in the sense that the characteristics of people (composition) and the nature and attributes of the place (context) act individually and collectively (Macintyre et al., 2002; Cummins et al., 2007). Further, it has been argued that these health divides between areas are 'political' in nature, influenced by the wider socio-political and macroeconomic context, for example economic recession and austerity (Schrecker and Bambra, 2015). In this chapter, the health gap between the most and the least deprived areas of Stockton-on-Tees is examined using validated measures of physical and general health. It also examines the contribution of compositional and contextual factors and their interaction in explaining this gap. Uniquely, this was done in a time of economic recession and austerity within the UK. The chapter will therefore be of interest not only to those who study health inequalities in the UK but also to the international public health research community who are tackling similar geographical inequalities in health in major urban settings (Bambra, 2016).

Understanding health and wellbeing

The World Health Organization defines health as 'a state of complete physical, mental and social wellbeing and not merely the absence of disease or infirmity' (WHO, 1995). With this holistic view of health and wellbeing, the primary focus shifts from a specific body part or symptoms of a disease to an overall performance of an individual. The holistic approach looks into the physical, emotional and social factors of an individual and explores how these factors in a collective way produce the health outcome. The principle of holistic approach is to understand how individual functions within their set of environmental and social characteristics. With this in the background, this chapter asserts the importance of the interaction between individual and collective characteristics. In addition, exploration of the determinants of health and wellbeing from a geographical perspective will also help understand the complex and dynamic nature of the social, political and economic factors that shape health and wellbeing (Nyman and Nilsen, 2016). This approach not only helps to understand the issue at an individual level but also looks at the differential exposures to the social determinants which lead to health inequalities. By assessing health and wellbeing from a macro perspective, it is possible to move beyond the traditional approach of individual subjectivity (La Placa et al., 2013). As argued by Knight and McNaught (2011), effective measures of health and wellbeing are able to demonstrate the dynamic construction of these states from an interplay of the individual and social structures at a macro-level.

Social determinants of health

The 'social determinants of health' are the collective set of conditions in which an individual is born, grows up, works and lives and which directly or indirectly affects their health. In their broadest form, they are identified as employment status, work and working environment, access to essential services (including health care), and housing and the living environment (Marmot, 2005; Bambra, 2011).

There is a strong research base that shows a relationship between unemployment and poor health (Warren et al., 2013; Beatty et al., 2017). Unemployment is an important life event, which not only induces stress, it is a primary determinant of health inequalities (Marmot et al., 2010; Marmot and Allen, 2014). Unemployment is associated with poor mental health conditions (Mattheys et al., 2016), and poor self-reported health and health damaging behaviours (Skalicka et al., 2009). The health impacts of unemployment are not limited to an individual, but can also extend to families (Bambra, 2011) and also contribute to geographical inequalities in health (Moller et al., 2013).

Work and working conditions also have strong relationships with health and health inequalities (Bambra, 2011). For example, exposure to hazardous chemicals (such as mercury and lead), vibrations (both hand-arm vibration and whole-body vibration with work which requires the use of hand-held power tools or who drive mobile machines) and physical load are associated increased risk of poor health. The psychosocial work environment (such as time pressure, job control and job security) also affects health (Bambra, 2011). Further, Bambra (2011) argues that the psychosocial work environment affects the social gradient among employees.

Access to essential services (including health care, goods and services) influences health and health inequalities from 'institutional mechanisms'. These services and health-affecting institutions (also referred to as 'opportunity structures'; for example, GP surgeries and fast food outlets) are socially constructed and can be of varied quality, availability and access (Macintyre et al., 2002; Sykes and Musterd, 2011).

Housing and the living environment are material determinants of health and wellbeing (Bambra, 2011). Housing issues (such as dampness, overcrowding and no heating) are negatively associated with health. Persistent exposure to housing problems results in poorer health conditions and exposure in the past could have health consequences in the present (Pevalin et al., 2017).

Geographical inequalities in health

Neighbourhoods that are the most deprived have worse health than those that are less deprived – this follows a socio-spatial gradient, with each increase in deprivation resulting in a decrease in average health. In England, the gap in average life expectancy between the most and least deprived areas is nine years for men and around seven years for women. Traditionally, geographical research drawing on the wider social determinants of health literature has tried to explain these differences in neighbourhood-level health by looking at compositional and contextual factors – and their interaction (Pickett and Pearl, 2001; Cummins et al., 2007). The compositional explanation asserts that the health of a given area is the result of the characteristics of the people who live there (demographic, behavioural and socioeconomic). The contextual explanation, on the other hand, argues that area-level health is determined by the nature of the place itself, in terms of its economic, social, cultural and physical environments.

The profile of the people within a community (demographic [age, sex, ethnicity], health-related behavioural [smoking, alcohol, physical activity, diet, drugs] and socioeconomic [income, education, occupation]) influences its health outcomes. Generally speaking, health deteriorates with age and health also varies by ethnicity/race. Smoking, alcohol, physical activity, diet and drugs – the five so-called 'lifestyle factors' or health behaviours, all influence health significantly. For example, smoking remains the most important preventable cause of mortality in the wealthy world. Alcohol-related deaths and diseases, as well as obesity, are on the increase, while exercise rates are in decline, and drugs are an increasingly important determinant of death among young people (Bambra et al., 2010). However, arguably of most importance is socioeconomic status. The literature suggests that there are several interacting pathways linking individual-level socioeconomic status and health: behavioural, material and psychosocial (Bartley, 2004). The 'materialist' explanation argues that it is income levels and what a decent or high income enables compared with a lower one, such as access to health-benefitting goods and services and limiting exposures to particular material risk factors. The 'behavioural-cultural' theory asserts that the causal mechanisms are higher rates of health-damaging behaviours in lower socioeconomic groups. The 'psychosocial' explanation focuses on the adverse biological consequences of psychological and social domination, and subordination, superiority and inferiority (for further detail see Chapter Six).

The contextual perspective asserts that differential exposure to the 'local geographical circumstances', brings about the differences in health status of the population (Pearce, 2015). Galster (2010) for example has proposed four specific, yet broad, mechanisms to describe the role of place in creating unequal health status: the social-interactive mechanism; the environmental mechanism; the geographical mechanism and the institutional mechanism. The social-interactive mechanism defines health inequalities as the outcome of the influence that one's social neighbourhood has in shaping the health-affecting norms, values and attitudes (Brannstrom and Rojas, 2012). The environmental mechanism deals with the socio-spatial distribution of health-damaging factors ('pathogens' such as violence and pollutants) and health-promoting factors ('salutogens' such as public parks and healing places), which have a distinct concentration pattern, the former being more common in the socially deprived areas and latter in less deprived neighbourhoods (Pearce, 2015). The geographical mechanism, on the other hand, explains that living in deprived locations over the long term, with limited or poor quality services, may lead to a vicious cycle of poverty and ill health (Hedman et al., 2015). Finally, institutional mechanisms seek to understand the health-affecting roles of institutions and services (also referred to as 'opportunity structures'; for example GP surgeries, fast food outlets) that are socially constructed and can be of varied quality, availability and access (Macintyre et al., 2002, Sykes and Musterd, 2011).

Macintyre and Ellaway (2009) have argued that a clear differentiation between compositional and contextual factors determining health inequalities is, in general sense impossible. It is because they are not mutually exclusive: the characteristics of individuals are influenced by the characteristics of the area. For example, compositional-level individual factors such as employment and job status of the people living in an area are influenced by the contextual-level characteristics of the local labour market, while these contextual factors are in turn influenced by the wider political and economic environment – with recessions and austerity again affecting local labour markets (Bambra, 2016). Moving away, then, from the conventional approach of focusing only on the contribution of compositional *or* contextual factors, Cummins et al. (2007) therefore argue for a 'relational approach' that accounts for the horizontal and vertical interaction between these factors – in addition to their individual contributions. This approach not only reconnects people and place but attempts to signify the importance of scale in understanding geographical health inequalities. It highlights the dynamic nature of place – how it is constructed and represented in research and how it is embedded in an individual's life. Place in this relational sense may not be defined by geographical administrative boundaries but by 'nodes in networks' (Horlings, 2016).

Recession, austerity and health inequalities

The financial crisis of 2007 – the worst since the Wall Street crash of 1929 – led to the onset of what has been called the 'Great Recession'. There had been several post-war financial downturns in Western European countries (for example the 1970s and 1990s) but none as serious, on economic and social grounds, as that which has affected the whole of Europe and the UK since 2008 (Ifanti et al., 2013). The UK had some austerity policies in hand such as tax reforms before the full crisis came into existence; this has been described by Blyth (2013) as 'pre-emptive tightening'. The crisis, though, accelerated after the imposition of austerity policies from 2010 onwards. UK austerity has been characterised by significant cuts to public service budgets, most notably in terms of local authority budgets, significant reductions in social security expenditure, alongside a strong emphasis on relying on a renewed market to repay the national deficit (Kitson et al., 2011). Though there have been strong voices against austerity, it remains in place and its impacts are ongoing (Baker, 2010). These funding and welfare cuts in the UK are geographically patterned and the worst hit areas are those that are already the most socially disadvantaged (Beatty and Fothergill, 2016). This has led to fears of widening deprivation and increases in health inequalities (Pearce, 2013; Bambra and Garthwaite, 2014; Beatty and Fothergill, 2016).

However, there is little by way of empirical assessment of the effects of austerity on inequalities in health (Pearce, 2013). The studies that do exist, however, have suggested a negative impact. For example, Niedzwiedz et al. (2016) found that reductions in spending levels and increased welfare conditionality adversely affected the mental health of disadvantaged social groups. Austerity measures have also affected vulnerable old-age adults, as a study by Loopstra et al. (2016) has noted that rising mortality rates among pensioners were linked to reductions in social spending and social care. Loopstra et al. (2015) also found that foodbank use is associated with cuts to local authority spending and central welfare spending. Across England there has been a widening inequalities in mental health since 2010 (Barr et al., 2015), with the largest increases in poor mental health (including suicides, self-reported mental health problems and anti-depressant prescription rates) in the most deprived areas (Barr et al., 2016).

Furthermore, as well as being few in number, the studies in the UK conducted to date which explore the extent of geographical health inequalities during austerity have also been conducted on a national scale and utilised national-level datasets. National-level statistics are often criticised for failing to represent and explain the proximal area-level situations or even the inequalities that persist between/in regional and local levels (Shouls et al., 1996; Cummins et al., 2005; Bambra, 2013). Those studies exploring different localities have also focused on local authority-level data rather than looking at a finer geographical scale such as neighbourhood or ward level. The indicators used have often been mortality rather than morbidity. This identifies a clear need for more localised studies that apply geographical theories to better understand the extent and causes of geographical inequalities in health in a time of austerity. Furthermore, focusing at a local scale provides us with a unique opportunity to get detailed primary information on health and the social determinants at a small geographical scale, which is not the case with secondary data (such as the census or Health Survey for England).

Methods

To understand the health of people living in the most and the least deprived areas of Stockton-on-Tees, a longitudinal survey was undertaken. The health gap in Stockton was examined using a stratified random sample of adults aged over 18, split between participants from the 20 most and 20 least deprived lower super output areas (LSOA). LSOAs are small areas of relatively even size, with around 1,500 people in each area; there are 32,484 LSOAs in England (DCLG, 2011). When studying deprivation status and relating it to health inequalities, LSOA is usually the preferred smallest spatial unit in England (Cairns-Nagi and Bambra, 2013). From 2010 the Index of Multiple Deprivation (IMD) scores for England was used to determine the 20 LSOAs in each of the extreme ends of deprivation within the borough. LSOA is the smallest geographical unit in England for which the IMD score is computed. IMD score is the key measure to identify area deprivation and its concentration in geographical units lower than local authorities in the England (Noble et al., 2006; Payne and Abel, 2012).

Survey recruitment

The final targeted sample size of 800 (400 in each group) was based on a conservative power calculation, derived from experience of previous health surveys in the same region of the UK (Warren et al., 2013). The sampling process utilised EQ5D (EQ5D is a part of EuroQol, which is a simple and generic health measure used in the clinical and economic appraisal) and SF8 (for detailed information on these indicators see the next section, 'Outcome variables', and Table 3.6), which assumed a 5% difference between the least and most deprived areas and the possible attrition in the follow-up surveys. Using a stratified random sampling technique (using 'R' statistical software program), a sample of 200 target households in each of the 40 LSOAs were created. Figure 3.1 shows the sampling strategy adopted for the study. For a detailed methodology, see Bhandari et al. (2017).

Figure 3.1: Sampling strategy for the survey

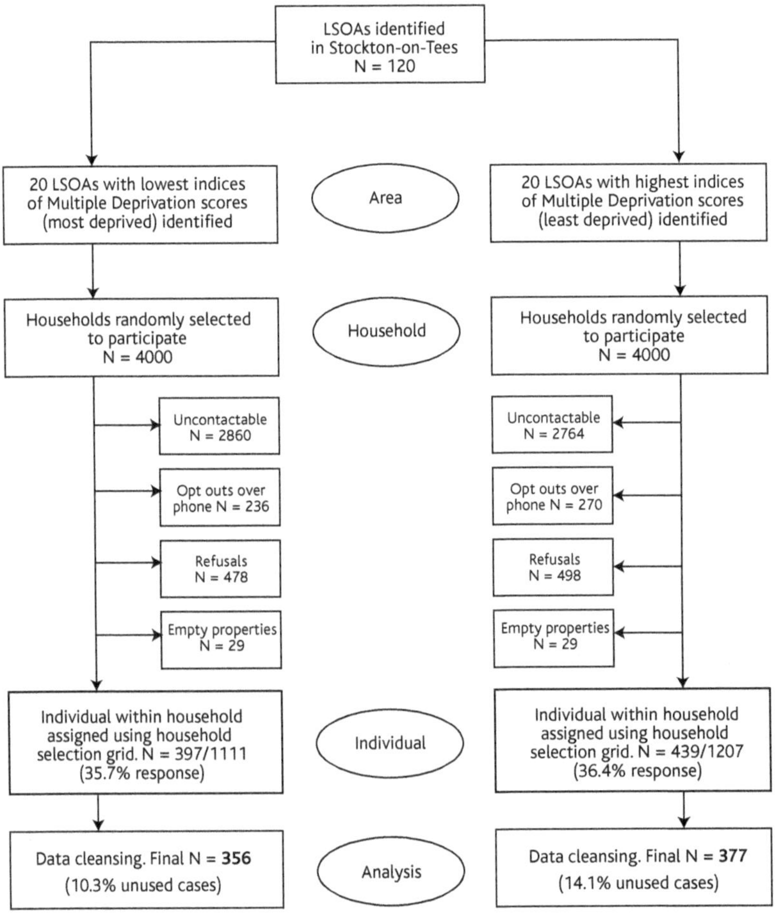

The baseline survey was conducted face-to-face and there were three follow up waves conducted by telephone (with the last one conducted 18 months after baseline). Table 3.1 presents a total number of survey participants in each wave and the dropout rates for each wave. In reaching the final wave, about half of the participants from the baseline cohort were retained, there was a higher rate of dropout in the least deprived areas which is typical of a longitudinal study (Eysenbach, 2005).

A data cleansing process was carried out and missing data were excluded for both outcome measures and predictor variables so that complete data were available for all cases allowing comparison between models. Table 3.1 summarises the number of participants that were included in the final analysis for each wave after dealing with the missing data. The rate of missing data was slightly over 12% for the baseline survey but it was 10% or less for all the follow-ups.

Outcome variables

The focus of my research was to assess inequalities in general and physical health among the most and least deprived neighbourhoods of Stockton-on-Tees. General health was assessed using EuroQol (EQ5D-VAS) and physical health was measured using 'quality metric short form (SF8)'. Both EuroQol and SF8 have been well-validated for use in the general population.

EuroQol consists of two parts: EQ5D questionnaire and the 'Visual Analogue Scale' (EQ5D-VAS), also known as health thermometer (EuroQol Research Foundation, 2016). EQ5D-VAS represents the perceived health status of the participant, which is measured on a scale of 0–100, 0 being the worst and 100 the best health state they can imagine (Warren et al., 2014).

Table 3.1: Total number of survey participants before and after data cleaning

	Least deprived		Complete data		Most deprived		Complete data		Total		Complete data	
	Total cases	%*	Cases	%	Total cases	%*	Cases	%	Total cases	%*	Cases	%
Baseline	439	–	356	81.1	397	–	377	95.0	836	–	733	87.7
6m	286	65	257	89.9	229	58	220	96.1	515	62	477	92.6
12m	260	59	238	91.5	218	55	205	94.0	478	57	443	92.7
18m	234	53	214	91.5	176	44	155	88.1	410	49	369	90.0

Note: * The percentages (%) represent the percentage of participants retained in the study relative to the number at baseline.

Using eight questions that focus on the health status of the participants during the last four weeks, SF8 produces two health scores: physical health score (SF8-PCS) and mental health score (SF8-MCS) (Warren et al., 2014). However, in this chapter, the analysis is limited to SF8-PCS only and one of the linked studies has used the SF8-MCS (see Chapter Six, this volume). The scores for this measure ranges between 0 and 100: the higher the score, the better the physical health state.

Statistical analysis

Multilevel modelling has been used as a way of determining the role of compositional factors, contextual factors and their interaction simultaneously (Curtis and Rees Jones, 1998; Duncan et al., 1998). MLM analysis was carried out to establish: (1) the magnitude of inequalities in general and physical health (as measured by EQ5D-VAS and SF8PCS); (2) the associations between compositional and contextual variables and the health outcomes; (3) relative explanatory contribution of the compositional and contextual variables and how this changed over time. The gap in the health outcomes between the participants from the most and least deprived LSOAs is labelled as 'Deprivation' in the results and tables.

Percentage reduction, percentage change for the specific model and percentage contribution of the categories of explanatory factors were computed for each health outcome as well as the indirect (interactive) contribution.

To explore the mean difference of the measures of health outcomes, multilevel models were applied. While doing so, age and gender were adjusted as the existing literature suggest a significant association of these factors with health inequalities (Graham, 2009) and it also controlled for the potential clustering within the LSOAs. The analysis started with the univariate analysis of the individual variables to filter out redundant variables (Hosmer et al., 2013; Agresti, 2015). Final models were obtained using likelihood ratio test to ensure no substantial information was lost due to variable selection (Verbeke and Molenberghs, 2000). The relative contribution of the variable categories was then calculated from the final model. Direct (sole contribution) and indirect (interactions) contributions of the explanatory variable categories were computed to explain the inequalities.

Results

Baseline characteristics

Table 3.2 shows the baseline socio-demographic information of the study participants that remained in the final analysis after excluding the missing data. These show that, in terms of gender, the sample has a higher proportion of women (60%) compared with the census data for Stockton for 2011 (51%). I also have an older population with 29% of the sample aged over 65 compared with about 16% in the 2011 census (ONS, 2013). However, in terms of socioeconomic status then the participants were broadly in keeping with the census as around 88% of households in the least deprived areas were owner occupied compared with 91% in the census. In the most deprived areas then 28% of the sample were owner occupiers compared with 38% recorded in the 2011 census. My modelling, therefore, adjusts for age and gender to take this into account. Table 3.3 shows the compositional factors. The

Table 3.2: Sociodemographic characteristics of the baseline sample

	Number (%)	
Variables	Least deprived	Most deprived
Age		
Under 25s	15 (4.0)	37 (10.4)
25–49	130 (34.5)	131 (36.7)
50–64	110 (29.2)	95 (26.6)
65 and over	122 (32.4)	94 (26.3)
Gender		
Male	162 (43.0)	146 (41.0)
Female	215 (57.0)	210 (59.0)
Marital status		
Married	221 (58.6)	90 (25.3)
Single	67 (17.8)	142 (39.9)
Divorced	39 (10.3)	58 (16.3)
Widowed	39 (10.3)	41 (11.5)
Ethnicity		
White	360 (95.5)	340 (95.8)
Asian or Asian British	10 (2.7)	0 (0.0)
Self-reported general health		
Good	280 (74.3)	174 (48.9)
Fair	79 (20.9)	119 (33.4)
Bad	18 (4.8)	63 (17.7)
Self-reported mental health problem	26 (6.9)	43 (12.0)

Table 3.3: Characteristics of the baseline sample: compositional characteristics

Material		
Highest Educational Level		
Higher or first degree	100 (26.5)	17 (4.8)
Higher diplomas/A-levels or equivalent	106 (28.1)	39 (10.9)
GCSE or equivalent	87 (23.1)	138 (38.8)
Entry level/no formal qualifications	84 (22.3)	162 (45.5)
Housing Tenure		
Own outright	193 (51.2)	61 (17.1)
Mortgage or loan	138 (36.6)	37 (10.4)
Rent	44 (11.7)	254 (71.3)
Live rent free	2 (0.5)	4 (1.1)
Household receipt of benefits	266 (70.6)	311 (87.4)
Household receipt of Housing Benefit	16 (4.2)	193 (54.2)
Workless household (at least one member out of work)	142 (37.7)	237 (66.6)
Current job skill type		
Professional	43 (11.3)	10 (2.8)
Unskilled	27 (7.1)	42 (11.8)
Work status		
Participant in paid employment	183 (48.5)	89 (25.0)
Retired	142 (37.5)	112 (31.4)
Unemployed*	53 (14.0)	156 (43.7)
Household annual income (mode)	£36400–£41600	£10400–£13000
Problems with damp in the home	10 (2.7)	94 (26.4)
Home is too dark	31 (8.2)	62 (17.4)
Home is not warm enough in winter	27 (7.2)	72 (20.2)
Home without double glazing	6 (1.6)	19 (5.3)
Own motor vehicle(s)	353 (93.6)	153 (43.0)
Psychosocial		
Lacking companionship		
Hardly ever	286 (75.9)	239 (67.1)
Some of the time	70 (18.6)	76 (21.3)
Often	21 (5.5)	40 (11.2)
Feeling left out		
Hardly ever	318 (84.4)	249 (69.9)
Some of the time	47 (12.4)	66 (18.5)
Often	12 (3.2)	41 (11.5)
Feeling isolated		
Hardly ever	310 (82.2)	255 (71.6)
Some of the time	54 (14.3)	60 (16.9)
Often	13 (3.4)	41 (11.5)

(continued)

Table 3.3: Characteristics of the baseline sample: compositional characteristics (continued)

Material		
Behavioural		
Respondents who smoke	39 (10.3)	132 (37)
Respondents who drink alcohol	297 (78.8)	210 (59.0)
Fruit/vegetable intake: average units (standard deviation)	4 (2.0)	2.8 (1.9)
Frequency of physical exercise		
Every day	113 (30.0)	128 (36.0)
Most days	65 (17.2)	44 (12.4)
Couple of times a week	78 (20.7)	42 (11.8)
Once a week	14 (3.7)	15 (4.2)
Less than once a week	13 (3.4)	14 (3.9)
Never	94 (24.9)	113 (31.7)

proportion of participants reporting housing issues was significantly higher in the most deprived areas (inadequate heating – 20% vs. 7%; dampness – 26% vs. 3%; darkness – 17% vs. 8%; and lack of double glazing – 5% vs. 2%). While smoking was more prevalent in the most deprived areas (37% vs. 10%), the use of alcohol was higher in the least deprived areas (79% vs. 59%). Table 3.4 presents the contextual neighbourhood-related factors reported by the survey participants from both areas. A higher proportion of participants from the most deprived areas reported noise problems (24% vs. 11%), pollution (13% vs. 3%) and crime (29% vs. 6%) in their neighbourhood. More than 12% of people from the most deprived areas felt unsafe walking alone in their neighbourhood after dark compared with less than 2% in the least deprived areas.

Table 3.4: Characteristics of the baseline sample: contextual factors

Variables	Number (%)	
Categories	Least deprived	Most deprived
Problems with neighbourhood noise	42 (11.1)	85 (23.9)
Problems with pollution	13 (3.4)	45 (12.6)
Problems with crime	24 (6.4)	105 (29.5)
Feeling unsafe walking alone after dark		
Very safe	207 (54.9)	107 (30.1)
Safe	141 (37.4)	132 (37.1)
Unsafe	23 (6.1)	73 (20.5)
Very unsafe	6 (1.6)	44 (12.4)

Stockton-on-Tees: the health divide

To explore the gap and relationship between area and the health outcomes, several multilevel models were fitted. Of the different models, the reference model (see Table 3.5) estimates the gaps in EQ5D-VAS and SF8PCS. For both health outcome measures and throughout the study period, there was a significant gap in physical and general health. People living in the least deprived areas had higher chances of having better general and physical health compared with those living in the most deprived areas. This supports the ongoing argument on the damaging effects of deprivation on people's health and wellbeing (Bambra and Garthwaite, 2015, Rahman et al., 2016, Stuckler et al., 2017).

Figure 3.2 shows the trend in estimated inequality gap in general and physical health between the areas. On average, people from the least deprived areas are likely to score more than 10 points higher on the EQ5D-VAS. Though no particular trend was observed with the general health measures, a steady increase in the gap between the two areas was observed with the physical health measure (SF8PCS). The estimate for SF8PCS increased from 4.76 (2.8, 6.73) during the baseline to 6.53 (4.42, 8.64) during the final wave, which is a 37% increase in the gap. When we correlate the findings presented in Table 3.4 and Figure 3.2, we can see that, over time, the people

Table 3.5: Trend of health inequalities in Stockton-on-Tees: estimates of fixed effects

Health measures	Parameter	Estimate (95% confidence interval)			
		Baseline	Wave 2	Wave 3	Wave 4
EQ5D-VAS	Intercept	71.85 (66.2, 77.47)	77.37 (71.1, 83.65)	77.02 (70, 83.33)	76.91 (70, 83.72)
	Deprivation	10.86 (5.89, 15.82)	10.41 (6.57, 14.26)	10.1 (6.69, 13.59)	10.96 (7.38, 14.5)
	Gender	−0.14 (−3.15, 2.87)	0.09 (−3.42, 3.59)	−1.93 (−5.44, 1.58)	−3.47 (−7.05, 0.12)
	Age	−0.15 (−0.24, −0.06)	−0.15 (−0.25, −0.04)	−0.1 (−0.20, 0.01)	−0.1 (−0.21, 0.01)
SF8PCS	Intercept	54.1 (51.51, 56.78)	51.1 (47.68, 54.4)	50.3 (46.79, 53.86)	50.36 (46, 54.38)
	Deprivation	4.76 (2.8, 6.73)	5.84 (3.71, 7.97)	6.48 (4.55, 8.42)	6.53 (4.42, 8.64)
	Gender	0.99 (−0.56, 2.54)	0.37 (−1.49, 2.23)	0.90 (−1.07, 2.87)	1.002 (−1.12, 3.12)
	Age	−0.17 (−0.2, −0.13)	−0.12 (−0.18, −0.07)	−0.11 (−0.17, −0.05)	−0.12 (−0.18, −0.05)

Figure 3.2: Trend of estimated inequality gap in EQ5D-VAS and SF8PCS scores between most and least deprived areas with 95% confidence interval

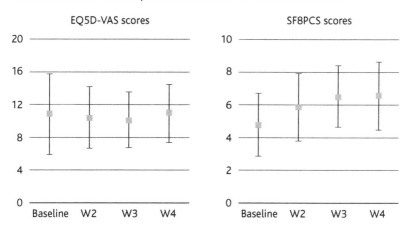

from the most deprived areas are not doing as well in physical health measures as their counterparts in the least deprived areas.

These findings support the argument that during a time of austerity, inequalities in health get wider (Abebe et al., 2016; Barr et al., 2017; Stuckler et al., 2017). A study by Abebe et al. (2016) has found that there was a significant increase in poor self-reported health during the recession and after the welfare cuts in the UK and they have highlighted its role in widening health gap. Bambra and Garthwaite (2015) have suggested that during a time of austerity, spatial health inequalities will increase and this will disproportionately affect the older industrial areas such as Stockton-on-Tees. More recently, compared with the post-financial crisis period, the general health of UK has slowly improved, albeit this improvements has left a trail of inequalities, with the most disadvantaged groups lagging behind (Beatty et al., 2017).

Explaining the Stockton-on-Tees health divide

After analysing the gap in general and physical health outcomes between the most and least deprived areas of Stockton-on-Tees, the next step was to explore the key compositional and contextual factors associated with this gap. Multilevel models were fitted for EQ5D-VAS and SF8PCS and for each wave. The associations between the health outcome measures and compositional and contextual factors are presented in Table 3.6. The relationship between health inequalities and the social determinants of health has been well established. This

Table 3.6: Association between health outcome measures and the explanatory variables (shaded blocks indicate the presence of significant association)

Factors	Variables*	EQ5D-VAS				SF8PCS			
		BL	W2	W3	W4	BL	W2	W3	W4
Material	Household income	■							■
	Household worklessness (Yes/No)		░						
	Paid employment (Yes/No)			░			■		
	Household benefits (Yes/No)							░	
	Housing benefit (Yes/No)								
	The house has double glazing (Yes/No)				■				
	The house is damp (Yes/No)								
Psycho-social	Lacking companionship								
	Happiness scale		■			■	■		■
	Frequency of feeling left out						░		
	Frequency of feeling isolated from others								
Behavioural	Frequency of physical exercise**				■	░			
	Alcohol use (Yes/No)						■	■	
	Alcohol Units								
	Alcohol consumption above recommended limit (Yes/No)				■				
Contextual/ Neighbourhood	Feeling unsafe walking alone after dark (Yes/No)								
	Neighbourhood noise (Yes/No)								
	Pollution/Environmental problems (Yes/No)								
	Neighbourhood crime (Yes/No)								
	Belongingness to the area (Yes/No)								
	Outdoor environment score-IMD								
	Crime score-IMD								

Notes: * For the Yes/No response variables, 'No' was the reference group; **Daily exercise was the reference category

Legend: ■ Positive association   ░ Negative association

study adds to the substantial evidence on the role of individual/ compositional (Marmot and Allen, 2014) and area level/contextual factors (Cummins et al., 2005) in creating the health gap. This was done by exploring the relative contributions of these determinants and further looking how this changed over time. Association between individual-level factors and health inequalities have been found which is consistent with previous research; for example, see Skalicka et al. (2009), Arber et al. (2014) and Pemberton et al. (2016).

Table 3.6 shows that having a higher household income, being in paid employment was positively associated with both the health outcome measures. Likewise, worklessness of an adult member, receipt of household and housing benefit were negatively associated with the health outcomes. Among the behavioural factors, people who are happier were more likely to have better general and physical health outcomes. However, frequency of feeling left-out, lacking of companionship and feeling isolated from others were all negatively associated with the health outcome measures. Compared with people who exercise daily, those exercising less frequently have lower EQ5D-VAS and SF8PCS scores. Interestingly, alcohol use was positively associated with the health outcome measures. People who felt belonging to their neighbourhood had better EQ5D-VAS scores (positive association). Feeling unsafe walking alone after dark, neighbourhood noise and pollution were all negatively associated with both EQ5D-VAS and SF8PCS scores. 'Crime scores' and 'outdoor living environment deprivation scores' (sub-domains of IMD) for IMD 2015 were significantly associated with lower SF8PCS scores.

The second part of model building process involved the exploration of the relative contribution of the variable categories from the final model. Direct (sole contribution) and indirect (interactions) contributions of the explanatory variable categories were computed to explain the inequalities. In this section, I will look into the percentage contribution of the various compositional and contextual factors to the health gap in Stockton-on-Tees borough, and explore who this contribution has changed over time. Figure 3.3 illustrates the approach.

Table 3.7 presents the standardised percentage contribution of the different categories to the gap in EQ5D-VAS. The percentage explanations of the final models were computed for each survey wave. Compared with the baseline survey, the percentage explanation of the health gap dropped in the subsequent follow-up surveys. The direct contribution refers to the unique share of a specific category in explaining the health inequalities gap. On the other hand, the indirect effect is the shared contribution of all the categories in explaining

Figure 3.3: Understanding geographical inequalities in health

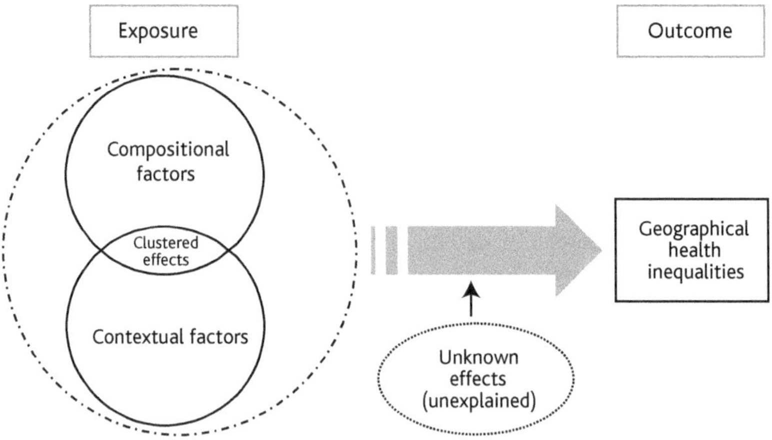

the health gap. The relative contribution was computed from the percentage explanation of the full model and the percentage change for each model. The relative contribution of a category was calculated, which subtracts the percentage change of the model without this specific category from the percentage change of the full model. The indirect contribution or *clustering effect* was computed in which the sum of the percentage contribution of each category was subtracted from the percentage explanation of the full model.

For all waves and for both health outcome measures, clustered effects were high indicating the importance of interaction between the compositional and contextual factors in explaining the gap in physical health between the people living in the most and the least deprived areas of Stockton-on-Tees.

Table 3.7: Relative contribution of different categories standardised to the total explained percentage of the full model for the gap in general and physical health measures

Category	EQ5D-VAS				SF8PCS scores			
	BL	W2	W3	W4	BL	W2	W3	W4
All compositional	57.8	35.1	52.7	68.6	46.6	25.7	54.2	54.8
Material	28.3	5.7	28.2	8.2	33.1	5.8	38.4	29.2
Psychosocial	1.0	14.9	14.4	28.9	0.4	11.4	4.3	0.8
Behavioural	6.0	9.9	2.4	28.5	5.1	0.3	8.1	15.8
Contextual	20.2	31.0	29.5	15.3	39.6	57.5	31.4	16.8
Clustered	44.6	38.4	44.6	19.1	21.7	25.0	17.9	27.5
Total explained	72.2	58.0	49.1	34.3	95.4	90.3	64.4	58.1
Total unexplained	27.8	42.0	50.9	65.7	4.6	9.7	35.6	41.9

Discussion

The results show that the health gap in terms of physical health slightly increased over the 18-month study period while the gap in self-rated general health remained constant. Further, in terms of how different factors explained the gap, the results suggest that the contributions of the individual-level compositional factors were more pronounced than the neighbourhood-level contextual factors. For both health measures and for each wave, all compositional factors combined had significant direct contributions, which were higher than the contribution of the contextual factors, such as neighbourhood noise, pollution and crime. Among the compositional factors and in most of the cases, material factors related to income and employment status of the household (such as household income, paid job, worklessness within the household, dampness in the house and lack of central heating) were the most important predictors of the health gap.

These findings match the qualitative findings from other research from the UK (Egan et al., 2015; Moffatt et al., 2016). In keeping with Pevalin et al. (2017) I have found that persistent exposure to housing problems resulted in poorer health conditions and the exposure in the past could have health consequences in the present. Likewise, a study from Norway found that material factors were the most important compositional factors in explaining the inequalities in mortality (Skalicka et al., 2009). The important contribution of household income to the physical health inequalities is also demonstrated by Arber et al. (2014). With my research findings, I agree on the existence of a two-way relationship between worklessness and poor health. For example, a research conducted in England by Pemberton et al. (2016) found that the current labour market does not appropriately cater to the job needs of the people with existing health conditions, resulting in them staying out of the active labour market. Using data from population surveys for England, a study by Moller et al. (2013) has attributed higher prevalence of morbidity (mental health problems and limiting long-term illness) and mortality with rising unemployment. The gap in unemployment between the most and the least deprived groups increased in the UK following the financial crisis and I agree with the argument of Moller et al. (2013) that this difference has disproportionately affected vulnerable families and communities. Worklessness within the household affects individuals and their families (Bambra, 2011).

This means austerity may well exacerbate existing health inequalities. For example, in his report on austerity in Teesside, Edwards (2012) highlighted a sharp rise and a high concentration of benefits claimants in the most deprived areas following the welfare cuts. The same report also highlighted the diminishing resources available to support the voluntary and community sector that are crucial in dealing with the issues (such as an increase in demand for advice and a penalty charge for 'under-occupation' also known as the 'bedroom tax') that can arise following dramatic welfare reform. The welfare changes mostly affected vulnerable families with low incomes, with members on out of work benefits, and/or who are long-term sick and disabled (Edwards et al., 2013). With more households from the deprived areas of Stockton-on-Tees facing economic hardships and the limited availability of collective resources and welfare support, the health of people from these households may suffer more, a concept known as *deprivation amplification*: area-level deprivation can amplify the health impacts of individual-level socioeconomic status (Macintyre, 2007; Bambra, 2016). The changing socioeconomic conditions of the households and that of the borough of Stockton-on-Tees as part of the welfare reforms when looked at in conjunction with the findings from my research could be correlated and used as an explanation of prevailing and/or widening health inequalities.

When compared with material and contextual factors, psychosocial and behavioural factors made relatively less contribution to the health inequality gap. Noticeably, people who had higher happiness scores were more likely to have higher scores for both health outcomes. These findings lend support to the argument of Friedli (2009) that happiness is a key element of general wellbeing. I agree with Veenhoven (2008) that happiness, as a compositional factor, is not just a predictor to better physical and mental wellbeing; it also has a strong correlation with contextual factors such as healthy living environment. Veenhoven (2008) further argues that happiness of an individual also depends on the wider socio-political context of the country – material wealth, political democracy, freedom and governance. Welfare reform and austerity were linked with a decrease in happiness score in Greece and Portugal (Blanchflower and Oswald, 2011), and as Veenhoven (2008) argues it is probable that the political context influences the happiness of individuals. Considering this alongside my findings that the average happiness scores decreased among the most deprived areas during the study period, I argue that the welfare cuts have negatively affected people's psychosocial wellbeing. Further, loneliness, which was assessed as feeling left out and/or isolated, was present in one or both forms in all the health inequalities models and made a significant negative contribution during each wave. These psychosocial factors often affect health from a behavioural pathway, for example, Lauder et al. (2006) have found lonely people had higher odds of adopting sedentary lifestyles and smoking. This could be the case among my survey participants as well because relatively more people from the most deprived areas reported of feeling lonely and left out compared with those from the least deprived areas (12% vs. 3%). Likewise, smoking (37% vs. 10%) and people who never did physical exercise (32% vs. 25) were also more prevalent in the most deprived areas. In addition, frequency of physical exercise was significantly associated with all health outcome measures and during each survey wave.

Throughout the 18-month study period, it was found that the participants who did less physical exercise had a higher likelihood of poorer general and physical health, which is consistent with studies conducted in Spain, Switzerland and England (Chatton and Kayser, 2013; Galan et al., 2013; Maheswaran et al., 2013). As argued by Warburton et al. (2006), there is a two-way relationship between health outcomes and physical exercise: poor health outcome could be the cause or the consequence of less physical exercise. My research involved older population and their health conditions could have an impact on the frequency of physical exercise. However, my research was not designed to explore the frequency of physical exercise as an outcome measure. Consumption of alcohol was, however, positively associated with better health outcomes (participants consuming alcohol could expect to have better general and physical health), which is similar to the finding by Powers and Young (2008). The linked study of mental health outcomes (see Chapter Six), found a similar relationship and that people who had better mental health outcomes and who consumed alcohol did so while socialising with family and friends. I agree that the social aspect of alcohol consumption could have provided protective psychosocial roles in the overall health and wellbeing of the participants (for example via decreased loneliness). This finding, however, contradicts much of the existing evidence base on the detrimental long-term effects of alcohol consumption (Rehm, 2011) – particularly problematic or binge drinking. These behavioural factors were significantly associated with the health gap but their contributions were mostly smaller than that of material and contextual factors. This indicates that attempts to reduce health inequalities by concentrating on behaviour and ignoring other factors are unlikely to be the most efficient or effective.

My research is one of the few studies looking at the relative contribution of contextual factors to the health divide. Ross and Mirowsky (2008) have argued that to correctly infer the contextual effects, multilevel modelling with adjustment of comprehensive individual characteristics is to be adopted in the study. People living in neighbourhoods where they felt unsafe walking alone after dark had higher chances of having significantly lower scores for both the health outcome measures included in this study. A longitudinal study conducted in Australia by Foster et al. (2016) has associated long-standing physical and mental health problems with the lower level of neighbourhood safety. The same study found a significant increase in recreational walking time with an increased perception of neighbourhood safety. I agree with Ruijsbroek et al. (2015) that the behavioural factors such as physical activities are often determined by contextual factors such as neighbourhood crime and feeling unsafe. Neighbourhood safety perception is a key feature of the contextual accounts of geographical health inequalities (Baum et al., 2009, Foster et al., 2016), with unsafe neighbourhoods particularly detrimental to people's general and physical health.

In my research, a higher proportion of survey participants from the most deprived areas reported the problems with pollution in their neighbourhood (12.6% vs. 3.4%) and neighbourhood noise (23.9% vs. 11.1%). The research findings suggest that the people living in areas with a higher level of neighbourhood noise and environmental problems can expect to have poorer physical and mental health outcomes. This is in keeping with a substantial body of literature which suggests an association between health inequalities and levels of outdoor air pollution (Marshall et al., 2009), with deprived areas being disproportionately and adversely affected. Marshall et al. (2009) has argued that neighbourhood pollution and environmental problems can have direct health impacts (cardiopulmonary morbidities such as chronic obstructive pulmonary disease – COPD) and indirect impacts through behavioural pathways (for example by limiting physical exercise). The disproportionate distribution of pollution and environmental problems between the most and the least deprived areas of Stockton-on-Tees could be linked to the health gap.

Most notably, though, this research shows the importance of the interaction of compositional and contextual variables, empirically supporting a relational view of health and place (Cummins et al., 2007). There were substantial indirect (clustered) effects for both health outcomes and for all waves, which is an indication of the interaction of the factors representing the different groups of explanatory variables. The clustered effects were as high as 44.6% for EQ5D-VAS (baseline and wave 3) and 27.5% for SF8PCS scores (wave 4). For both outcome measures, the combined analysis explains the highest percentage of the health gap, which demonstrates the important interaction between the individual-level material and contextual environmental factors in causing the health gap. A study by De Clercq et al. (2012) among Flemish communities has revealed a complex interaction between individual material factors and the neighbourhood context to produce health inequalities. These findings lend support to the idea of the 'mutually reinforcing' nature of compositional and contextual factors, it also justifies the need of 'relational approach' in understanding the contribution of individual- and area-level factors (Cummins et al., 2007).

In this study, the secondary data sources used to measure context were based on fixed administrative boundaries and they had little influence on the health gap. However, the contextual factors from the survey measured at an individual level made a significant contribution to the health inequalities gap. This may be because individuals have relatively dynamic and fluid area definitions. They were not confined to the LSOAs of the study but to how participants viewed the relational structure of the neighbourhoods they felt that they belonged to and therefore there was variation by individual (Bernard et al., 2007; Horlings, 2016). This level of data is not usually available at a national or regional scale, which validates the relational approach that was adopted at a local level.

This survey started after the onset of austerity programme in the UK the timeline for the role-out of some specific welfare reform programmes are still underway. In this context, this study will be unable to show direct links of these programmes to health gap. It was, however, able to explore changes during the current period. While my research questions were concerned with the inequalities in general and physical health over time, I also wanted to explore if there was any link between austerity and the health gap. The longitudinal survey has highlighted the existence of a significant and almost constant gap in general health over time while the inequalities gap in physical health was increasing, with the most deprived areas having constantly declining average scores. There was a noticeable gap between the two areas for material and contextual factors: level of unemployment, not in paid jobs, receipt of benefits, worklessness in the household, housing tenure, household annual income, neighbourhood noise, neighbourhood pollution, crime and feeling safe walking out after dark. These findings add to the existing literature on how the global financial crisis of 2008 and the austerity that followed has caused, helped sustain or even widen the local inequalities in general and physical health (Nunn, 2016; Barr et al., 2017; Basu et al., 2017;

Ruckert and Labonte, 2017). Regarding the post-2010 period, Barr et al. (2017) have further argued that the increasing trend of inequalities is due to the 2008 financial crisis and resulting politics of austerity. As part of austerity, several large-scale health-promotion policies were reversed (Taylor-Robinson and Gosling, 2011; Barr and Taylor-Robinson, 2014; Loopstra et al., 2016) and the welfare sector received major budget cuts. Existing evidence suggesting that the impacts of welfare reform are more damaging to the poorest parts of society (Pearce, 2013), could be the explanation for the widening gap in physical health in Stockton-on-Tees.

Conclusion

The work presented in this chapter contributes towards understanding the geographical health divide during the time of austerity. Exploiting the power of longitudinal data, this chapter has revealed the causal relationships between different compositional and contextual factors with the geographical health divide in Stockton-on-Tees. This research has shown the extent to which 'place' and its attributes matter for health inequalities; these contextual factors either contribute directly or interact with compositional factors in the creation of the health gap between the most and the least deprived neighbourhoods. The results presented in this chapter reinforce the need to understand composition and context of health inequalities from a relational perspective. The study has also found some damaging effects of austerity on physical health. Against a backdrop of continued austerity and further changes in welfare programmes (for example, the shift to universal credit), it is crucial that researchers and policy makers consider their adverse consequences for health and wellbeing.

References

Abebe, D. S., Tøge, A. G. and Dahl, E. (2016) Individual-level changes in self-rated health before and during the economic crisis in Europe. *International Journal for Equity in Health*, 15, 1

Agresti, A. (2015) *Foundations of linear and generalized linear models*, New Jersey, John Wiley & Sons

Arber, S., Fenn, K. and Meadows, R. (2014) Subjective financial well-being, income and health inequalities in mid and later life in Britain. *Social Science & Medicine*, 100, 12–20

Baker, A. (2010) *Austerity in the UK: Why it is not common sense but politically driven nonsense.* Centre for Progressive Economics. www.qub.ie/schools/SchoolofPoliticsInternationalStudiesandPhilosophy/FileStore/Stafffiles/AndrewBaker/Filetoupload,224825,en.pdf

Bambra, C. (2011) *Work, worklessness, and the political economy of health,* Oxford, Oxford University Press

Bambra, C. (ed.) (2013) *'All in it together'? Health inequalities, austerity and the 'great recession',* London: Demos Collection

Bambra, C. (2016) *Health divides: where you live can kill you,* Bristol, UK, Policy Press

Bambra, C. and Garthwaite, K. (2014) Welfare and Austerity. *Inquiry into Health Equity in the North of England.* Department of Geography, Durham University and Fuse: UKCRC Centre for Excellence in Translational Research in Public Health

Bambra, C. and Garthwaite, K. (2015) Austerity, welfare reform and the English health divide. *Area,* 47, 341–343

Barr, B. and Taylor-Robinson, D. (2014) Poor areas lose out most in new NHS budget allocation. *BMJ : British Medical Journal,* 348

Barr, B., Kinderman, P. and Whitehead, M. (2015) Trends in mental health inequalities in England during a period of recession, austerity and welfare reform 2004 to 2013. *Soc Sci Med,* 147, 324–31

Barr, B., Higgerson, J. and Whitehead, M. (2017) Investigating the impact of the English health inequalities strategy: time trend analysis. *BMJ,* 358

Barr, B., Taylor-Robinson, D., Stuckler, D., Loopstra, R., Reeves, A. and Whitehead, M. (2016) 'First, do no harm': are disability assessments associated with adverse trends in mental health? A longitudinal ecological study. *J. Epidemiol. Community Health,* 70, 339–45

Bartley, M. (2004) *Health inequality: An introduction to theories, concepts and methods,* Cambridge, Polity Press in association with Blackwell

Basu, S., Carney, M. and Kenworthy, N. J. (2017) Ten years after the financial crisis: The long reach of austerity and its global impacts on health. *Social Science & Medicine,* 187: 203–207

Baum, F. E., Ziersch, A. M., Zhang, G. Y. and Osborne, K. (2009) Do perceived neighbourhood cohesion and safety contribute to neighbourhood differences in health? *Health & Place,* 15, 925–934

Beatty, C. and Fothergill, S. (2016) The Uneven Impact of Welfare Reform: The financial losses to places and people. Sheffield: Sheffield Hallam University

Beatty, C., Fothergill, S. and Gore, T. (2017) The real level of unemployment 2017. Project Report. Sheffield: Sheffield Hallam University

Bernard, P., Charafeddine, R., Frohlich, K. L., Daniel, M., Kestens, Y. and Potvin, L. (2007) Health inequalities and place: a theoretical conception of neighbourhood. *Social Science & Medicine*, 65, 1839–1852

Bhandari, R., Kasim, A., Warren, J., Akhter, N. and Bambra, C. (2017) Geographical inequalities in health in a time of austerity: Baseline findings from the Stockton-on-Tees cohort study. *Health & Place*, 48, 111–122

Blanchflower, D. G. and Oswald, A. J. (2011) *International happiness.* National Bureau of Economic Research

Blyth, M. (2013) Austerity: The history of a dangerous idea. Oxford/ New York: Oxford University Press

Brannstrom, L. and Rojas, Y. (2012) Rethinking the Long-Term Consequences of Growing Up in a Disadvantaged Neighbourhood: Lessons from Sweden. *Housing Studies*, 27, 729–747

Cairns-Nagi, J. M. and Bambra, C. (2013) Defying the odds: a mixed-methods study of health resilience in deprived areas of England. *Soc Sci Med*, 91, 229–37

Chatton, A. and Kayser, B. (2013) Self-reported health, physical activity and socio-economic status of middle-aged and elderly participants to a popular road running race in Switzerland: better off than the general population? *Swiss Med. Wkly.*, 143, w13710

Cummins, S., Stafford, M., Macintyre, S., Marmot, M. and Ellaway, A. (2005) Neighbourhood environment and its association with self rated health: evidence from Scotland and England. *Journal of Epidemiology and Community Health*, 59, 207–213

Cummins, S., Curtis, S., Diez-Roux, A. V. and Macintyre, S. (2007) Understanding and representing 'place' in health research: a relational approach. *Soc Sci Med*, 65, 1825–38

Curtis, S. and Rees Jones, I. (1998) Is there a place for geography in the analysis of health inequality? *Sociology of Health & Illness*, 20, 645–672

De Clercq, B., Vyncke, V., Hublet, A., Elgar, F. J., Ravens-Sieberer, U., Currie, C., Hooghe, M., Leven, A. and Maes, L. (2012) Social capital and social inequality in adolescents' health in 601 Flemish communities: A multilevel analysis. *Social Science & Medicine*, 74, 202–210

DCLG (Dept for Communities and Local Government) (2011) *The English Indices of Deprivation 2010* www.gov.uk/government/uploads/ system/uploads/attachment_data/file/6871/1871208.pdf

Duncan, C., Jones, K. and Moon, G. (1998) Context, composition and heterogeneity: using multilevel models in health research. *Social Science & Medicine*, 46, 97–117

Edwards, P. (2012) *The Impact of Welfare Reform in Stockton*. Durham: Institute for Local Governance

Edwards, P., Jarvis, A., Crow, R., Crawshaw, P., Shaw, K., Irving, A. and Whisker, A. (2013) *The Impact of Welfare Reform in the North East*. Durham: Institute for Local Governance

Egan, M., Lawson, L., Kearns, A., Conway, E. and Neary, J. (2015) Neighbourhood demolition, relocation and health. A qualitative longitudinal study of housing-led urban regeneration in Glasgow, UK. *Health & Place*, 33, 101–108

Euroqol Research Foundation. (2016) *EQ-5D Nomenclature*. www.euroqol.org/about-eq-5d/eq-5d-nomenclature.html

Eysenbach, G. (2005) The law of attrition. *J. Med. Internet Res.*, 7, e11

Foster, S., Hooper, P., Knuiman, M., Christian, H., Bull, F. and Giles-Corti, B. (2016) Safe RESIDential Environments? A longitudinal analysis of the influence of crime-related safety on walking. *Int J Behav Nutr Phys Act*, 13, 22

Friedli, L. (2009) *Mental health, resilience and inequalities*. Copenhagen: WHO Regional Office for Europe

Galan, I., Boix, R., Medrano, M. J., Ramos, P., Rivera, F., Pastor-Barriuso, R. and Moreno, C. (2013) Physical activity and self-reported health status among adolescents: a cross-sectional population-based study. *BMJ open*, 3

Galster, G. C. (2010) The mechanism(s) of neighbourhood effects: Theory, evidence, and policy implications. *Neighbourhood effects research: New perspectives.* Springer

Graham, H. (2009) *Understanding health inequalities*. 2nd ed. Maidenhead: McGraw-Hill Open University Press

Hedman, L., Manley, D., Van Ham, M. and Osth, J. (2015) Cumulative exposure to disadvantage and the intergenerational transmission of neighbourhood effects. *J Econ Geogr*, 15, 195–215

Horlings, L. G. (2016) Connecting people to place: sustainable place-shaping practices as transformative power. *Current Opinion in Environmental Sustainability*, 20, 32–40

Hosmer, D. W., Lemeshow, S. and Sturdivant, R. X. (2013) *Applied logistic regression*, John Wiley & Sons

Ifanti, A. A., Argyriou, A. A., Kalofonou, F. H. and Kalofonos, H. P. (2013) Financial crisis and austerity measures in Greece: their impact on health promotion policies and public health care. *Health Policy*, 113, 8–12

Kitson, M., Martin, R. and Tyler, P. (2011) The geographies of austerity. *Cambridge Journal of Regions, Economy and Society*, 4, 289–302

Knight, A. and McNaught, A. (2011) *Understanding wellbeing: An introduction for students and practitioners of health and social care*, Lantern

La Placa, V., McNaught, A. and Knight, A. (2013) Discourse on wellbeing in research and practice. *International Journal of Wellbeing*, 3, 116–125

Lauder, W., Mummery, K., Jones, M. and Caperchione, C. (2006) A comparison of health behaviours in lonely and non-lonely populations. *Psychol. Health Med.*, 11, 233–45

Loopstra, R., McKee, M., Katikireddi, S. V., Taylor-Robinson, D., Barr, B. and Stuckler, D. (2016) Austerity and old-age mortality in England: a longitudinal cross-local area analysis, 2007–2013. *J. R. Soc. Med.*, 109, 109–116

Loopstra, R., Reeves, A., Taylor-Robinson, D., Barr, B., McKee, M. and Stuckler, D. (2015) Austerity, sanctions, and the rise of food banks in the UK. *BMJ*, 350, h1775

Macintyre, S. (2007) Deprivation amplification revisited; or, is it always true that poorer places have poorer access to resources for healthy diets and physical activity? *International Journal of Behavioral Nutrition and Physical Activity*, 4, 32

Macintyre, S. and Ellaway, A. (2009) Neighbourhood influences on health. In: Graham, H. (ed.) *Understanding health inequalities.* Second ed.: McGraw-Hill International

Macintyre, S., Ellaway, A. and Cummins, S. (2002) Place effects on health: how can we conceptualise, operationalise and measure them? *Soc Sci Med*, 55, 125–39

Maheswaran, H., Petrou, S., Rees, K. and Stranges, S. (2013) Estimating EQ-5D utility values for major health behavioural risk factors in England. *Journal of Epidemiology and Community Health*, 67, 172–180

Marmot, M. (2005) Social determinants of health inequalities. *The Lancet*, 365, 1099–1104

Marmot, M., Allen, J., Goldblatt, P., Boyce, T., McNeish, D., Grady, M. and Geddes, I. (2010) Fair society, healthy lives. *Strategic review of health inequalities in England post-2010.* London: UCL Institute for Health Equity

Marmot, M. and Allen, J. J. (2014) Social Determinants of Health Equity. *American Journal of Public Health*, 104, S517-S519

Marshall, J. D., Brauer, M. and Frank, L. D. (2009) Healthy neighborhoods: walkability and air pollution. *Environ. Health Perspect.*, 117, 1752–9

Mattheys, K., Bambra, C., Warren, J., Kasim, A. and Akhter, N. (2016) Inequalities in mental health and well-being in a time of austerity: Baseline findings from the Stockton-on-Tees cohort study. *SSM – Population Health*, 2, 350–359

Moffatt, S., Lawson, S., Patterson, R., Holding, E., Dennison, A., Sowden, S. and Brown, J. (2016) A qualitative study of the impact of the UK 'bedroom tax'. *J Public Health (Oxf)*, 38, 197–205

Moller, H., Haigh, F., Harwood, C., Kinsella, T. and Pope, D. (2013) Rising unemployment and increasing spatial health inequalities in England: further extension of the North–South divide. *Journal of Public Health*, 35, 313–321

Niedzwiedz, C. L., Mitchell, R. J., Shortt, N. K. and Pearce, J. R. (2016) Social protection spending and inequalities in depressive symptoms across Europe. *Soc. Psychiatry Psychiatr. Epidemiol.*, 51, 1005–14

Noble, M., Wright, G., Smith, G. and Dibben, C. (2006) Measuring Multiple Deprivation at the Small-Area Level. *Environment and Planning A*, 38, 169–185

Nunn, A. (2016) The production and reproduction of inequality in the UK in times of austerity. *British Politics*, 11, 469–487

Nyman, C. and Nilsen, A. (2016) Perspectives on health and well-being in social sciences. *Int J Qual Stud Health Well-being*, 11, 31468

ONS (Office for National Statistics) (2013) Usual resident population. In: Office for National Statistics (ed.). Nomis

Payne, R. A. and Abel, G. A. (2012) UK indices of multiple deprivation: a way to make comparisons across constituent countries easier. *Health Statistics Quarterly*, 22

Pearce, J. (2013) Commentary: Financial crisis, austerity policies, and geographical inequalities in health'. *Environment and Planning A*, 45, 2030–2045

Pearce, J. (2015) Invited commentary: history of place, life course, and health inequalities-historical geographic information systems and epidemiologic research. *Am. J. Epidemiol.*, 181, 26–9

Pemberton, S., Fahmy, E., Sutton, E. and Bell, K. (2016) Navigating the stigmatised identities of poverty in austere times: Resisting and responding to narratives of personal failure. *Crit Soc Policy*, 36, 21–37

Pevalin, D. J., Reeves, A., Baker, E. and Bentley, R. (2017) The impact of persistent poor housing conditions on mental health: A longitudinal population-based study. *Prev. Med.*, 105, 304–310

Pickett, K. E. and Pearl, M. (2001) Multilevel analyses of neighbourhood socioeconomic context and health outcomes: a critical review. *Journal of Epidemiology and Community Health*, 55, 111–122

Powers, J. R. and Young, A. F. (2008) Longitudinal analysis of alcohol consumption and health of middle-aged women in Australia. *Addiction*, 103, 424–32

Public Health England (2015) *Stockton-on-Tees: Health Profile 2015* www.apho.org.uk/resource/item.aspx?RID=171624

Rahman, M. M., Khan, H. T. A. and Hafford-Letchfield, T. (2016) Correlates of Socioeconomic Status and the Health of Older People in the United Kingdom: A Review. *Illness, Crisis & Loss*, 24, 195–216

Rehm, J. (2011) The risks associated with alcohol use and alcoholism. *Alcohol Res Health*, 34, 135–43

Ross, C. E. and Mirowsky, J. (2008) Neighborhood socioeconomic status and health: Context or composition? *City Community*, 7, 163–179

Ruckert, A. and Labonte, R. (2017) Health inequities in the age of austerity: The need for social protection policies. *Soc Sci Med*, 187, 306–311

Ruijsbroek, A., Droomers, M., Groenewegen, P. P., Hardyns, W. and Stronks, K. (2015) Social safety, self-rated general health and physical activity: Changes in area crime, area safety feelings and the role of social cohesion. *Health & Place*, 31, 39–45

Schrecker, T. and Bambra, C. (2015) *How politics makes us sick : neoliberal epidemics*, Houndmills, Basingstoke, Hampshire; New York, NY, Palgrave Macmillan

Shouls, S., Congdon, P. and Curtis, S. (1996) Modelling inequality in reported long term illness in the UK: combining individual and area characteristics. *Journal of Epidemiology and Community Health*, 50, 366–376

Skalicka, V., Van Lenthe, F., Bambra, C., Krokstad, S. and Mackenbach, J. (2009) Material, psychosocial, behavioural and biomedical factors in the explanation of relative socio-economic inequalities in mortality: evidence from the HUNT study. *Int J Epidemiol*, 38, 1272–84

Stuckler, D., Reeves, A., Loopstra, R., Karanikolos, M. and McKee, M. (2017) Austerity and health: the impact in the UK and Europe. *Eur. J. Public Health*, 27, 18–21

Sykes, B. and Musterd, S. (2011) Examining Neighbourhood and School Effects Simultaneously: What Does the Dutch Evidence Show? *Urban Stud*, 48, 1307–1331

Taylor-Robinson, D. and Gosling, R. (2011) Local authority budget cuts and health inequalities. *BMJ*, 342

Veenhoven, R. (2008) Healthy happiness: effects of happiness on physical health and the consequences for preventive health care. *Journal of Happiness Studies*, 9, 449–469

Verbeke, G. and Molenberghs, G. (2000) *Linear mixed models for longitudinal data*. New York: Springer-Verlag

Warburton, D. E., Nicol, C. W. and Bredin, S. S. (2006) Health benefits of physical activity: the evidence. *CMAJ*, 174, 801–9

Warren, J., Garthwaite, K. and Bambra, C. (2013) A health problem? Health and employability in the UK labour market. *Disability Benefits, Welfare Reform and Employment Policy.* Springer

Warren, J., Bambra, C., Kasim, A., Garthwaite, K., Mason, J. and Booth, M. (2014) Prospective pilot evaluation of the effectiveness and cost-utility of a health first case management service for long-term Incapacity Benefit recipients. *Journal of Public Health*, 36, 117–125

WHO (World Health Organization) (1995) Constitution of the world health organization

WHO (World Health Organization) (2016) Life expectancy data by country. *Global Health Observatory data repository*

FOUR

How the Other Half Live

Kayleigh Garthwaite

Introduction

This chapter examines how people living in two socially contrasting areas of Stockton-on-Tees experience, explain and understand the stark health inequalities in their town. Drawing on extensive ethnographic observations and over 100 qualitative interviews, documentary research, and photographic data with people living in one of the most and one of the least deprived neighbourhoods, this chapter emphasises the importance of stigma, place and perception in people's everyday lives at a time of austerity. It focuses on three key themes: lay perspectives on inequalities, place and its meaning(s), and the relationship between austerity, family life and health. The chapter emphasises the importance of conducting ethnographic research across two socially contrasting neighbourhoods; explores how explanations for health inequalities, experiences of place, stigma, social networks and communities, and family life are all affected by austerity and cuts to the social security safety net; and it concludes by arguing for a prioritisation of listening to, and working to understand, the experiences of communities experiencing the brunt of health inequalities, especially important at a time of austerity.

Considerable research attention has been paid to identify and explain how health and place interrelate, and the resultant impact on health inequalities (Sloggett and Joshi, 1994; Curtis and Rees Jones, 1998; Macintyre et al., 2002; Bernard et al., 2007; Bambra, 2016; among others). Geographical research has been dominated by the debate between compositional (population characteristics of people living in particular areas including demographic, health behaviours and individual-level socioeconomic status) and contextual (area-level factors including the social, economic and physical environment) explanations. This academic debate – about the causes and complexities of geographical inequalities in health – could benefit from lay perspectives on health and place and the causes of health inequalities, particularly from people living in the most and least deprived communities.

Research by Popay et al. (2003), Macintyre et al. (2005) and Davidson et al. (2006; 2008) has examined lay perspectives in socioeconomically contrasting areas of cities across northern England and Scotland. Other studies (such as Blaxter, 1997; Parry et al., 2007; Mackenzie et al., 2017) have examined the perspectives of people living in the most deprived areas. These studies have employed mixed methodologies, including surveys, focus groups and in-depth interviews; however, ethnographic research which explores the everyday lived realities of health inequalities is notably absent. Davidson et al. (2008: 168) have recognised this gap in the literature, and noted how 'even fewer studies have specifically focused on the relationships between the types of place people reside in, and their experiences of, and attitudes to, health inequalities'.

This chapter, in keeping with Popay (Popay et al., 2003), Macintyre (Macintyre et al., 2005) and Davidson (2006, 2008), presents research that directly explores the lived experience of, and perspectives on, geographical inequalities in health of people from socioeconomically contrasting areas. Following Backett (1992: 257) in her research into lay health moralities in middle-class families, the key purpose of this study was to 'develop understandings of how beliefs and behaviours which may have implications for health are part of the fabric of daily life'. In particular, this study focused on people's everyday awareness and understanding of living in a place with severe health inequalities, and to question how this might be affected during a time of austerity (as outlined in Chapter One).

This chapter examines how people living in two socially contrasting areas of Stockton-on-Tees experience, explain and understand the stark health inequalities in their town. Through detailed ethnographic observation between November 2013 and September 2017, this chapter emphasises the importance of stigma, place and perception in people's everyday lives at a time of austerity. It explores how explanations for health inequalities, together with experiences of place, social networks and communities, are all affected by austerity and cuts to the social security safety net. There can also be a significant impact on family life for people residing in the two contrasting areas. This chapter concludes by arguing for a prioritisation of listening to, and working to understand, the experiences of communities living with the brunt of health inequalities; especially important at a time of ongoing austerity and cuts to the social security safety net.

Researching lived experience of health inequalities in Stockton-on-Tees

Studying health inequalities through ethnography allows people's lived experiences to be studied in everyday contexts, by following a flexible research design, with participant observation and relatively informal conversations forming a central part of the research process. Undertaking participant observation of a particular place involves the researcher walking or driving through local places to observe social environments and happenings (Pink et al., 2010: 3). Routine daily activities across the two field sites were observed in public places that made seeking informed consent unfeasible. The researcher's casual conversations with residents in local places were included as non-verbatim data in observation notes.

Town Centre ward is the most deprived in the borough and is the 17th most deprived ward in England (Smith et al., 2015). The ward particularly experiences health, disability and employment deprivation. Statistics show 27.1% of economically active people are unemployed and 10.2% are receiving out of work benefits. Only 22% of residents own a house, which is significantly lower than the borough average of 69%. The majority (53%) live in socially rented accommodation and 23% live in private rented accommodation. In the 2011 census, 12% of people reported that they were in bad or very bad health, much higher than the borough average of 6.3%. Further, 26.5% of people have a long-term health problem or disability; this is higher than the borough average of 19.0%. Poor quality housing, takeaway shops, convenience stores selling low quality food, betting and pawn shops, and a pub where all drinks cost £1 are all plentiful in the most deprived area. There has, however, been a recent £38 million regeneration of High Street, which has been much discussed by participants throughout the research. Fieldwork in Town Centre ward began in November 2013, with participant observation and interviews carried out in a Trussell Trust foodbank (Garthwaite, 2016a), Citizens Advice Bureau, children and family centres, community centres, gardening clubs, cafes and coffee mornings alongside engagement with charities, events and services in the area.

From March 2014, participant observation began in Hartburn, the third least deprived ward out of the 26 in the borough, and one of the least deprived wards in England. The unemployment rate here is 5.1%, lower than the average for England and Wales of 7.6% and the Stockton-on-Tees average of 9.6%. Only 1.2% of people in the Hartburn ward are receiving out of work benefits. Statistics show 92% of residents own a house outright or are buying it with a mortgage; only 1% live in socially rented accommodation and 6% live in private rented accommodation; both are much lower than the borough averages of 17% and 13% respectively. Only 4.3% of people reported that they were in bad or very bad health; this is lower than the borough average of 6.3%, and 19.2% of people have a long-term health problem or disability. The area is characterised by manicured green space, flower beds, attractive period houses and independent businesses such as a delicatessen, a dog grooming parlour and a florist. Observations and interviews here took place at coffee mornings, yoga classes, cafes, churches, mother and toddler meetings, a credit union and community centres.

In total, 124 qualitative interviews, including eight ethnographic walking interviews, were completed across both areas between 2014 and 2017, alongside detailed participant observation, field notes, documentary research and photographic data. To ensure a varied sample, in-depth interview participants were sampled across these locations to include variation in age, gender, occupation and marital status. Participants were recruited by a mix of approaches; they were asked following ethnographic observation, and sometimes acted as gatekeepers with snowballing approaches used to recruit others. Topics covered during the in-depth interviews included (but were not limited to) area perceptions, health and health inequalities, austerity and welfare reform, social networks, community, employment, leisure activities and social security benefits receipt. Interviews that were arranged to take place in people's homes were recorded and transcribed verbatim. The age range of the overall sample varied from 16 to 78 years old and was almost equally split in terms of men and women. Ethnographic observations captured a wider age range.

Participation was voluntary, confidential and secured by either verbal or written informed consent where possible. Interviews were transcribed verbatim and the transcripts produced included references to both field notes made and photographs taken. Data were fully anonymised before transcripts were analysed thematically, using open coding to identify initial categories. Data were then further broken down into sub-themes, allowing me to then compare and contrast data in a detailed manner. Thematic content analysis was used to analyse the data and extract relevant relationships between study ethnographic observation and interview results. In this way participants' verbal accounts and non-verbal behaviours could be analysed and coded in one dataset to give a fuller picture. Although NVivo 10 software was used to facilitate and organise data thematically, the process of analysis has involved moving between these NVivo 'nodes' and full transcripts to ensure that the richness of transcripts was not lost.

Findings

This chapter focuses on three key themes that emerged from the research. First, lay perspectives on inequalities in both areas is examined. Here, there is a focus on people's everyday awareness and understanding of living in a place with severe health inequalities, and how this might be affected at a time of austerity (for a fuller exploration, see Garthwaite and Bambra, 2017). Second, place and its meaning(s) for residents living in both the most and least deprived areas will be explored, including a discussion of identity making and community networks. Finally, the relationship between austerity, family life and health in both areas will be explored.

1. Lay perspectives on health inequalities

Participants displayed opinions that fluctuated between a variety of converging and contrasting explanations. Three years of ethnographic observation in both areas generated explanations which initially focused closely on behavioural and individualised factors, while 124 qualitative interviews subsequently revealed more nuanced justifications, which prioritised more structural, material and psychosocial influences. Inequalities in healthcare, including access, the importance of judgemental attitudes and perceived place stigma were then offered as explanations for the stark gap in spatial inequalities in the area. Notions of fatalism, linked to (a lack of) choice, control and fear of the future were common reasons given for inequalities across all participants. Following Backett (1992: 257) in her research into lay health moralities in middle-class families, the key purpose in taking an ethnographic approach was to 'develop understandings of how beliefs and behaviours which may have implications for health are part of the fabric of daily life'.

The importance of lay knowledge has emerged as being central to knowledge and understanding surrounding health inequalities (Blaxter, 1997; Popay et al., 1998, 2003; Backett-Millburn et al., 2003; Macintyre et al., 2005; Davidson et al., 2006, 2008; Elliot et al., 2015, among others). As Davidson et al. (2008: 1368) and others (Blaxter, 1997; Backett-Milburn et al., 2003; Macintyre et al., 2005) have recognised, very few studies have directly explored lay understandings of the causes of health inequalities in general. Further, there has been even less attention dedicated to exploring the relationships between where people live, and their experiences of – and attitudes towards – health inequalities, with a focus on lay understandings of health inequalities at a time of austerity being relatively absent (see Mackenzie et al., 2016 for a notable exception). Ethnographic methods have also been underutilised in this regard.

Beyond lifestyle choice

Explanations that centred on behaviour and education were mostly found in the perspectives of people in the least deprived area, and particularly during ethnographic observation. This tended to be linked to the transmission of generational family values. Katie, 41, worked in marketing and lived in the more affluent suburb with her husband and two children. Katie placed an emphasis on the importance of cultural values and aspirations of education, but also accepts that the "odds are stacked against you" if you're living in one of the most deprived areas:

> 'You're talking a lot about [a] third generation of people who've never had a job. You learn from your parents, you learn your principles and values and everything. Everyone's looking for the fast and easy way round everything, it's just not realistic and they just forget about education. It goes right back to even at the beginning, if you're in a shit school and there's people with all different needs, the odds are stacked against you, and then if you're feeding your kids crap right at the beginning, it's like what's going on? So I can see why people aren't living longer, and like the smoking thing, I mean I've smoked and as soon as I found out I was pregnant I stopped, and now I wouldn't dream of it. But I suppose if you live where everybody is smoking around you, it's just what you do, isn't it?'

The following field notes extract identifies how fieldwork observations and conversations tended to centre on 'hard' (Macintyre, 1997) behavioural explanations.

FIELD NOTES
9 June 2015
It's my first day of the credit union that's been set up by some of the people I've come to know in Hartburn. Heather invited me into the back room for a coffee and offered to introduce me to the

others who I don't know, who are looking fairly suspicious of me to be honest. I get sat next to a serious looking woman, Jennifer, and Kathryn comes to join us and starts explaining about the project. Jennifer looked at me as if I was stupid and simply said: "Well it's all about behaviour, isn't it?" She seemed horrified that a £1 million grant was being used to investigate something that she believed could be explained away by faulty behaviour. I said obviously behaviour is part of the whole story, but actually isn't the major factor in the gap in life expectancy according to our survey findings – income, education, housing and quite frankly money are more important. She doesn't look convinced: "I would imagine behaviour is the most important" she said, and turned around to talk to someone else.

In contrast to findings from Popay et al. (2003) and Macintyre et al. (2005) though, participants in this study living in the most deprived areas also recognised that income, housing and stress were all factors in explaining the severe health inequalities in Stockton-on-Tees. Glen, a chef working on a zero hours contract, lived in a deprived area a couple of miles outside of the town centre. He believed the gap in life expectancy was linked to lower stress and higher income levels in the more affluent areas of town. Despite this, he also linked the difference to the behaviour and lifestyles of people living in the most deprived areas:

> 'I think it's cos them in Hartburn have jobs and they have loads of money. They've got good work and they've got good living. And I think some of these in the town centre they just go around getting drunk, being homeless. It's a lifestyle choice, it gets them out of it for a couple of days, y'know?'

Participants from the more deprived areas in Davidson et al.'s (2008) study discussed how deprivation was 'written in the body' in terms of premature ageing. Our findings (Garthwaite and Bambra, 2017) show that participants across both the most and least deprived areas recognised how poverty can have an impact on people's health and bodies, both physically and mentally. In an in-depth interview with Steph, 42, a welfare rights adviser who lived in one of the least deprived areas, she expressed her "shock" at how the combination of multiple traumatic incidences, such as bereavement, sexual abuse, domestic violence and ill health, can affect people physically:

'I suppose you know anecdotally which areas have more concentrations of poor health but sometimes it shocks me how much it ages people. I think they look old, you can see it in their faces the way they are and I think that's sad. They tell me their date of birth and I think "God you're my age", or a few years older and I think what is it that's so different about us, that we look so different? But then a lot of people I deal with, they've had not just one kind of traumatic thing happen to them, they might have had two or three things that would be almost kind of nobody I know in my friendship circle has had that happen to them, but that person has had like multiple.'

Living in the least deprived area, Catherine, 65, initially spoke during ethnographic encounters of how smoking and obesity were key factors in explaining the large gap in life expectancy, but during an in-depth interview she also identified how psychosocial factors can play a role in explaining the health inequalities within the area:

'Smoking, obesity ... but the overriding thing is that they don't seem happy. I really would say that the most notable thing is they're not going round with big smiles on their face, happy jolly people. They're miserable. So that would come back to the mental health issues, wouldn't it? It would wear you down.'

The impact of these cumulative traumas can then further widen pre-existing health inequalities, and perhaps go some way to understanding ideas of fatalism, choice and hope that participants felt helped to explain the gap in life expectancy in Stockton-on-Tees.

Fatalism, choice and opportunity in a time of austerity

Notions of fatalism linked to (a lack of) choice, control and opportunity were common reasons given for inequalities across all participants, but more often from those living in the least deprived areas. Heather, 72, a trustee of various mental health and addiction charities, felt fatalism was key to explaining the gap in life expectancy within the borough:

'People feel stuck, don't they? People don't feel that any effort they make is going to make a difference where out there in the affluent areas we know that efforts we make will make a difference. There's an element … it isn't so much confidence, well it is confidence but it's also a bit fatalistic, "Well whatever I'm doing doesn't matter," and I think that's why people don't bother with healthy living. "Well do I want to be here?" Y'know if you've developed lots and lots of poor health, what's the joy of living to 100? And I guess, but I don't know, I guess it's a sense of "Well whatever I do won't make a difference" for myself or anyone else. It's about drive isn't it, and have they ever had drive in the Town Centre? Because people who have drive have got out.'

Heather strongly associated this sense of fatalism with the geographical boundaries of Town Centre ward and the perceived culture among people living there that combined to create an overall sense of hopelessness or lack of control. Carol, 68, was a former health visitor who worked within deprived communities nearby for over 40 years. Living in the least deprived area, Carol agreed that difficulties in thinking about the future may lead to "impulsive behaviour" which she defined as drug taking and smoking:

'When you've got this impulsive behaviour, not thinking about tomorrow, then you don't care very much about the future of your health, either. You're thinking about today. And a lot of these people who I worked with, who aren't going to live very long, actually just getting through today, and they don't care about 20 years' time or 10 years' time. Sometimes today is so awful for them.'

Here, Carol recognises that everyday life can be filled with multiple and complex issues, making it impossible to plan and even imagine a future. Carol, and others across both in-depth interviews and ethnographic observation, regularly referred to the notion of 'luck' for helping to explain the differences between their situation and those living in the most deprived area. "We're kind of a lucky generation really, I think," was often offered as a justification, generally from the older participants who were now retired. Luck was also used as an explanation for the good health that people in the least deprived area experienced.

For people living in the least deprived area, conversations would focus on the regular trips to the theatre, language courses, horse riding, ukulele classes, dining out and frequent holidays. In contrast, people living in the most deprived area often tried to find free things to do, such as go for a walk with their children in the local park, or sit in High Street on a sunny day, watching the water fountains that had recently been installed as part of a £38 million regeneration of the town centre. People across the least deprived area made full use of the local groups and activities that were often free to access, including ones specifically aimed at people who lived in the most deprived areas, such as Sure Start. Heather, speaking about the weekly coffee morning she helps to run, recognised this as being a particular factor in explaining the gap in life expectancy in the area:

> 'I think people, well you know the people come here, particularly as helpers, they're very active, y'know, walking groups, the community choir, volunteering, the gym. And there are things like cycling groups and walking groups that are provided by the council, but they tend to be taken up by folk like us. We fill them up.'

Ethnographic observations were carried out across various clubs, groups and initiatives aimed at improving the health and wellbeing of people living in the most deprived areas. Due to cuts to local authority budgets, several services and clubs that the researcher became involved with had to be closed due to funding constraints – for instance, a weekly walking group was forced to cease a few months after the researcher joined. Often, such groups would be poorly attended; a notable example being a credit union set up by those living in the least deprived area but situated within a church on one of the most deprived streets in the town. To date, only members of the congregation had signed up to use it, and there was a sense of frustration and incomprehension as to why people living on the doorstep were not engaging with it. But in spending time in the most deprived area, it became clear that one possible explanation for the reluctance to engage with services such as the credit union was a perceived sense of being subject to judgement and stigma.

Importance of judgement and attitude

Participants in the most deprived areas described a hardening of attitudes towards people living in low-income areas. Living in the most deprived area, Lauren, 33, identified the struggles she had with judgemental attitudes, and the effect this could have on accessing support:

'I think for me it's people's attitudes when you go and seek help. I think if you've never experienced it, someone looking down their nose at you because you don't work, or you've got depression, whatever if may be, because you need something from society, you know financially or medically. You'd think nurses and doctors and receptionists, you'd think they'd be nice to you but what I found, and I would say ... I would assume that people who are on the bad end of the health gap may feel the same, is that people's attitudes towards you are awful, it makes you not want to ask for help. All the time this message is that you're bad – it's on the telly, you're not a worthy person so at what point do you not access things because you feel it yourself?'

For Lauren, these attitudes were strongly linked to so-called 'poverty porn' television programmes which depict a certain lifestyle of benefits receipt or living on a low income. 'Poverty porn' has 'been used to critique documentary television in post-recession Britain which focuses on people in poverty as a political diversionary entertainment' (Jensen, 2014: 2.6). This genre of television depicts people as lazy, criminal, violent, undisciplined and shameless, playing into the media and government rhetoric about people living on a low income. The impact of 'poverty porn' is particularly relevant given the second series of Love Productions' 'Benefits Street' was set on Kingston Road in the deprived Portrack and Tilery wards, next to Town Centre. The significance of 'not speaking the same cultural language' as patients and the potential resultant impact on health inequalities was reinforced by Town Centre GP Dr Harrison who spoke of the importance of the health service:

'I can give you the example of doctors, you know you've come into a fancy building here, which is intimidating for people. I speak with a posh voice, I'm wearing a tie which puts a certain barrier up. But also many doctors live in the wealthier parts of town. So they live in this very precious enclave, they drive in in a car, [they're] protected, sealed in with air conditioning, they're listening to Radio 4, they're parking it, coming into their own safety environment which is very different to the environment people live in, they're seeing people, then they're going home. Occasionally they might do a home visit but they're not using ... they're not really understanding where people are coming from, they will never really understand the financial constraints on people – and it isn't just doctors, it's nurses, it's health visitors, it's midwives, it's the whole health infrastructure, it's receptionists as well and they can often act as a barrier. We might say "How on earth do they still continue to smoke? Don't they know it's bad for them? I've invited them three times to come and they haven't come," so you get these kind of … these attitudes, and then of course you get organisational culture where people talk about it in the tearoom and it reinforces those attitudes and you then get a kind of "them" and "us", patient-blaming culture and it widens health inequalities.'

The attitudes described by Dr Harrison have become progressively more noticeable amidst ongoing austerity and reforms to the social security system, he felt, and it was clear in the perspectives of those living in the most deprived area that they agreed with this. Naomi, 36, a recovering heroin addict, had a range of physical and mental health problems, including gastrointestinal issues, depression and anxiety. Naomi identified a stigmatising and judgemental attitude attached to her accessing the local pharmacy for her methadone:

> 'Every day I go to the chemist and it's supervised, I have to drink it. In the Stockton area everyone knows what you're going in for, no matter how well you're dressed, they still know what you're going in for so you get the funny looks. People look at you up and down and you know what they're thinking and that gets you down.'

The health implications are clear, with such attitudes possibly having an impact on mental health and wellbeing, as Naomi suggests.

2. Place-based stigma

Residents across both areas identified what made their neighbourhood desirable or health promoting. This was related to the composition of the physical environment, perceptions of safety and fear, and finally, narratives of disgust and how this influenced engagement within a particular space.

Living in Stockton-on-Tees is therefore regularly associated with stigmatising conceptions of poverty and welfare dependency. Here, I explore how territorial stigma can affect residents' interactions with the environment and their social networks, including their identity and 'sense of place'. This is also closely linked to political- and meda-driven ideology, which vilifies deprived communities and its residents (Hancock and Mooney, 2013). Interestingly, notions of community were most commonly associated with the least deprived area and were interestingly linked to the 'poverty porn' TV show 'Benefits Street', which was set in Stockton-on-Tees. Territorial stigma was present in the narratives of residents in both areas. This stigma was related to perceptions of risk and danger in the environment – for instance, in the form of nearby sex work, drug dealing, and also hazardous chemicals from the nearby industries (see also Bush et al., 2001).

(Dis)engagement with the environment

Following a £38 million regeneration programme, Stockton High Street now features independent shops, regular farmers markets, fountains and art installations. This has resulted in it winning a 2016 Great British High Street of the Year 'Rising Star' award. Despite this progression, residents from both areas were critical of the town's rejuvenation, and felt efforts to improve the area were "a waste of money, [as it is] still the same people" living in the area (field notes, 16/4/15). Living in the least deprived area, Fiona, 42, who rarely visited the town centre, said:

> 'I don't know if it's like sticking a plaster over it really. I don't know how we change and become an affluent town. It's gone too far.'

As Slater and Hannigan (2017: 9) have contended, 'it should not be assumed that any investment is uniformly positive. The appropriate question to ask, rather, is, "To what extent is any investment in stigmatized territories in the interests of their residents?"' This sentiment is evident when speaking to Denise, 49, living in the most deprived area:

> 'What they've done with the High Street, it's amazing. That fountain, it's unrecognisable. They're [the empty shops] all coffee shops now, it's nice but it's no good if you can't afford a coffee.'

It was evident in Denise's narrative that despite living in close proximity to the town, she felt excluded by her inability to participate in the newly regenerated space. Participants living in the least deprived area also spoke about their feelings of segregation between their area and the town centre, typically related to the physical environment. Residents living in the most affluent area discussed the importance of what they perceived to be familial values and a child-centred lifestyle in Hartburn. Abundance of green space, proximity to a 'good school', and local amenities such as libraries and playgroups were cited as the most important health-protecting features of the area. Living in the least deprived area, Jessica, 41, a journalist who was married with two children, described the importance of the physical environment to her and her family:

> '… it's ever so green, everyone had their own home and a garden front and back, they planted cherry blossom trees when these were first built and it gives a lovely burst of colour. Our gardens here are really big, that was a huge pulling point. And you can be walking here, everywhere, I feel very much like we're in a village. The parks you can walk to, the primary [school] and also the Oaktree [Centre] is up there with all the playgroups, we used to amble up there so you can easily walk and that for us was a big, big extra pulling point. I think we've got pretty much all that we would ever need just here.'

Many participants in Hartburn described how the physical space was conducive to a healthy lifestyle – there were parks to exercise in and few takeaway shops selling unhealthy food – which contrasted with the myriad of fast food outlets and lack of green space in the town centre. Andy, 43, from Hartburn, explained how the environment of the town motivated him when he was exercising:

> 'I think Hartburn has that feeling, you do see people out exercising. I go for a run maybe three times a week, on a weekend I do quite a big loop and end up going in the High Street, but I do see quite a few people out in Hartburn having a run, and when I get to the town centre there's no one. And part of my motivation is I run past all of the chip shops, and there's a road called King George Street and I probably run past 20 different fast food [shops], and I just think for those to survive they're obviously having custom.'

In contrast, Town Centre was associated with unhealthy behaviours and an environment that promoted obesity, drug and alcohol addiction, and smoking. Living in Hartburn, Katie, 41, drew attention to a difference between Hartburn and Town Centre:

> 'You don't really see people smoking as well round here, very rarely, even outside the pubs. Further into town you go, everyone's vaping or smoking, and obviously if you've got a pound pub in your town like Stockton then you're not really ... you're just fuelling the fire, aren't you, really.'

Aside from physical health behaviours, participants residing in the most deprived areas described negative ways in which their mental health could be affected – in terms of feelings of self-worth, for example – when faced with the inequalities present in their area. Residing just outside of Town Centre, Naomi, 36, said:

> 'You can see certain people looking down their nose at you, just by the way you dress, your accent, even cos even though we're from the same town they always seem to have a better accent than you, they pronounce their words properly so straight away you're different, they turn their nose up ... even when you're in a shop as well – it's not very often I'll go in Marks and Spencer's but if there's a sale on I will go in cos there are some nice clothes in there, and you can see them looking at you ... nah, I don't like it.'

Laura, 33, was a full-time carer to her two sons who were diagnosed with autism. Despite growing up in nearby Hartburn, and now living in one of the borough's most deprived wards, she described a sense of belonging to Town Centre that she did not associate with her birthplace:

> 'D'you know what, I feel comfortable in the town. If I go to Hartburn shops I feel uncomfortable, I feel like I don't fit there ... I just don't feel like I want to be there, but I go to town and I see loads of people from all these different places, they're sitting round the fountain and I can hear all these different accents and languages and it reminds me of being away at uni. Going away to uni was such an eye opener to me and when I came back to Stockton there were people seeking asylum, and it looked different. Different types of shops opened, and I love all that, I love seeing a

Polish shop or, you know, different places to eat, so I love being in town and I like the atmosphere.'

Although in Laura's account there is an appreciation of the diversity in Town Centre, for other participants, this led to feelings of fear and negative perceptions of the area. These perceptions were almost always linked to perceived negative behaviour and characteristics of the people, rather than being attributed to the particular place and space, and were also linked to wider concerns over criminality and safety.

Safety and fear

Residents in both the most and least deprived areas regularly associated safety concerns with living in Town Centre, while Hartburn was seen as "a different world" (field notes, 16/4/15) where affluence and success were more easily reachable. Stockton town centre was regularly described as "Tattooville", "a ghetto", "Dickensian", "scummy" and "grotty". In contrast, Hartburn was described as "idyllic", "beautiful", "ideal" and "a dream". Tim, 69, living in the least deprived area, discussed what he believed was the presence of anti-social behaviour which led to him and his wife avoiding the town:

'The people you see when you go in, the drunkenness if you go in later in the day, probably the drugs as well playing a part, the language as you're walking around … it's not a pleasant experience to go because you've got to go to the bank or whatever.'

Living in Hartburn with her husband and two children for over nine years, Jessica agreed, and commented:

'I don't like going in [to town] because it makes me sad. I feel as though I look different and I feel very, very conscious of that. My bag I hold that extra bit tightly without actually even meaning to do it. And then I'm thinking "Why is it there are so many young people in town with babies and pushchairs, and other groups of young people who obviously aren't at work or at college?" And it makes me think about their lives, and why aren't they doing that? There's almost this air of sadness. There's this whole kind of underclass of people I guess, who are there, who exist but who almost people can go past without ever really seeing them. And you do, you know there is this big change and big disparity in people, but you don't have to see it if you don't want to. Yet they're so near us, it's miles away, if that.'

Jessica identified how she looks physically different from people who she sees in the town centre, resulting in feelings of fear, sadness and disbelief at the vast inequality in the area. Such a perspective was not limited to those living in the more affluent parts of town. Peter, the manager of a drug and alcohol treatment service in the town centre, emphasised the existence of "no-go areas" in the town, which were perceived as too risky and unsafe to enter:

'I mean, if you talk to anyone in the area and say "Do you go down Harley Road?" they don't. They keep away from the area, in effect it's causing … I suppose you could say a ghetto.'

Fears over safety were also linked to the presence of sex workers in the area. Melinda, 44, lived in what she termed "Stockton's red-light district", a street just outside of the town centre, with her two children. She said:

'You don't feel safe letting your children out, not even in the daylight really. I spent years paying for them to go to theatre school after school just so they weren't on the streets. When they were younger and were just playing on the street [that was ok], but when they got older and wanted to go to the next street, where I couldn't see them that was the period when I said "No, you've got to do activities somewhere safer," and that was a big overdraft for me. I complained about it quite a lot because I'm not really very understanding of the kind of people that use that kind of service, so I was quite concerned it was bringing predatory threats into my neighbourhood.'

Safety concerns were less frequent in nearby Hartburn, but were very much on the agenda for residents, as the following field notes extract shows.

FIELD NOTES
26 June 2014
Trish, the chatty local police community support officer, has come to the coffee morning today to give us the monthly crime report. We

all gather round and lean in to make sure we don't miss anything. Normally, we hear about garages that have been broken into, or damage to cars parked in driveways. There's a buzz today as we talk about it, and Patricia tells me there was some vandalism in the village last night – a dozen 'youths', tipping wheelie bins over, and wrecking someone's fence. They have been hanging around until late at night, 11pm, and it's intimidating. Everyone is talking about it, and they think police have now caught them. 'They're the ones who should know better, they're not the rough ones,' Patricia said, and everyone nodded in agreement.

Criminality would be associated with a distinct 'Other', rather than those living in the more affluent area. Although connotations of crime, drug use, and health-reducing behaviour such as smoking and drinking alcohol were associated with Town Centre, so, too, was the idea that a sense of community was present – more so than in the least deprived area – as the following section explores.

Community and social networks

When asked about health and what might protect it or damage it, participants across both areas discussed the importance of community and social networks. Living in the least deprived area, Trisha, 54, a healthcare practitioner, described what she termed a "community feel" in the most deprived areas:

> 'I often think in Stockton [town centre] people have a network of friends and they sort of help each other, and certainly where I work in the deprived areas there's a definite community spirit, more so than in the affluent areas. Like my parents who've always lived in Hartburn, they hardly ever see their neighbours, you know they're not in and out of each other's houses, which they prefer. Yes, if they had a problem the neighbour would be there and they'd help, but certainly where I work when I'm out visiting the neighbour will be coming around, knocking on the door visiting. There's definitely a community feel.'

Although community was perceived to be more present in the most deprived parts of town, those living in Hartburn emphasised the quality of their social environment, and what they believed constituted a "good neighbourhood" – the presence of families, having relatively similar socioeconomic capital, and sharing similar values and lifestyles, especially regarding bringing up children. Katie, living with her husband and two children in Hartburn, said "we have standards round here … it was our choice, it was a definite choice to move here and raise our kids and I'm happy with it". Andrew agreed, focusing on education and safety of the environment as factors for deciding to relocate to his childhood home of Hartburn:

> 'I like the fact that both my kids can play out, I think it's a safe environment. I just think it's a child-friendly place to grow up, and I think as far as going out, either cycling or playing football, I don't think you have an excuse [not to] around here.'

For those living in the most deprived ward, Town Centre, taking part in leisure activities was rare, largely due to a combination of financial and time constraints. Further, the 'work' involved in living in poverty is substantial (Lister, 2015), with regular meetings at the Jobcentre, Citizens Advice Bureau, visits to the housing office, alongside childcare and negotiating (often precarious) employment, meaning there is less time to take part in leisure activities. In contrast, those living in the least deprived area were highly active, engaging in language courses, music lessons, exercise classes, regular holidays and coffee mornings.

The maintenance of community in the most deprived areas becomes increasingly difficult with housing demolition, and the construction of housing and services aimed at a more affluent class of resident is becoming increasingly common. Within Stockton town centre, the Victoria estate, labelled a 'sink estate' by local media (Blackburn, 2014), had been fully demolished during the period the fieldwork was undertaken, and was being transformed into an 'urban village'. A dispersal of current residents has taken place, with people being removed from their communities, thus rupturing pre-existing social networks and ties.

Those in the most deprived area would retreat from the public realm into the private sphere in response to perceived threats related to territorial stigmatisation, as Naomi's earlier comments show. This was also linked to racial tension in and around the town centre. Denise, 49, did not engage with the town centre very frequently, as she believed it had "changed beyond words" since she recently moved back into the area after living outside of the borough for five years:

'Hell of a change, really, I can't say for better or for worse. It's gone from druggies and drunks to Africans, it scared the life out of me when I come back here.'

Here, we can see a shift in blame for feelings of unsafety from the "druggies and drunks" to what Denise terms "Africans". Stockton-on-Tees has the fourth highest population of asylum seekers per head of population in the UK (*The Economist*, 2016), many of whom are housed in and around Town Centre. This was a topic discussed across both research sites, and ethnographic observation witnessed a steady increase of people seeking asylum in Town Centre, particularly at the foodbank and in High Street. Katie was keen to explain that although she had friends from Kenya, she felt that the placement of asylum seekers and immigrants caused tension and division:

'We have a lot of immigrants but we drop them directly into Stockton town centre. I understand why because it's the cheapest place for rent and things, but what ends up happening is you just end up creating these areas of like, erm, you know, one type of ethnicity, and it creates division.'

Disassociating himself from Stockton as a place, Glen, living on an estate in Town Centre ward, readily distanced himself from the 'Others' he believed were living there:

KG: 'And do you like Stockton as a place to live?'
GK: 'Naw … naw wouldn't want to live in Stockton.'
TK: 'Well this is classed as Stockton, Glen! [laughs]'
GK: 'I like round this area where we are – there's too many different colours and types of people in Town Centre, if you see what I mean.'

Glen's wife Tracey pointed out that they were living in Stockton, but for Glen the ethnic diversity in Town Centre meant that he was keen to detach himself from the place, which he viewed as "dirty" and "not for us".

It is clear that classed moral undertones of respectability and what constituted a 'good' area were at play when considering residents' relationships and opinions on their local area. This theme could also be found when considering family life in austerity.

3. Family life and everyday austerity

Third, the relationship between family life and austerity was a key theme throughout the research. Those living in the most deprived area had an ever-present relationship with austerity in the form of visits to a foodbank, fuel poverty, debt and poor housing. This could then have a subsequent effect on mental health (Garthwaite et al., 2015). Living in the least deprived area, austerity was something that people had largely been unaffected by in the way that those in the most deprived area had. However, participants described decisions that they had taken as a family – for example, husbands moving to other parts of the country to work away, avoiding foreign holidays, consciously shopping in cheaper supermarkets, and taking separate holidays to avoid childcare costs – often with a moral undertone of making the 'right' choice, and 'making do' in times of austerity.

Everyday austerity in Town Centre

Participants from both areas were asked about the impacts of austerity on their own lives, as well as on Stockton as a place. In Town Centre, austerity manifested itself in the form of visits to the foodbank (Garthwaite, 2016a, 2016b), zero hours contract employment, visits to Citizens Advice Bureau and everyday budgeting practices. Constant worry and hardship was therefore a common (yet unsurprising) theme found in the experiences of people living through austerity in the most deprived area. Simon, 52, was a volunteer at the foodbank after using it three times himself. Currently unemployed, he described the daily struggles he had in making his Employment and Support Allowance of £146.20 per fortnight cover his bills, debt and food expenditure:

> 'I get a big bag of spuds for £2.75 and that lasts for two weeks, if you've got potatoes you can always have chips. Beans, tomatoes is a good one, buy spices every week then you can mix things together. I've had pasta and beans before with spices, mix it in, it's not the best of things to be eating but at least it's a meal. Porridge is good cos with porridge you don't need milk, milk is a luxury. Things like that, just things that'll spread.'

The following extract from my field notes highlights the difficulties of managing during austerity for families.

FIELD NOTES

24 January 2014

Today I met Kim, a single mother with two daughters, aged nine and eleven. She was teary, emotional and embarrassed from the moment she sat down with me. She was not working due to depression and anxiety, and was receiving JSA [Jobseeker's Allowance] whilst she waited for the outcome of her ESA [Employment and Support Allowance] appeal. Kim had been sanctioned by the Jobcentre as she was required to apply for 17 jobs between 24/12/13 and 31/12/13 (Christmas period). She hadn't been able to achieve this so she had been sanctioned. She now had no income whatsoever for herself and two kids. She has donated to the food bank before and her kids go to the youth group in the church. She was particularly struggling with energy costs – her kids switch the TV on all the time, leave lights on, have long baths, plug straighteners in. She doesn't nag them to stop as 'kids shouldn't have to worry about things like that'. She recently changed her electricity payment meter – the old meter charged 38p per day for gas and electric even when not in use – the new one, thankfully, does not, and won't run out if you only have 1p on the meter whereas the old one did. Kim said: 'I want what everybody else has. Weekends away with the kids, things like that. I want to earn my own money to get the luxuries I want, to feel I've earned it.'

Laura spoke about how she managed everyday budgeting practices for herself and her two sons after her partner at the time lost his job. Like Kim, a complex negotiation of relying on family members, selling things to raise extra cash and cutting back were common:

'We could not live off what we were getting. I wasn't looking for work and I wasn't going to pretend that I was so I wasn't getting Jobseeker's [Allowance]. He lost his job so was getting Jobseeker's for us as a unit but not for me. My dad bought all our food shopping out of his DLA [Disability Living Allowance] because he had cancer. My mum and dad were eating scrambled eggs and beans on toast because they were funding themselves and us. Cos I couldn't … rent was most important, bills came after that and there was absolutely nothing left. Once you've paid for nappies and the other things that babies need … I sold everything. People would buy the boys presents and they went straight on eBay. I sold all my clothes. I just left a few things. I sold all my photography equipment that I'd bought for next to nothing, I took my rings round ...'

Naomi, 36, described how she would manage her food shopping, and spoke about the difficulty of getting paid her benefits once every fortnight:

'Well we normally, what we do in the first, we, we fill up our cupboards, like, with tinned stuff, noodles things like that, fill up the freezer with, like, chicken, there's always meat, vegetables, chips, stuff like that and I've just been paid so I've filled up the cupboards now, but when you get to the end of the week you see it all go, all the fresh stuff's gone and it's really hard to keep some money in your account for the following week cos if something happens and you need some cash for summat, y'know, you've got to take it out for something else. A long time ago I got paid weekly and you wouldn't have needed a foodbank, I think really if they could they should pay people weekly.'

Many struggled to buy their children school uniforms, Christmas and birthday presents, and treating them to days out or holidays. Single mother Anna, 51, spoke of how she was unable to buy treats for her 11-year-old daughter:

'There has been a dramatic change particularly for my daughter. [Before] she could have the games machines, I could afford to buy them, but that's all completely gone now. I really struggle to buy Holly anything which is such a shame, I mean she does understand and I am good at explaining it to her but it's really tough when all her friends have got that kind of stuff and I just can't provide it.'

A continual battle of getting into debt, stretching food out as much as possible and selling items to receive extra cash were commonplace among interviewees in the most deprived area.

"We cut our cloth accordingly": middle-class experiences of austerity

Tyler (2015) has argued that the increasingly precarious conditions brought on by neoliberalism has an impact not only on the working classes, but also on some members of the middle classes. Participants in Hartburn spoke about "cutting back" and "being sensible". In Hartburn, austerity was visible through redundancy, tightening spending practices and library closures. The emotional impact of austerity was highlighted for people who were working in professions such as welfare rights advisers, district nurses and foodbank volunteers. Derek, 64, was retired from his job in the local chemical industry. He volunteered weekly at a local foodbank, 15 minutes' walk away from his home. Derek said:

> 'When I see people in the High Street, you can see they have nothing [because of] the shoes they wear. People who help out at the foodbank, I know one who has electrician's tape to keep his shoe on. Now I've often thought of going to Windsor's or somewhere and buying him a pair of trainers but I know that would be an insult. So, yeah, austerity has affected me badly really, not financially but emotionally very much so. If I go on holiday I feel guilty about going away, I really do.'

Steph, 42, living in Hartburn, differentiated her family's experiences between general cost of living and the effects of austerity. However, she was aware that austerity would affect them in certain ways, such as the closure of public services. Steph said:

> 'I wouldn't say it's affected us in terms of day to day spending, everyone has to tighten their belt but I think that's more to do with the cost of living that's not austerity, rising fuel and food prices and everything like that, everyone's experiencing that. But I think in terms of austerity and government cuts to services, I think it'll affect people like us when the libraries close, and if it affects like the park being maintained and things like that. I mean you can see it in the streets can't you, roads not getting repaired, massive holes in the road. I don't know, what else are we seeing? Libraries is the one ... because the middle classes use the libraries don't they?'

This was echoed by Harriet, 41, who also lived in Hartburn with her husband and three children. When asked if austerity had affected her, Harriet said:

'Well … I'm a big saver, I really don't like spending. Even though everything's become a bit tighter, I'm always so cautious. That's why we don't have Sky, that's why we don't have gym memberships, they're luxuries as I see it. My phone is my husband's old phone, I'm on a pay-as-you-go and I'm happy with that.'

Andy, 43, from Hartburn emphasised how he and his friends were not affluent, but instead "everyone here lives within their means":

'We've got friends who are teachers, friends who are doing well in the police force, and yeah all of these have got other stresses in their lives. But I don't think financially anyone's ever struggled. It's not as though anyone ever has these plush holidays, it's not as though they're driving round in a £30,000 car. I think we're all survivors, we're all able to manage on a day-to-day basis. Have the odd meal out, have the odd night out all of us. But I think generally at the end of each month there's a small bit of cash left in our bank account. Whereas I always think it must be hard when you watch these programmes and see people with a handful of change in their pocket at the end of each month, they can only afford milk today and that's all. I don't think any people in Hartburn have probably reached that stage yet. I think Hartburn is one of those places where everyone here lives within their means. I mean I don't know anybody who has a huge overdraft, second houses, like really taking chances with money. I think we're quite cautious, certainly the people I know are. We might not have the Rolls Royces and the Porsches on the drive, but it isn't as though we're in the courts pleading poverty and ending up in administration.'

Katie said that austerity had led to her "making sacrifices" for herself and her family, but she was reluctant to discuss this with others as they may perceive her as "whinging":

'Definitely but I would definitely never whinge on to anyone cos they would never believe it. I mean I don't have new clothes, we don't go out, if we go out we do freebie things most of the time … we just go on walks, or like I say if the kids have got like … we go to the seaside a lot, we go to Saltburn and Sands End and things, but we'll try and … I mean we do go to the pictures but it's really rare as it's so expensive, to me it's a bit of a luxury. What else do we do? Well we used to go out a bit more, we used to go out for meals more as a family but it's just one of the things that had to be scrapped, can't do it. Go out on bike rides, erm … that's about it, really. Swimming, kids go swimming a lot, that's quite cheap. I'll do things like I'll make some popcorn, I'll get sugary sweets and we'll buy a video off Virgin for £2.49 and we'll close the curtains and make a big thing of it, have a cinema night, erm, and then I feel the kids are not missing out on something.'

Discussion and conclusions

This study has outlined lay perspectives on the experiences, understandings and explanations of health inequalities in two geographically close but socioeconomically distant areas of a post-industrial town in the North East of England.

First, conversations and observations in both the most and least deprived areas generated explanations which initially focused closely on behaviour and individualised factors, suggesting smoking, alcohol and the consumption of unhealthy food were root causes of the gap in life expectancy within their area. In-depth interviews revealed more nuanced justifications, for both groups, which prioritised altogether more structural, material and psychosocial factors, such as income, housing, happiness and community networks. These categories were neither separate nor distinct, and participants often displayed opinions that fluctuated between a variety of explanations.

Ethnographic observation generated explanations which initially focused closely on behaviour and individualised factors – 'hard' explanations (Macintyre, 1997), while qualitative interviews prioritised more structural, material and psychosocial influences – the 'soft' explanations as put forward by Macintyre (1997). Inequalities in healthcare, including access, the importance of judgemental attitudes and perceived stigma were then offered as explanations for the stark gap in spatial inequalities in the area. These lay perspectives link to the wider academic literature on health and place with compositional factors privileged over contextual ones.

A notable difference between the previous work by Popay et al. (2003), Macintyre et al. (2005) and Davidson et al. (2008) and this study is the context of austerity measures and cuts to the social security safety net which do not affect all groups or neighbourhoods equally. The importance of this context is evident when we consider the deeply divisive rhetoric between 'shirkers', 'skivers', 'workers' and 'scroungers' being applied to people living on a low income (Garthwaite, 2011) and the emergence of a 'new welfare commonsense' as identified by Jensen (2014). The idea of 'commonsense' relies heavily on the welfare-dependent and deceptive benefit 'scrounger' who is then portrayed as a figure of social disgust by politicians and the media. This thereby enables the state to retreat from providing basic levels of welfare support with reliance on charity instead becoming the norm for many in the most deprived neighbourhoods (Garthwaite, 2016b).

The resultant judgemental attitudes towards people living in low-income areas can then have negative impacts on people's (often already poor) mental health, with the ensuing stigma preventing them from seeking further help and support. Seabrooke and Thomsen (2016: 253) identify key 'story sets' from their analysis of British and Danish newspaper narratives on austerity. Two of the most popular notions in a UK context are 'scroungers' and 'living beyond our means'. As the findings in this chapter have shown, both themes were important ones in the context of the fieldwork undertaken in Stockton-on-Tees.

Second, place-based stigma was found in accounts of people living in both the most and least deprived areas. Such a 'blemish of place' (Wacquant, 2007) can then have impacts on residents in a number of ways, disrupting their sense of identity and social interactions, while also constraining their access to other neighbourhoods (Keene and Padilla, 2014; Wutich et al., 2014). The concept of territorial stigmatisation forged by Loïc Wacquant (for example, 2007, 2008) is defined as 'not a static condition or a neutral process, but a consequential and injurious form of action through collective representation fastened on place' (Wacquant et al., 2014: 1270). Territorial stigmatisation can then 'exacerbate existing inequality for these populations, often leading to considerable consequences for their well-being' (Collins et al., 2016: 169). Slater and Hannigan (2017: 5) describes how we are witnessing 'a phenomenon of spatial disgrace' distinct from other forms of stigmatisation – such as that associated with poverty, race or unemployment – exerting very real and deleterious effects. For Pearce (2012: 1922), 'a comprehensive conceptualisation of the ways in which place-based stigmatisation can shape population health through the concentration of poverty and ill health, as well as the likely institutional discrimination that leads to inadequate service provision, has not been fully realised'.

It is important to emphasise that territorial stigma is not always a direct result of living in a deprived place. Thomas (2016: 1) found that young people in post-industrial Merthyr Tydfil could 'resist stigma by Othering certain districts and social groups'. Research in deprived communities in North East England shows similar findings; in order to engage in identification (with 'the ordinary') and disidentification (from 'the undeserving') participants constructed ostensible 'Others'; an 'underclass' situated financially, culturally, socially and morally below them (Shildrick and MacDonald, 2013: 299). Reducing place-based stigma, and its capacity to both negatively affect one's health and reinforce social inequalities (Keene and Padilla, 2014), should therefore involve contesting popular discourses about stigmatised places which are promoted in political rhetoric and mass media representation.

Third, the relationship between family life and austerity was a constant throughout the interviews and ethnographic observation. Research by Hall (2017: 305) on the everyday experiences of austerity for families living in Greater Manchester found that 'Although not all families or family members have felt themselves to be personally impacted by current austerity measures, all describe living "in it" as a social condition.' Hall (2017: 303) also comments how 'the experience of austerity, like all elements of social life, is characterised by difference; austerity impacts on individuals, families and communities in different ways'. The findings presented here echo Hall's findings, and suggest that for those not affected financially, austerity had an emotional affect on some participants living in the more affluent area.

People living in Hartburn were keen to emphasise how they "lived within their means" – a common theme found in reporting of austerity measure in the UK and beyond (Seabrooke and Thomsen, 2016). A common narrative within the mass media focuses on the notion that if you are spending more than you are making, or if you are unable to pay off your debts, you must save in order to do so (see Seabrooke, 2010). In contrast, those living in Town Centre faced the 'sharp end' (O'Hara, 2015) of austerity, and were unable to find money for everyday necessities such as food, fuel, clothing and rent. They described daily budgeting practices such as shopping in multiple supermarkets, despite the time and effort this costs. Other practices such as selling personal items, getting into debt and borrowing from friends and family were often reported. In this sense, 'living within their means' was taken to the extreme.

Finally, what is needed is the approach of 'empathetic ethnographers' (Garthwaite et al., 2016). We must prioritise listening to, and working to understand, the experiences of communities experiencing the brunt of health inequalities; especially important at a time of austerity.

References

Backett, K. 1992. The construction of health knowledge in middle class families. *Health Education Research*, 7, 4, pp. 497–507.

Backett-Milburn, K., Cunningham-Burley, S. and Davis, J. (2003) Contrasting lives, contrasting views? Understandings of health inequalities from children in differing social circumstances. *Social Science & Medicine*, 57, 4, pp. 613–623.

Bambra, C. (2016) *Health divides: Where you live can kill you*. Bristol: Policy Press.

Bernard, P., Charafeddine, R., Frohlich, K.L., Daniel, M., Kestens, Y. and Potvin, L. 2007. Health inequalities and place: a theoretical conception of neighbourhood. *Social Science & Medicine*, 65(9), pp. 1839–1852.

Blackburn, M. (2014) Stockton's run-down Victoria Estate could be replaced by exclusive retirement village. *The Gazette*, 3 November, http://www.gazettelive.co.uk/news/teesside-news/stocktons-run-down-victoria-estate-could-8041048 (accessed 3/10/17).

Blaxter, M. (1997) Whose fault is it? People's own conceptions of the reasons for health inequalities. *Social Science & Medicine*, 44, 6, 747–756.

Bush, J., Moffatt, S. and Dunn, C. (2001) 'Even the birds round here cough': stigma, air pollution and health in Teesside. *Health & Place*, 7, 1, pp. 47–56.

Collins, A. B., Parashar, S., Closson, K., Turje, R. B., Strike, C. and McNeil, R. (2016) Navigating identity, territorial stigma, and HIV care services in Vancouver, Canada: A qualitative study. *Health & Place*, 40, pp. 169–177.

Curtis, S. and Rees Jones, I., 1998. Is there a place for geography in the analysis of health inequality? *Sociology of Health & Illness*, 20(5), pp. 645–672.

Davidson, R., Kitzinger, J. and Hunt, K. (2006) The wealthy get healthy, the poor get poorly? Lay perceptions of health inequalities. *Social Science & Medicine*, 62, 9, pp. 2171–2182.

Davidson, R., Mitchell, R. and Hunt, K. (2008) Location, location, location: The role of experience of disadvantage in lay perceptions of area inequalities in health. *Health & Place*, 14, 2, pp. 167–181.

Elliott, E., Popay, J. and Williams, G. 2015. Knowledge of the everyday: confronting the causes of health inequalities. In K. E. Smith, C. Bambra and S. E. Hill (eds) *Health inequalities: Critical perspectives.* Oxford: Oxford University Press, pp. 222–237.

Garthwaite, K. (2011) 'The language of shirkers and scroungers?' Talking about illness, disability and coalition welfare reform. *Disability & Society*, 26, 3, pp. 369–372.

Garthwaite, K. (2016a) *Hunger Pains: life inside foodbank Britain.* Bristol: Policy Press.

Garthwaite, K. (2016b) Stigma, shame and 'people like us': an ethnographic study of foodbank use in the UK. *Journal of Poverty and Social Justice*, 24, 3, pp. 277–289.

Garthwaite, K. and Bambra, C. (2017) "How the other half live": Lay perspectives on health inequalities in an age of austerity. *Social Science & Medicine*, 187, pp. 268–275.

Garthwaite, K., Smith, K. E., Bambra, C., and Pearce, J. (2016) Desperately Seeking Reductions in Health Inequalities: Perspectives of UK researchers on past, present and future directions in health inequalities research. *Sociology of Health & Illness*, 38, 3, pp. 459–478.

Hall, S. M. (2017) Personal, relational and intimate geographies of austerity: ethical and empirical considerations. *Area*, 49, 3, pp. 303–310.

Hancock, L. and Mooney, G. (2013) "Welfare ghettos" and the "broken society": Territorial stigmatization in the contemporary UK. *Housing, Theory and Society*, 30, 1, pp. 46–64.

Jensen, T. (2014) Welfare commonsense, poverty porn and doxosophy. *Sociological Research Online*, 19(3), p. 3.

Keene, D. E., and Padilla, M. B. (2014) Spatial stigma and health inequality. *Critical Public Health*, 24, 4, pp. 392–404.

Lister, R. (2015) "'To count for nothing": poverty beyond the statistics'. *Journal of the British Academy*, 3, pp. 139–65.

Macintyre, S. (1997) The Black Report and beyond: what are the issues? *Social Science & Medicine*, 44, 6, pp. 723–745.

Macintyre, S., Ellaway, A. and Cummins, S. (2002) Place effects on health: How can we conceptualise, operationalise and measure them? *Social Science & Medicine*, 55, 1, pp. 125–139.

Macintyre, S., McKay, L. and Ellaway, A. (2005) Are rich people or poor people more likely to be ill? Lay perceptions, by social class and neighbourhood, of inequalities in health. *Social Science & Medicine*, 60, 2, pp. 313–317.

Mackenzie, M., Collins, C. E., Connolly, J., Doyle, M. and McCartney, G. (2017) Working-class discourses of politics, policy and health: 'I don't smoke; I don't drink. The only thing wrong with me is my health'. *Policy & Politics*, 45, 2, pp. 231–249.

O'Hara, M. (2015) Austerity bites: A journey to the sharp end of cuts in the UK. Policy Press.

Parry, J., Mathers, J., Laburn-Peart, C., Orford, J. and Dalton, S. (2007) Improving health in deprived communities: What can residents teach us? *Critical Public Health*, 17, 2, pp. 123–136.

Pearce, J. (2012) The 'blemish of place': stigma, geography and health inequalities. A commentary on Tabuchi, Fukuhara & Iso. *Social Science & Medicine*, 75, 11, pp. 1921–1924.

Pink, S., Hubbard, P., O'Neill, M., and Radley, A. (2010) Walking across disciplines: from ethnography to arts practice. *Visual Studies*, 25, 1, pp. 1–7.

Popay, J., Williams, G., Thomas, C. and Gatrell, T. (1998) Theorising inequalities in health: the place of lay knowledge. *Sociology of Health & Illness*, 20, 5, pp. 619–644.

Popay, J., Bennett, S., Thomas, C., Williams, G., Gatrell, A. and Bostock, L. (2003) Beyond 'beer, fags, egg and chips'? Exploring lay understandings of social inequalities in health. *Sociology of Health & Illness*, 25, 1, pp. 1–23.

Seabrooke, L. (2010) What do I get? The everyday politics of expectations and the subprime crisis. *New Political Economy*, 15, 1, pp. 49–68.

Seabrooke, L. and Thomsen, R. R. (2016) Making sense of austerity: Everyday narratives in Denmark and the United Kingdom. *Politics*, 36, 3, pp. 250–261.

Shildrick, T. and MacDonald, R. (2013) Poverty talk: how people experiencing poverty deny their poverty and why they blame 'the poor'. *The Sociological Review*, 61, 2, pp. 285–303.

Slater, T. and Hannigan, J. (2017) Territorial stigmatization: Symbolic defamation and the contemporary metropolis. London: SAGE Publications Ltd.

Sloggett, A. and Joshi, H. (1994) Higher mortality in deprived areas: community or personal disadvantage? *British Medical Journal*, 309, 6967, pp. 1470–1474.

Smith, T., Noble, M., Noble, S., Wright, G., McLennan, D. and Plunkett, E. (2015) *The English indices of deprivation 2015*. London: Department for Communities and Local Government.

The Economist (2016) Marginal benefits: Asylum-seekers are sent to the poorest parts of Britain. What happens next? (13 February) www.economist.com/britain/2016/02/13/marginal-benefits

Thomas, G. (2016) 'It's not that bad': Stigma, health, and place in a post-industrial community. Health & Place, 38, pp.1–7.

Tyler, I. (2015) Classificatory struggles: class, culture and inequality in neoliberal times. *The Sociological Review*, 63, 2, pp. 493–511.

Wacquant, L. (2007) Territorial stigmatization in the age of advanced marginality. Thesis Eleven, 91, 1, pp. 66–77.

Wacquant, L. (2008) Urban outcasts: a comparative sociology of advanced marginality Cambridge: Polity Press.

Wacquant, L., Slater, T. and Pereira, V. B. (2014) Territorial stigmatization in action. *Environment and Planning A*, 46, 6, pp. 1270–1280.

Wutich, A., Ruth, A., Brewis, A. and Boone, C. (2014) Stigmatized neighborhoods, social bonding, and health. *Medical Anthropology Quarterly*, 28, 4, pp. 556–577.

FIVE

Divided Lives

Kate Mattheys

Introduction

This chapter considers how inequalities in mental health are affected by austerity, providing a qualitative account of the *human price* of government policy. Engaging with debates about inequalities in mental health, it uses interview data from people experiencing mental health problems in the most and the least deprived neighbourhoods of Stockton-on-Tees, to show how people experience austerity and inequality in their everyday lives. Austerity measures are shown to have a damaging impact on communities in the most deprived areas while leaving those from less deprived areas relatively unscathed. It documents how people's lived experiences have been shaped by austerity, and how long-standing structural inequalities have been compounded by deeply regressive policies which are shown to be having a damaging impact on the mental health of those affected by them, causing a chronic level of stress that has a relentless influence on their everyday lives. Although government rhetoric highlighted how we were 'all responsible' for fixing the national debt, this chapter shows how it is those on the lowest incomes and living in the most deprived communities who are paying the highest price.

While dealing with mental health problems was challenging for everybody in this study (regardless of their background and the areas they came from), there were key differences in their lives and in the day-to-day difficulties that they faced. These included differences in income and financial stability, employment and the environments that people were living in. All were discussed in relation to their impacts on mental health. Austerity, and in particular the 'welfare reform' programme, are shown to have disproportionately affected those living in the most deprived areas. This is because austerity has been regressive, overwhelmingly targeting those on the lowest incomes (Hills, 2014). The impact of these cuts has been pervasive, cutting across people's financial, emotional and social lives. For those already dealing with issues related to their mental health, these policies are creating additional and unnecessary levels of distress, undermining well-being and leading to emotional harm. This is aggravating inequalities in mental health in a place which already had the highest health inequalities in England Public Health England (2015).

Background

Mental health follows a social gradient in the same way as physical health (Marmot, 2010). The higher a household's income, the lower the likelihood of the individual in that household having mental health problems (McManus et al., 2009). We are not all equally likely to experience poor mental health. There is a strong evidence base for the link between mental health and material deprivation, low income and socioeconomic status (Williams, 2002; Melzer et al., 2009). The effects of living in poverty, including the impact of low income, debt, unemployment, poor working conditions (including insecure employment and zero hours contracts), housing, and living in areas with high levels of deprivation can all have negative impacts on people's mental health (Rogers and Pilgrim, 2003). Additionally, people who are experiencing mental distress are at increased risk of poverty, due, for instance, to discrimination in the workplace preventing people from being able to secure and maintain employment (Evans-Lacko et al., 2013). Between 30% and 40% of people who report having mental health problems such as depression or anxiety in England are not in employment (Mental Health Taskforce, 2016), while between 85% and 95% of people who have been labelled with schizophrenia are not in paid work (NICE, 2015). Some people are unable to work as a result of their mental and physical health. Discrimination and a lack of appropriate employment opportunities also play a role. When people with mental health problems are in employment, they are over-represented in insecure, low-paid work (Mental Health Taskforce, 2016). These types of precarious jobs have been shown to have as damaging an impact on mental health as being out of work (Kim and von dem Knesebeck, 2015).

Despite strong links between social inequality and mental health, in the past 30 years the dominant position in public health has been to adopt approaches that focus solely on the individual (Morrow, 2013). These approaches are pathologising and ignore the wider contexts in which people are living (Beresford, 2005). Despite clear research linking mental health problems to intersecting social and structural inequalities such as poverty and racism, these social and structural determinants are often marginalised (Morrow, 2013). Social perspectives provide an alternative to the dominant medical models. Although there is no clear definition of a social model of mental health (Tew, 2005), these approaches recognise the role of broader social and environmental factors (Beresford et al., 2010). This includes, for instance, the impact of income, employment and the environments in which people are living. Social models of mental health do not position people as outsiders with abnormal experiences, but instead as people who are responding to experiences and trauma in their lives. There is a strong degree of support for more socially oriented models from mental health service users (Beresford et al., 2010). These recognise the social and structural determinants of mental health and accept that experiences of inequality and oppression can contribute to poor mental health.

Since 2010, research at a national level has shown that inequalities in mental health (the gap in mental health between people from different socioeconomic backgrounds and between people from more and less deprived areas) has worsened in the UK (Barr et al., 2015a). People living in more deprived areas have seen the largest increases in poor mental health (Barr et al., 2015b). Worsening mental health has been linked to the programme of 'welfare reform' that has included numerous and significant cuts in social security. These cuts have led to increasing financial hardship for those on the lowest incomes, and the increasing financial insecurity has affected mental well-being (Barr et al., 2015b). The effects of austerity have not been distributed evenly, either spatially or socially (Bambra and Garthwaite, 2015). The most affected areas have included the older industrial areas such as the North East of England (Beatty and Fothergill, 2016). Further, those on the lowest incomes have been affected most by the cuts in social security as the cuts have fallen most heavily on this group of people (Hills, 2014).

Qualitative studies have identified the negative mental health impact of worsening financial situations and increasing insecurity (Pemberton et al., 2014). Cuts in social security have led to chronic worry, stress and anxiety for people (Patrick, 2015), and this stress created by the social security system has been reported as an endless and unremitting pressure (Garthwaite et al., 2015). This has been accompanied by damning political and media portrayals of people who are in receipt of out-of-work and ill-health-related benefits (Pemberton et al., 2014). This includes people increasingly positioned as to blame for being unable to work, with a divisive rhetoric applied between the 'shirkers' and 'strivers' (Garthwaite, 2011). Within this context we have seen the rise of the so-called 'poverty porn' programmes on television, including 'Benefits Street', 'Benefits Britain: Life on the Dole' and the 'The Great British Benefits Handout'. Overwhelmingly these shows portray people in a negative light. Such critical depictions have been found to have a damaging impact on mental health (Garthwaite, 2014).

This chapter will present findings from qualitative research exploring differences in the lives and the experiences of austerity among people with mental health problems living in more and less deprived areas of Stockton-on-Tees. Although there is a social gradient in mental health, experiences of mental health problems still exist across the social spectrum. People's experiences of austerity are likely to be different between those from different socioeconomic backgrounds (Bambra, 2016). The interviews explored these differences in experience. Alongside the inequalities that are the focus of this chapter, it is important to acknowledge that other experiences were also discussed during the interviews. People talked about the importance of traumatic experiences – such as abuse, grief and loss – they had faced in their lives and which they felt contributed towards their experiences of mental distress. However, for those who were dealing with poverty, factors such as worsening financial situations and relentless benefits assessments served to compound these issues, creating additional levels of strain in people's lives. The inequalities in their lives and their relationship with mental health is the focus of this chapter. A key point is that dealing with complex and multiple issues compounded the challenges faced by some of the people in the study. So, some were not only dealing with mental health problems, they also faced the challenges of managing on a reduced income, of being unable to work and of increased chronic stress as a result of welfare cuts. Although participants were surviving they were faced with numerous challenges in their lives. Austerity measures such as the welfare cuts were exacerbating the difficulties faced by those on low incomes. While participants from all of the groups had experienced difficulties with their mental health, their lives, and the challenges they faced, were often very different. This had an impact on their mental health and on the strategies they used to navigate this.

Methodology

This research developed out of the findings from the longitudinal household survey exploring inequalities in physical and mental health between people from the most and least deprived areas of Stockton-on-Tees (discussed in Chapter Six). Qualitative semi-structured interviews were undertaken with people from the survey who self-identified as having mental health problems. Additional interviews were undertaken with people with mental health problems who were accessing support from the local Citizens Advice Bureau (CAB), in order to capture the specific experiences of people who were being supported with welfare advice. The participants in the survey who self-reported as having mental health problems formed the sampling frame of participants to take part in the semi-structured interviews. A sample of 17 participants, mixed between those from the most and least deprived areas of Stockton-on-Tees and the CAB was drawn to undertake further interviews, using a theoretical sampling approach. There were ten women and seven men in the sample. Five participants were recruited from the most and seven from the least deprived areas of Stockton-on-Tees, and five participants from the CAB. Ages ranged between 27 and 62 years, although the majority of participants were in their forties and fifties. In the most deprived/CAB groups, two participants were in paid employment, two participants were in receipt of Job Seeker's Allowance (JSA); six participants received either Employment and Support Allowance (ESA) or Incapacity Benefit (IB); and four participants received Disability Living Allowance (DLA)/Personal Independence Payments (PIP). In the least deprived group, four participants were in paid employment, one participant was in receipt of JSA, and two participants were recently retired. The interviews took place in a six-month period between March and September 2015. A thematic analysis was used to interpret the findings.

Findings: inequality and mental health

In this section, key themes around the relationship between material inequalities and mental health are explored. First, the impact of increasing financial hardship in the more deprived areas is discussed. This is then contrasted with the relatively comfortable financial situations of those in the least deprived areas. People's experiences of the impact of austerity on their day-to-day lives are explored, including the impact of the social security system, and the cuts, on mental health. The differences in people's experiences of employment and the relationship between employment and physical and mental health are explored. The chapter concludes by considering the impact of different living environments – the role of place – on mental health.

Increasing hardship: struggling to get by in the more deprived areas

> 'You're living week to week. Food's gone mad, gas has gone mad, electric has gone mad.' (Jimmy, 47)

Materialist explanations of health inequalities focus on the impacts of poverty, relative deprivation and processes of social exclusion on health outcomes (including mental health) and life expectancy (Shaw et al., 2006). They link income, and lack of resources and power, to the continuing gap in health. There were large differences in the financial situations of people from the least deprived areas, those from the most deprived areas and CAB. The participants from the most deprived areas talked about their material circumstances as having worsened significantly in recent years. Financial insecurity was a significant issue in people's lives; they talked about the challenges in trying to get by and the ongoing stress.

Between 2010 and 2015, people on low incomes faced worsening material circumstances across the UK (MacInnes et al., 2015). Increases in the cost of living (including the cost of food, fuel and rent) have had a more substantial impact on people on low incomes, as these items represent a much larger proportion of expenditure. Almost a fifth of the population is now unable to afford three or more items from a list of everyday items such as a washing machine, car or a healthy meal (MacInnes et al., 2015). Paul was a 27-year-old man who lived with his partner in a socially rented flat. He had grown up in Stockton-on-Tees and had strong ties to the area. Paul had type 1 diabetes and mental health problems and was not currently able to work as a result of his ill-health. He described the struggle of getting by day to day. Paying for even basic bills, such as heating and electricity, was a weekly challenge:

> 'It is hard, because when you're thinking of the electric you can't think "I'll put this on that," because you never know how much you're going to use. And you try and keep some back, but then you run out of something like food and you've got to dip into that, and then the leccie [electricity] runs out and … so you're just going round and round.' (Paul, 27)

For Paul, alongside the other participants in the study, financial worries affected their mental health by increasing levels of stress and anxiety. This increased stress compounded the difficulties that people were already facing as a result of dealing with mental health problems. The uncertainty of how to make ends meet, and whether they were going to be able to pay their bills that month, or even have enough to buy food had a chronic impact. Generally it was the participants who were reliant on out-of-work or ill-health-related benefits who were in the most difficult financial situations. However there were also participants employed in low-paid jobs who were struggling to cope financially. This reflects increasing levels of in-work poverty in the UK: a record high of 55% of people in poverty are now in working households (JRF, 2016). Since 2007/08 household incomes have risen more slowly than prices for virtually everyone in the UK (aside from the wealthiest, who have managed to fare well from the global financial crisis), leading to declining living standards for many (Hirsh, 2015). This is particularly the case for low-income households of working age (Belfield et al., 2015). Claire was a 49-year-old woman who lived with her husband and worked part-time on a minimum wage in a local community centre. She spoke of the day-to-day difficulties in managing the costs of daily living:

> 'I think it's still bad, like bills and that, they've gone up a hell of a lot … it's absolutely horrendous… Your money doesn't go as far as it used to. And the wages don't go up much to compensate. I think it's definitely harder, we're struggling.' (Claire, 49)

The people who were in receipt of either JSA, or ESA, or had been affected by some of the other cuts such as the bedroom tax, were often in challenging financial situations. Laura and her husband were both in receipt of ill-health-related benefits, and had been affected by the bedroom tax and a requirement to now pay council tax. Laura also had a 17-year-old son living at home. While 16–19 years olds from low-income households could previously receive Education Maintenance Allowance (EMA) to attend further education, in 2010 this payment was abolished. Combined, the welfare cuts that the family had experienced were having a really significant impact on their finances. Laura spoke about some of the challenges in getting by on a reduced income.

> 'When me son's at college, we have to pay for him. When me niece went she got about thirty pound a week, but they don't get it now. He walks to college and we give him money for his dinner. And so that's coming out of

what you get. We only get paid fortnightly, so you find that when you've paid all your bills at the end of it, you're like Oh my god I've only got a hundred pound to live on for a fortnight. You know, it's hard. It's hard to budget your money. You're always looking for the cheapest shop. Where once over you could think Ah right, I'll just go to Asda and do me shopping there, you can't now. Cause you think, a loaf of bread in there's £1.50, I could go to Aldi and get two loaves for that price. So you're dropping between shops, you know.' (Laura, 53)

As with Laura, the people who were struggling financially adopted a variety of methods and strategies to cope with this. Many of these strategies involved 'doing without'. Other findings have identified that managing on benefits involves strategies such as shopping in the reduced aisles in supermarkets, 'shopping around', and pawning items in difficult times (Patrick, 2015). Similar findings are presented here. Participants talked about the cyclical nature of food consumption and having to do without groceries to make sure they were able to pay for other outgoings. Peter had coeliac disease and received some food items on prescription. He talked about the need to make do with what was in the house because he did not have any money to buy food:

'Last fortnight was good because I had money for food. This fortnight I don't. So whatever's in the cupboard, and whatever me girlfriend helps us out with, like I get pizza bases off the chemist, and she's going to pick them up for me, I got tomato puree, I got cheese. So that's it, we're having pizza for tea. It's hand to mouth.' (Peter, 47)

Participants also spoke of strategies such as using catalogues as this meant that, although more expensive in the long run, they could spread the cost of more expensive household goods into more manageable weekly payments. The 'poverty premium' is a term to describe how people on low incomes need to pay more for essential goods and services (Davies et al., 2016). This includes, for instance, the need to use higher-cost credit to buy goods because people do not have the money to buy items outright. As an example of these inflated costs, a washing machine at a well-known high street retailer costs £435 to buy outright. The same washing machine, paid for by weekly instalments over a 3 year period, would cost the customer £975 (at an interest rate of 69.9%). For people who don't have the savings, or income, to be able to buy these items outright, they often have no choice but to pay these rates:

> 'It's a case of get it on the never never. I say that but it's catalogue, my friend's got a catalogue.' (Alison, 50)

Although people had strategies they used to try and deal with a lack of money, and carefully budgeted their finances, there often simply was not enough to get by. This was a source of significant stress.

Managing comfortably: financial stability in the least deprived areas

Finances were not an issue that came up naturally in the interviews with people in the less deprived areas. While they did not perceive themselves as being 'wealthy', they talked about being comfortable financially. Money was not a source of stress to them. Dennis was a 57-year-old man who lived with his wife in his own home in one of the more affluent areas of Stockton-on-Tees. He spoke of how he felt that the cost of living had improved recently:

> 'I've found in recent months the petrol is down, and that's had a knock-on effect on gas and electricity, and I've found that gas and electricity is cheaper than it was maybe two years ago. So I think it's quite cheap now, inflation is next to nothing anyway. So yeah I find it very comfortable.' (Dennis, 57)

Participants in the least deprived areas used their income to pay for goods and activities that might help their mental health, and that would give them a break from their daily lives. Holidays were discussed as important as they gave people an opportunity to get away and take some 'time out'. Participants also frequently spoke about going on trips out for the day, hobbies, going out for meals and drinks with family and friends. They had the financial means to be able to do this. James spoke about the different hobbies that were important to him:

> 'I love getting out and about, love walking, love camping …
> I love motorbikes, passionate about motorbikes … love touring, Scotland, Wales, Spain, France. Me and a few of the lads go over. So I'm passionate about bikes, love cars, love engines, love speed, love going to see the motorbikes

race … What else do I do? Work, gym, bike, walking, beer.' (James, 47)

For James, the ability to get out into the countryside and be outdoors was really important for his mental health. He talked about how he would often take himself away on his bike for the weekend if he was having a bad time and needed some solitude. He could afford to do this. Having enough income also, crucially, gave people the means to resolve situations that were damaging their mental health, such as taking early retirement or dropping down to part-time employment. This was more possible for the participants who were in their fifties and sixties. Dennis had taken early retirement from HM Revenues & Customs (HMRC) as a result of the stress that he had been under at work, and was in a financial situation where he could afford to do this. It was damaging his mental health and as he was in a position where he could afford to retire early, he took that option:

'I mean, it's very stressful in HMRC. It was very stressful. So I said "I can do without this, I can get out. I've done 39 years." That's what I did, took early retirement in May last year.' (Dennis, 57)

This ability – to be able to escape from a harmful work situation – was not an available option to those living in the more deprived areas.

Being dragged down: the negative mental health impacts of the social security system

For those participants who were managing on a low income, a lack of money, and the stress that this caused, was a recurrent theme. The stress involved in not having enough money was particularly present for those who were in receipt of out-of-work or ill-health-related benefits. This was linked to anxiety around not knowing when (or if) benefits were going to be paid, and the ongoing stress around how to get by financially if benefits were not paid. This was presented as a relentless, ongoing stress that people had to contend with. They discussed how when one benefit was stopped, this often had a knock-on effect on other benefits. This uncertainty and relentlessness often aggravated the difficulties that people were already facing with their mental health. Jimmy was a 47-year-old man who lived with his wife and two children. He was in receipt of ill-health-related benefits and talked about the pressure he had been placed under since 2010:

'The minute the Conservative government came in, there was no let up. With the pressure. Four years. I worked it out the other day, so in that four year, well it's a blur to me really. Cause I'm still enduring it.' (Jimmy, 47)

Stress was particularly spoken about in relation to ESA and the Work Capability Assessment (WCA), the assessment that tests people's eligibility for this benefit. The WCA was introduced by the previous Labour administration; however, since 2010 its implementation has seen greater conditionality (with significant cuts to eligibility and entitlement) and more stringent medical tests. This is despite ongoing controversy and a five-year review process (Daguerre and Etherington, 2014). Previous claimants and any new claimants are assessed via the WCA. People can also be reassessed at intervals to identify if they are still eligible for the benefit. Since its initial implementation there has been an ongoing and substantial criticism of the WCA, with arguments that it is both unfair and lacks credibility: nearly 40% of appeals lead to decisions being overturned (Barr et al., 2015a). Mental health charities have repeatedly voiced alarm that the process is damaging people's mental health, concerns which have been supported by academic research finding a link between reassessments via the WCA and an increase in suicides, self-reported mental health problems and prescriptions in anti-depressant use (Barr et al., 2015a). Debra was 55 years old and lived alone in the town centre. She was facing an upcoming reassessment for ESA and had been informed that she would be being taken off it and would need to appeal. She discussed how this worry was affecting her mental health:

'I'm terrified. It's absolutely eating me up. How the hell am I going to manage? Because they'll automatically put me on Jobseeker's Allowance. How on earth am I going to manage? If I start thinking about it I'll end up in tears. And shaking. It has brought on some dreadful panic attacks thinking about this coming up.' (Debra, 55)

The processes involved in ESA were highlighted as being particularly stressful. Participants talked of a relentless process of failing medicals, challenging decisions, passing the appeals and then being sent for a reassessment within a very short period of time. There was no respite from this. Some participants kept going with this process of assessment and appeals (particularly those who were being given advocacy support), whereas others had felt unable to keep appealing. Andy talked about the process of assessment for ESA and how, because he had attended the medical on his own, he was seen as able to work and told his was no longer eligible to receive ESA. He had tried to appeal but "gave up" in the end, despite feeling this was the wrong decision:

> 'I was on ESA. Usually people take people with them [to the assessment] you know, but I didn't want to, I wanted to be on me own. They thought I was all right to get there on me own and that's how they put it. They just didn't listen. I appealed, I tried to appeal, and in the end I just give up and went back on the dole.' (Andy, 46)

One of the key ways in which the benefits system aggravated the difficulties participants were experiencing with their mental health was through increased levels of stress. This included being mandated to attend courses or certain activities, such as the Work Programme, as a requirement of receipt of benefits. This was often very challenging for participants who were struggling with their mental health and who had difficulties dealing with these situations. Jimmy had been on the Work Programme, which he was mandated to attend as a condition of receiving ESA. Jimmy reflected on the difficulties involved in this and the impact on his mental health:

> 'I've just been on a two-year work programme, which was compulsory, but I used to turn up and my brain would be elsewhere, in a terrible state. And that just finished in January, I had two year of that. And that was like pressure that I just didn't need. Of turning in. I'm all anxious and stressed and going in different environments that I'm not used to.' (Jimmy, 47)

Increasing conditionality has been one of the key features of the 'welfare reform' programme, and has included an increase in sanctioning. Under this process, claimants can be refused benefits for periods at a time when they do not comply with rules relating to job seeking (O'Hara, 2013). For instance, failure to attend a Jobcentre appointment can lead to an initial four-week sanction, in which the JSA benefit is suspended; any further error within the next year will lead to a 13-week sanction. There was a significant increase in the numbers of JSA sanctions given between 2010 and 2014, with over 800,000 applied in that period (Lupton, 2015). Effectively sanctioning leaves people without an income, forcing people into financial hardship. The severity of the cuts, including the increase in rates of sanctions, has been linked to increased suicide rates in the UK (Barr et al., 2015b). In 2013, the suicide rate was at a 13-year high, with the region most affected being the North East (ONS, 2015). Andy talked about suicides in his local neighbourhood and attributed this to the rise in sanctions:

> 'I think nine people in the last few months have jumped in that river, local people. Out of all of them, I think one was an accident. All the rest, it's just that bad around here … People aren't coping.' (Andy, 46)

Being caught up in the benefits system put many in a situation where they were powerless about the decisions being made about them. Alison spoke of the stress involved in this, although she remained committed to fighting unfair decisions. She spoke of the 'fear of the brown envelope', a theme identified in other research (Garthwaite, 2014):

> 'It's really, really got me so down and depressed. Regarding the benefit changes and having to fight for it. And then them realising you should have stayed on that one. Some people give in and they say "Ok, whatever." No. If that's right, then I'll fight for it. But it's dragged me down so much, because then you get into debt more, and you get more into this and have to find extra for that. It's hard, and when you're not well anyway. I dread them brown envelopes coming, I put them to one side and then I look away. It makes you feel sick inside, with everything. And with the pain all the time as well, that doesn't help. But what can you do?' (Alison, 50)

Narratives of powerlessness were present in discussions around a host of agencies, including housing, social services, GPs and the police. Negative encounters with formal agencies were repeated often. While there was at times a sense of helplessness in their narratives, people nevertheless responded to this lack of power with the resources that were available to them. Anger was a common response. Participants reported anger at the government and the benefits system and the impact that this had on their daily lives. They were also angry at the labelling and stigmatisation of them by the government and the media, and the impact this had on their self-esteem. Jimmy spoke about the media portrayal of people who are not in work and the rise of the so-called 'poverty porn' on television:

> 'It seems that now we're under attack from all angles. You just watch the television and see what's happening. How people on the dole are portrayed. It's entertainment to see a girl drunk and shouting and swearing at two in the afternoon, 'cause that's what all people do on the dole. From 'Benefits Street' to refugees with six bedrooms.' (Jimmy, 47)

He went on to describe the impact of this and the feelings of shame that he had subsequently experienced:

> 'You know, I don't tell people that I don't work and stuff like that … you wouldn't dream of telling anybody that you're on the dole. You'd just make something up. Anything's better than saying you're on the dole. Believe me, when I'm in the garden with my kids, and my neighbour comes home from work, I can see that he hates me. When he sees that stuff on the telly and he sees me in the garden with my kids, it just reinforces what they're saying. That we're just lazy.' (Jimmy, 47)

The employment divide: work, health and mental health

The evidence base on employment and health suggests that being out of work negatively affects health and leads to worsening mental health (Bambra, 2016). However, insecure, poor-quality employment is also a risk factor for mental health (WHO/CGF, 2014): insecure employment can be equally as bad for health as unemployment (Kim and von dem Knesebeck, 2015). Participants from the most deprived areas and the CAB generally had employment trajectories of insecure, low-paid work. Although the majority of these participants were not in paid employment at the time of the interviews, none of them fitted into dominant neoliberal stereotypes of being part of an 'underclass' who had never worked. Participants had lengthy employment histories and wanted to be in work if they were able (some, as a result of their physical and mental ill-health, were not able to work). Paul spoke about his extensive employment history:

> 'Me first job was a paper round … after that, I went to college. Me next job was B&Q, I was on the tills about

a year and a half, I worked in the garden department …
I worked for Bells, and I worked at Zanzibar, one of
the nightclubs. It's now closed down. I cleaned for
Middlesbrough council … I used to be a youth worker …
I had that job for about six months before government cuts
and stuff closed it down.' (Paul, 27)

Claire was still in part-time employment, although as a result of her
deteriorating health she was unsure how long she would be able to
stay in work. Claire had stopped working for a period when her
children were young in order to care for them. She spoke about the
shop and production jobs she had had in the past and the insecurity
of those roles:

'I've done a lot of shop work, filling shelves, on the till.
I've worked at the crisp factory. I've worked at Frankie D's,
it's not that now, it's Sainsbury's… I've worked at Tesco's as
well. I didn't work for a lot of years because of my children.
I had no one to mind them… I was made redundant from
Tesco's, that was why I left there. I liked that job but it
closed down and I lost my job.' (Claire, 49)

Claire had then trained to become a teaching assistant; however, the
lack of permanent jobs meant that she had been unable to continue
in that career. She talked about the difficulties of being employed by
an agency:

'I was working for an agency, and they were reluctant to
take you on because of money. So I was shoved all over
the place. And they were putting me further and further
away, and you were supposed to get paid for your bus fares
but only so much. I had to get a taxi to one, 'cause it was
the other side of Middlesbrough and I couldn't get to it by
bus. But they were messing me about … I couldn't get a
permanent job and like I say, I started at the community
centre.' (Claire, 49)

As in other studies, for participants who were not able to work as
a result of ill-health or disability, they spoke about their illness or
disability as determining their relationship with the labour market
(for example, Pemberton et al., 2014). Their employment histories
often involved unskilled or manual work. For the participants who

had developed physical health problems, this had meant that they were often then unable to continue in previous roles when their health problems had become too severe (for example, labourer). Lily had previously been a care worker for severely disabled people. She had loved her job; however; her physical health problems had affected her ability to work and she had to leave. Lily developed lumbar spondylosis, a degenerative disease of the spine. It was very painful and Lily was on the waiting list for operations to her neck and back. Lily spoke of having to leave employment:

> 'The last project, when I was finished, were two old gentlemen in Hartlepool. Both with severe epilepsy. But you see, when they had seizures, you don't just stand there and watch them have the seizure. You get down, and if I get down I can't get back up again, so what good would I be. So, you know, that was the end of my career.' (Lily, 60)

The participants who had chronic physical health problems spoke of how these interacted with their mental health. These narratives were more present in participants from the more deprived areas. Participants spoke about their health being cyclical (about having 'good' days and 'bad' days). When their physical health was bad, this often affected their mental health, and vice versa: the one would aggravate the other. Coping with pain appeared to have a particularly detrimental impact. Claire was living with significant pain on a daily basis as a result of fibromyalgia. She described the interaction with her mental health and how this affected her:

> 'I get depressed, bit worse now because of the fibromyalgia. I think it's because I am coping with the pain. It all came to a head and I thought I can't go on like this. I didn't want to go on because of the pain and that, I thought I can't cope. I had a bit of a breakdown and I went to the doctor's and he put me on the amitriptyline, just one then, to block some of the pain. It does affect me a lot. The depression has been brought on again because of this.' (Claire, 49)

The participants who were not in employment missed working and wanted to be in work, discussing the social benefits of working, doing something they felt was 'productive', and the benefit of having more income. Paul discussed how he missed the financial freedom that working had given him:

'I enjoyed getting up, going to work, coming home, having me tea. End of the month, a thousand pound or so, paid the rent, paid tax and stuff, and I was still coming out with like six or seven hundred pound a month … It's more freedom. Nowadays, it's like, you're on the dole, being on the dole it's like a lifestyle, and it's a big come-down from work. It's a big shock to the system. When you're depressed and things like that, and you lose your job, it makes you anxious thinking how am I going to live, how am I going to afford this, and, that's another thing that doesn't help with depression and that either.' (Paul, 27)

Participants in the least deprived areas generally reported more secure employment histories; for instance, with long careers in the public sector. James, who came from a working-class background, described his initial employment history after leaving school:

'Having that work ethic from me dad, and that council estate upbringing, I'd do anything. I did loads of jobs, worked in shops, worked for friends, did gardening jobs, went down to London for a bit on a building site. And then I worked with severely disabled kids, at this college.' (James, 47)

After a year working with disabled children, James was subsequently recruited by the police, and remained in the police force for almost 30 years:

'The Metropolitan Police were recruiting all over the country … I saw the girl from the Met in the job centre, it was about 1986 … She said "Come down to London"… So I went, did five years down there. I transferred back up here in 1992 … And that was it, I bounced around doing different jobs in the police, and then went into the CID [criminal investigation department]-type role in 1998 … And I've been pretty much doing that since then.' (James, 47)

Although these participants reported more secure employment histories, some also reported increasing job insecurity, increasing pressures and changing demands at work. For this group of people, austerity was particularly felt in relation to its impact on the working environment, including the impact of reduced budgets and increased workloads. This gave people significant stress. Dennis discussed the impact of austerity on his work at HMRC:

> 'There's been a push in recent years, I can sum it up as more for less. So they wanted more money bringing in for less resource being put into it. So what you found was, since 2010, it's very political, there was more justification of the jobs, which is fair enough, but in return for investing a billion in the service they expect five billion back. So it was tough going. Very tough. A lot of people have found it very stressful. I've left friends there who are in a bad way, they're not happy. I've got one friend who I've been seeing in the summer, she's off work, with stress, she's going through what I went through a couple of years ago.' (Dennis, 57)

Psychosocial factors relating to work environments have all been shown to be damaging to mental health (for example, Brunner and Marmot, 2006). As participants in the interviews were generally older, they were often able to report on changing demands at work over a period of many years in the same agency. Employment was cited more often as affecting mental health for participants in the least deprived areas (for participants in the most deprived areas, employment appeared to have a greater impact on their physical, as opposed to mental, health). Brenda talks about her changing role at work, initially the Department for Health and Social Security which then merged into Jobcentre Plus:

> 'I used to work for the benefits side of things, the helping caring side of it, you know, making sure that people's benefits were there, not all about finding people jobs. But then they did the merger a few years ago, so I jumped before I got pushed. I went into Jobcentre because I could have ended up anywhere ... I've done it for too long. The job's changed so much. You get the impression that you're not there to help people any more, you're there to do a business.' (Brenda, 56)

The interviews revealed a complex relationship between employment and its impact on mental health. Participants who were not in paid employment missed work and missed the benefits that work had provided. In particular for participants from the least deprived areas, issues relating to the work environment, such as work-related stress, were spoken about as having an impact on their mental health. This supports other research suggesting that psychosocial work factors, such as a lack of control at work, may affect mental health (Brunner and Marmot, 2006; Finne et al., 2014; Niedhammer et al., 2015). Notably, the work environment was one area in which austerity had an impact on people from the less deprived areas. For some this had led them to make decisions to remove themselves from the stress, such as reducing their employment to part-time working or taking early retirement. Having greater financial stability gave people the choice to make those decisions.

Whereas work had an impact on mental health in the less deprived areas, it more frequently had a physical health effect on people living in more deprived areas. Many of the participants wanted to work and missed the economic and social benefits that working had given them; however, sometimes paid work was not a viable option. There was no evidence of a 'culture of worklessness' that has been represented in dominant narratives (Pantazis, 2016). This perspective places the blame for being out of work on 'faulty' behaviours and attitudes; people out of work are seen as those who 'won't work' rather than as people who in fact face multiple barriers in accessing paid work (Bambra, 2011). Without exception, the participants in this study who were not in employment faced numerous difficulties in accessing work. This included significant barriers posed by chronic health problems and a lack of suitable jobs to apply for. The lack of employment opportunities is borne out by the data. Office for National Statistics job density profiles for 2014 showed there were 0.73 jobs per working-age resident in the local authority, meaning that there were not enough jobs for the number of people looking for them (Nomis, 2015). Participants presented extensive employment histories and no culture of being 'workshy' or 'idle'.

The difference place makes: mental health and home

> 'Everyone's got their own different opinions of it and that, but to me, it's where I was born and it's where I live, it's where I grew up. To me it's home.' (Paul, 27)

This final section considers the differences in the living environments of people in different areas of Stockton-on-Tees, and any associated impact on their mental health. Most participants (from all groups) had very strong ties to Stockton-on-Tees, having been born there and lived in the borough for most, if not all, of their lives. As a result they had a strong sense of belonging to Stockton and to their communities. In the least deprived areas, most participants had lived in the same home for a long time; apart from one participant they all owned their home (either buying it with the help of a mortgage or owning it outright). There was more fluctuation in the more deprived areas and with the participants from the CAB: some participants had lived in the property a long time while others had moved in relatively recently. Most participants in these two groups were renting their current home. Participants from the deprived areas (and from the CAB) had lived in Stockton-on-Tees for most of their lives, often in the same ward. Their own personal identity was connected with the place where they had lived and grown up. Places can be seen to have specific identities, made up of a history, a geography, industry and culture, and these 'biographies of place' (Warren and Garthwaite, 2014; Warren, 2017) were at times reflected in the personal biographies of participants. Laura spoke of her connection to the neighbourhood she came from:

> 'I was brought up on Norton Grange. And then got married, moved around a bit, but always in Norton. Been in here about eight year now … Me mam and dad always lived in Norton. So did [her husband's] parents. So we've always, like, been in Norton.' (Laura, 53)

Despite the strong ties that people had with the places they lived, there were key differences between those from the least deprived areas, the most deprived areas and the CAB. People in the more deprived areas were dealing with problems with housing, crime, and social problems such as drug and alcohol abuse, while those living in less deprived areas did not face these difficulties with their living environments. Curtis (2010) discusses the importance of the physical environment in terms of 'therapeutic landscapes' and 'landscapes of risk'. Therapeutic landscapes are the landscapes people live in that may benefit mental health. Conversely, landscapes of risk describe places that are damaging to mental health, where persistent exposure to poverty and harmful physical surroundings (such as poor-quality housing, pollution and run-down neighbourhoods) may contribute to increased mental ill-health (Curtis, 2010).

This was a theme in which, alongside the differences between people living in the most and least deprived areas, there was also a difference between participants from the most deprived areas and those who had been recruited via the CAB (who generally lived in relatively deprived areas; however they did not live in the *most* deprived areas of the local authority). While some participants from the CAB discussed problems in their living environments, generally they perceived the streets they lived on as being relatively safe spaces. The concern about neighbourhood safety was cited as important by many participants in the interviews (regardless of whether they came from the most or least deprived areas) and also feeds into more psychosocial models of the determinants of mental health (for example, Marmot and Wilkinson, 2006): people wanted to live in places that felt safe, both for themselves and for their families. The reason for feeling positive (or negative) about the home environment often concerned how safe it was perceived to be:

> 'It's a nice quiet area. And it's good for the kids, because the kids can all play out the front and there's always some mum have got their eye on them all.' (Alison, 50)

However in the most deprived areas, participants talked more frequently about social problems, in particular about the difficulties of living in proximity to drug and alcohol abuse, problems with noise and crime. Paul talked about the lack of safe green spaces in the neighbourhood for his family:

> 'When the bairn's here, she's like "Can I go and play out?" Like, the little park bit around there, we only allow her to stay there, we don't like her going on the field … The amount of needles we've found on that field. We don't want the bairn going over there, like falling, and pricking herself on one of them.' (Paul, 27)

Along with several other participants in the most deprived group, Paul was also living in a home that had structural problems with damp and was in a poor condition. Paul was in the process of applying to move and spoke of the problems with his flat:

> 'It's getting worse. The windows are knackered. It's like damp and stuff on the floor so we've had to pull all the carpet up, that's why there's no carpet. The flat itself, when there's loads of traffic, it shakes. It vibrates for about half an hour. It's horrible, absolutely horrible.' (Paul, 27)

Problems with living environments could at times have a significant impact on participants' mental health. However, the environmental and social problems that people in the deprived areas were dealing with were largely absent in the narratives of those from the least deprived areas. They lived in areas that they perceived as relatively safe, where crime was not a significant problem, where they had enough space that they did not have to deal with noise from neighbours. Although some spoke of how the sense of community was not 'what it once was', there was no sense of the physical environment having a damaging impact on participants' mental health. The 'therapeutic landscapes' (Gesler, 1992) literature discusses the potentially beneficial impact of certain natural environments on mental health, such as access to woodland or the coast. James had lived in Ingleby Barwick, one of the least deprived areas, for over 15 years with his wife and daughter. He talked about the area and reflected on how it was safe, affordable and met his family's needs, although he would have preferred to live somewhere more aesthetically attractive:

> 'We moved to Ingleby Barwick. The houses are cheaper over there so that's why we've stayed. It's not ideal but it does. Thousands of brand new houses, just stacked up on top of each other, so it's not like an olde worlde place with lots of character about it. It's just a brand new housing estate. It's dry and it's warm and it serves its purpose. And it's cheap enough. And there's no crime up there really. And the kids are all right.' (James, 47)

James went on to discuss his ideal home, in the countryside in North Yorkshire:

> 'I'd like a static caravan, maybe in Swainby … the views are stunning. You come out on your veranda with a cup of tea on a morning and there's like rabbits and deer and stuff, no traffic, no horrible people. I could probably see meself finishing up in one of them, checking out of society, sat there on my meditation cushion with my incense sticks and my little Buddha. Grow old out there.' (James, 47)

For James, as with some of the other participants, access to green spaces, woodland and more 'therapeutic landscapes' (Gesler, 1992) were reflected on as being important for their mental health. However although these participants were living in some of the least deprived areas of the local authority, they generally spoke of having to travel to benefit from more 'therapeutic' environments. The home environment, for participants in the least deprived areas, was beneficial because it did not have those features of deprived environments, such as crime, which could have such a detrimental impact on people living in the most deprived areas.

Summary

This chapter has explored differences in the lives of people experiencing mental health problems in more and less deprived areas of Stockton-on-Tees. There were key differences in people's lives, and experiences, across a range of different areas. This included employment, finances and the physical environments that people were living in. People living in the least deprived parts of the local authority have a good quality of life, adequate income, decent jobs and live in communities that are safe and relatively protected from crime. Financial stability gives people more power: to live in environments free from crime, to not have to worry on a daily basis about money, to be able to access opportunities and activities that benefit wellbeing, and to break away from situations that are harmful to their mental health. The people interviewed in the less deprived areas were still dealing with mental health problems and talked about how challenging this could be at times. Coping with mental distress was hard for everybody, regardless of their background. However there were additional pressures placed on those who were managing on low incomes and living in the more deprived areas of Stockton-on-Tees.

Poverty affects mental health. This includes the impact of living on a low income, the benefits system, unemployment/insecure employment, deprived housing and living in communities in which there is crime and other social issues. Poverty prevents people from being able to engage in normal everyday life and constrains the choices that people have. While people have agency to make their own decisions, and do so, those choices become increasingly limited when people are facing material hardship. Participants in the most deprived areas spoke of struggling financially and of finding it increasingly difficult to make ends meet. The stress that came about from a lack of money had a detrimental effect on their mental health. The findings support the consistent evidence base showing the link between factors relating to material deprivation and their impact on mental health, including low income (Melzer et al., 2009), unemployment and underemployment (Rogers and Pilgrim, 2003) and living in areas with high levels of deprivation (Curtis, 2010). Material deprivation compounds and exacerbates the difficulties people are facing with their mental health, leading to chronic emotional strain. Poverty presents significant financial and psychosocial challenges to those who are forced to deal with its effects.

This study has found that features of the austerity programme, in particular the welfare cuts, are disproportionately affecting those on the lowest incomes. While narratives about austerity were largely absent from the accounts of people living in less deprived parts of Stockton, they were pervasive in the lives of those from the CAB group and most deprived areas. These were people (and communities) who had already been dealing with issues relating to poverty and deprivation in their lives. Austerity had served to exacerbate and compound those issues. The relentlessness and rigidity of the benefits system aggravated the problems people had with their mental health, creating uncertainty and chronic stress. Since 2010 the series of cuts in welfare and in public spending has affected social inequality in the local authority, and is ultimately having an impact on the mental health of the people who are bearing the brunt of those spending cuts. For those on the lowest incomes, they have been placed under greater financial hardship; they have faced significantly more stress as a result, and this has had an inevitable impact on their mental health.

Politically the programme of austerity measures were outlined as an economic necessity, as a need to balance the £103.9 billion budget deficit held by the UK in 2009/10 (Lupton, 2015). However, Hall et al. (2013) argue that in reality austerity has been a project to justify the ideological aims of the government. This has included a move towards shrinking the role of the state and a further restructuring of the state along market lines. The post-war welfare state was developed with the principle of trying to ensure that people had sufficient income at times when they were unable to work (in childhood, old age, unemployment or as a result of sickness); it is based on the idea that benefits and services should go to people according to their need (as opposed to whether they can pay for it) (Hills, 2014). These principles are being eroded, with dominant narratives increasingly attributing poverty to individual choice and individual responsibility, removing the responsibility of the state to ensure that its citizens do not have to live in poverty. These narratives have permeated public discourses, with increasingly stigmatising rhetoric and media representations all leading to a hardening of perceptions of people who live in poverty (PSE UK, 2013). Social safety nets are being removed to such an extent that people are increasingly left without enough income to be able to meet even basic necessities. This is not acceptable. Poverty is a social – and a political – problem.

A continuation of these regressive measures is likely to lead to growing inequalities, and lives that are even further separated by social division. Planned changes in social security include further reforms to Housing Benefit and the imminent rollout of Universal Credit, a benefit that is best understood as a repackaging of six means-tested existing working-age benefits (Beatty and Fothergill, 2016). The government is currently moving forward with the implementation of Universal Credit, despite widespread and significant concerns about its design and implementation. Failures throughout the implementation period mean that the rollout is five years behind schedule. Claimants must wait for a minimum of six weeks for a first payment (although typically residents in some areas are waiting for 12–13 weeks), effectively leaving them without any income at all in this period (Butler, 2017). As a result, rent arrears have skyrocketed in the areas in which it has been tested and people have been forced into debt and significant financial hardship. Concerns have been so vocal and widespread that the chief executive of Citizens Advice argued that this is 'a disaster waiting to happen' (Cowburn, 2017). If the rollout continues as planned, this is likely to have a severe impact.

Issues relating to poverty and deprivation are central determinants of poor mental health. People on the lowest incomes are faced with daily – and often insurmountable – challenges in meeting even the most basic of needs. Life on a low income creates chronic stress, which has a significant impact on mental health and wellbeing. In continuing with policies that regressively target those on the lowest incomes, this is likely to lead to a widening of the gap in mental health and wellbeing. Unequal societies are unhealthy ones (Wilkinson and Pickett, 2010). It is only by addressing social inequality, and raising the living standards of those on the lowest incomes, that inequalities in mental health can begin to narrow.

References

Bambra, C. (2011) *Work, Worklessness and the Political Economy of Health.* Oxford: Oxford University Press

Bambra, C. (2016) *Health Divides: Where You Live Can Kill You.* Bristol: Policy Press

Bambra, C. and Garthwaite, K.A. (2015) Austerity, Welfare Reform and the English Health Divide. *Area* 47: 341–343

Barr, B., Kinderman, P., and Whitehead, P. (2015a) Trends in mental health inequalities in England during a period of recession, austerity and welfare reform 2004–2013. *Social Science and Medicine* 147: 324–331

Barr, B., Taylor-Robinson, D., Stuckler, D., Loodstra, R., Reeves, A., Whitehead, M. (2015b) 'First, do no harm': are disability assessments associated with adverse trends in mental health? A longitudinal ecological study. *Journal of Epidemology and Community Health*, 0: 1–7

Beatty, C and Fothergill, S. (2016) *The Uneven Impact of Welfare Reform. The Financial Losses to Places and People.* Centre for Regional Economic and Social Research: Sheffield Hallam University www.shu.ac.uk/research/cresr/sites/shu.ac.uk/files/welfare-reform-2016_1.pdf

Belfield, C., Cribb, J., Hood, A., and Joyce, R. (2015) *Living Standards, Poverty and Inequality in the UK 2015.* London: Institute for Fiscal Studies

Beresford, P. (2005) Social approaches to madness and distress: user perspectives and user knowledge. In J.Tew (Ed) 2005. *Social Perspectives in Mental Health: Developing social models to understand and work with mental distress.* London: Jessica Kingsley Publishers

Beresford, P., Nettle, M., and Perring, R. (2010) *Towards a Social Model of Madness and Distress? Exploring what Service Users Say.* York: Joseph Rowntree Foundation

Brunner, E and Marmot, M. (2006) Social organisation, stress and health. In Marmot, M and Wilkinson, R. (2006) *Social Determinants of Health.* Oxford: Oxford University Press

Butler, P. (2017) Universal credit: why is it a problem and can the system be fixed? *The Guardian*, 2 October

Cowburn, A. (2017) Universal Credit delays leave claimants to 'drop off a cliff' in rent arrears, hear MPs. *Independent*, 13 September

Curtis, S. (2010) *Space, Place and Mental Health.* Surrey: Ashgate Publishing Ltd

Daguerre, A and Etherington, D. (2014) *Welfare Reform in the UK under the Conservative-led coalition government: ruptures and continuities.* http://workfare.org.uk/images/uploads/docs/Welfare_Reform_in_the_UK_PubReady.pdf

Davies, S., Finney, A., and Harfree, Y. (2016) Paying to be Poor: Uncovering the Scale and Nature of the Poverty Premium. www.bristol.ac.uk/media-library/sites/geography/pfrc/pfrc1615-poverty-premium-report.pdf

Evans-Lacko, S., Knapp, M., McCrone, P., Thornicroft, G., and Mojtabai, R. (2013) The Mental Health Consequences of the Recession: Economic Hardship and Employment of People with Mental Health Problems in 27 European Countries. *PLoS ONE* 8(7): e69792

Finne, L. B., Christensen, J. O., and Knardahl, S. (2014) Psychological and Social Work Factors as Predictors of Mental Distress: A Prospective Study. *PLoS ONE* 9(7): e102514

Garthwaite, K. A. (2011) 'The language of shirkers and scroungers?' Talking about illness, disability and the coalition welfare reform. *Disability & Society* 26(3): 369–372

Garthwaite, K. A. (2014) Fear of the Brown Envelope: exploring welfare reform with long term sickness benefits recipients. *Social Policy and Administration* 48: 782–798

Garthwaite, K. A., Collins, P. J., and Bambra, C. (2015) Food for Thought: An ethnographic study of negotiating ill-health and food insecurity in a UK food bank. *Social Science and Medicine* 132: 38–44

Gesler, W. M. (1992) Therapeutic landscapes: Medical issues in light of the new cultural geography. *Social Science & Medicine* 34(7): 735–746

Hall, S., Massey, D., and Rustin, M. (2013) After Neoliberalism: analysing the present. *Soundings: A Journal of Politics and Culture* 53: 8–22

Hills, J. (2014) *Good Times Bad Times: The welfare myth of them and us.* Bristol: Policy Press

Hirsch, D. (2015) *A Minimum Income Standard for the UK in 2015.* Joseph Rowntree Foundation

JRF (Joseph Rowntree Foundation) (2016) Monitoring Poverty and Social Exclusion www.jrf.org.uk/press/work-poverty-hits-record-high-housing-crisis-fuels-insecurity

Kim, T.J and von dem Knesebeck, O. (2015) Is an insecure job better for health than having no job at all? A systematic review of studies investigating the health-related risks of both job insecurity and unemployment. *BMC Public Health* 15: 985

Lupton, R. (2015) The Coalition's Social Policy Record: Policy, Spending and Outcomes 2010–2015. http://sticerd.lse.ac.uk/dps/case/spcc/RR04.pdf

MacInnes, T., Tinson, A., Hughes, C., Born, T. B., and Aldridge, H. (2015) *Monitoring Poverty and Social Exclusion 2015.* Joseph Rowntree Foundation

Marmot, M. (2010) *Fair Society, Healthy Lives: The Marmot Review.* London: University College

Marmot, M. and Wilkinson, R. (2006) *Social Determinants of Health.* Oxford: Oxford University Press

McManus, S., Meltzer, H., Brugha, T. S., Bebbington, P. E., and Jenkins, R. (2009) *Adult psychiatric morbidity in England, 2007: results of a household survey.* The NHS Information Centre for health and social care

Melzer, D., Fryers, T., and Jenkins, R. (2009) *Social Inequalities and the Distribution of the Common Mental Disorders.* Maudsley Monographs. Hove: Psychology Press

Mental Health Taskforce (2016) *The Five Year Forward View for Mental Health.* www.england.nhs.uk/wp-content/uploads/2016/02/Mental-Health-Taskforce-FYFV-final.pdf

Morrow, M. (2013) Recovery: Progressive Paradigm or Neoliberal Smokescreen? In B. A. Le Francois, R Menzies and G Reaume (Eds) *Mad Matters. A Critical Reader in Canadian Mad Studies.* Toronto: Canadian Scholars Press Inc

NICE (National Institute for Clinical Excellence) (2015) *Psychosis and schizophrenia in adults.* National Institute for Health and Care Excellence www.nice.org.uk/guidance/qs80/chapter/quality-statement-5-supported-employment-programmes

Niedhammer, I., Lesuffleur, T., Algava, E., and Chastang, J. F. (2015) Classic and emergent psychosocial work factors and mental health. *Occupational Medicine* 65 (2): 126–134

Nomis (2015) *Labour Market Profile – Stockton-on-Tees.* www.nomisweb.co.uk/reports/lmp/la/1946157063/report.aspx

O'Hara, M. (2013) *Austerity Bites: a journey to the sharp end of the cuts in the UK.* Bristol: Policy Press

ONS (Office for National Statistics) (2015) *Suicides in the United Kingdom, 2013 Registrations* www.ons.gov.uk/ons/dcp171778_395145.pdf

Pantazis, C. (2016) Policies and Discourses of Poverty during a Time of Recession and Austerity. *Critical Social Policy* 36(1): 3–20

Patrick, R. (2015) Rhetoric and Reality: Exploring lived experiences of welfare reform under the coalition. In L. Foster, A. Brunton, C. Deeming and T. Haux (Eds) *In Defence of Welfare 2.* Social Policy Association

Pemberton, S., Sutton, E., Fahmy, E., Bell, K. (2014) *Life on a Low Income in Austere Times.* ESRC: PSE UK. www.poverty.ac.uk/sites/default/files/attachments/Life%20on%20a%20low%20income%20in%20austere%20times_final_report.pdf

PSE UK (2013) *The Impoverishment of the UK.* ESRC. www.poverty.ac.uk/sites/default/files/attachments/The_Impoverishment_of_the_UK_PSE_UK_first_results_summary_report_March_28.pdf

Public Health England (2015) Stockton-on-Tees Health Profile 2015. APHO, www.apho.org.uk/resource/item.aspx?RID=50336

Rogers, A., and Pilgrim, D. (2003) *Mental Health and Inequality.* Hampshire: Palgrave Macmillan

Shaw, M., Dorling, D., and Smith, G. D. (2006) Poverty, social exclusion and minorities. In Marmot, M. and Wilkinson, R. (Eds) *Social Determinants of Health*. Oxford: Oxford University Press

Tew, J. (2005) Power relations, social order and mental distress. In J. Tew (Ed) *Social Perspectives in Mental Health: Developing Social Models to Understand and Work with Mental Distress*. London: Jessica Kingsley Publishers

Warren, J. (2017) *Industrial Teesside Lives and Legacies: A Post-Industrial Geography*. London: Palgrave

Warren, J., and Garthwaite, K. (2014) Biographies of Place: Challenging Official Spatial Constructions of Sickness and Disability. In K. Soldatic, A. Roulstone and H. Morgan (Eds) *Disability – Spaces and Places of Policy Exclusion*. London: Routledge, pp. 115–129

WHO (World Health Organization)/CGF (Calouste Gulbenkian Foundation) (2014) *Social Determinants of Mental Health*. Geneva: WHO

Wilkinson, R. and Pickett, K. (2010) *The Spirit Level: Why Equality is Better for Everyone*. London: Penguin

Williams, J. (2002) Social inequalities and mental health. In C. Newnes, G. Holmes and C. Dunn (eds) *This is Madness: A Critical Look at Psychiatry and the Future of Mental Health* Services. Ross on Wye: PCCS Books

SIX

Minding the Gap

*Nasima Akhter, Kate Mattheys,
Jon Warren and Adetayo Kasim*

Introduction

This chapter examines inequalities in mental health in Stockton-on-Tees using survey data. It engages with key debates around the causes of socioeconomic inequalities in mental health by examining the extent and underpinning determinants of the gap in mental health and wellbeing between the most and least deprived neighbourhoods of Stockton-on-Tees. Using data from the longitudinal household survey, it establishes the extent of inequalities in mental health and wellbeing in Stockton-on-Tees and examines the explanatory role of behavioural, psychosocial and material factors in explaining this gap. Longitudinal time trend analysis also examines the effects of austerity and welfare reform on this gap and on the contribution of the underpinning determinants. The results indicate that there is a significant gap in mental health and wellbeing between the most and least deprived neighbourhoods of Stockton-on-Tees and, in contrast to the majority of public health practice and discourse, it is material and psychosocial factors that are the major explanations of the health gap – not behavioural factors. However, there were few changes in these relationships overtime. The chapter discusses the implications of the findings for mental health policy and practice in the context of further likely exacerbation during prolonged austerity.

The Great Recession

Recessions are period of temporary economic decline (technically defined as two consecutive quarters of negative growth in gross domestic product: Oxford Dictionaries [2012]). The 2007/08 economic crisis affected most countries around the world. Economic recessions are accompanied by a rise in unemployment, decline in income, unmanageable debts, precarious job environment, stress, and consequently higher prevalence of mental health problems, substance misuse and an increase in suicides. The 2007/08 crisis also resulted in increased bankruptcies, downward trends in stock markets, increased unemployment and housing repossessions. According to the International Labour Organization, worldwide the number of jobless people increased to 212 million in 2009 compared to about 34 million jobless people in 2007 (Chang et al., 2013). The post-2007 economic decline has been longer, wider and deeper than earlier recessions (for example, the 1930s Great Depression) and is commonly known as the 'Great Recession'. The International Monetary Fund (IMF) has stated that this Great Recession is the worst experienced in the global economy for 60 years (Gamble, 2009).

The effect of the recession varied by country as a result of social safety nets and the policy measures taken. International responses varied and the UK responded with policies of austerity (Reeves et al., 2013). In an attempt to reduce public deficits, large cuts were made to central and local government budgets, health care system, welfare services and social security benefits (Reeves et al., 2013; Kitson et al., 2011). Reeves et al. (2013) compared policies across European countries between 2009–11 to assess how the UK fared with rest of the Europe (Reeves et al., 2013). They found that the UK had the third most extensive austerity policy among other European countries. There have been a raft of 'welfare reforms' initiated in the UK, with many individuals affected by multiple cuts. Consequently, the UK had a large rise in unemployment and a strong association was evident between unemployment rates and increased rates of suicide in males. For example, Knapp (2012) reported that more than 2.7 million people were unemployed with over 860,000 of them being unemployed for more than a year. The average household debt was high and rising (Knapp, 2012). Between 2009 and 2011, the UK experienced a reduction of 2.5% public expenditure (equivalent to about £245 per capita). At this time of increased unemployment, there were also considerable cuts to social security with those on the lowest incomes who have been most heavily affected (Reeves et al., 2013). It is also the most deprived local authorities that have been hardest hit by the cuts (Beatty and Fothergill, 2016). Since 2010 the North East as a region has lost £966 million (O'Donoghue, 2016). Previous international research on welfare changes has shown that where welfare services are cut, this has a detrimental impact on the health of the poorest (Shaw et al., 2005; Blakely et al., 2008). This chapter discusses the effect of post-recession austerity on neighbourhood inequalities in mental health in Stockton-on-Tees using data from our longitudinal household survey.

Inequalities in mental health

Mental health is a crucial element of the overall wellbeing of individuals, societies and countries (Box 6.1), and deprivation in various forms can be detrimental to it. Positive mental health promotes wellbeing so that individuals can realize their abilities, are able to cope with normal stresses of life, to work productively and to contribute to their community (WHO, 2003). There is ample evidence that mental health and social position are inversely associated and even follows a social gradient (Murali and Oyebode, 2004; Reiss, 2013; Delgadillo et al., 2016; Marmot, 2017). The 2001 World Health Report, for example, shows that in high-income countries the prevalence of mental health problems such as depression and anxiety was 1.5 to 2 times higher among the most deprived than their most affluent counterpart (WHO, 2001).

Box 6.1: Mental health

Concepts of mental health include subjective well-being, perceived self-efficacy, autonomy, competence, intergenerational dependence and recognition of the ability to realize one's intellectual and emotional potential. It has also been defined as a state of well-being whereby individuals recognize their abilities, are able to cope with the normal stresses of life, work productively and fruitfully, and make a contribution to their communities. Mental health is about enhancing competencies of individuals and communities and enabling them to achieve their self-determined goals. (WHO, 2003: 7)

Poverty and deprivation have wide-ranging impacts. Poverty acts as a constraint for many of the material conditions of life. This includes leading to limited access to adequate housing, inability to access good nutrition, constrained opportunities to participate in society and reduced access to goods and services (Shaw et al., 2006; Bambra, 2016). Poorer health and higher rates of mortality are found in almost all studies of neighbourhoods characterised by poverty and unemployment, and the link between income and health is evidenced in the vast majority of studies in this area (Bambra, 2016; Bartley, 2016). The stress associated with life on a low income – such as insecure work, financial difficulties, and living in areas with high levels of deprivation – also appears to have particularly damaging effects on mental and physical health (Marmot and Wilkinson, 2006; Thoits, 2010).

While poverty and health are inversely associated, economic hardship due to crisis such as recession has an additional mental health impact (Friedli, 2009). The 2008 global recession had both short and long-term negative impacts on mental health, particularly on key groups such as disabled people and those experiencing mental distress (Frasquilho et al., 2016). The effects of economic hardship are widespread, negatively affecting many aspects of wellbeing and functioning (Barnes et al., 2017). Following the 2008 recession, worldwide an excess of 4,884 suicides were observed in 2009; these would not have occurred if the trend in 2000–07 had continued (Corcoran et al., 2015). A rise in suicide attempts or self-harm was also evident in Ireland, Greece, Spain and Italy (Hawton et al., 2016). In the longer term, an excess of 4,750 suicides in the US, 1,000 suicides in England (Corcoran et al., 2015), and 680 suicides in Spain were observed over the next three years (2008–10). Although suicide is often reported, it is only tip of the iceberg. Both self-harm and non-fatal negative effects on wellbeing follow a gradient of socioeconomic deprivation (Hawton et al., 2016).

The long-term public health impacts of recession varied between countries as a result of their respective policy measures (Hawton et al., 2016; Ruckert and Labonté, 2017). Stuckler and Basu (2013) argue that it is *how* the state responds to economic crises that determines their impact on health. Where social safety nets are reduced for instance, economic shocks can rapidly turn into health crises (Stuckler and Basu, 2013). Conversely, economic stimulus can have a protective effect on the harm caused by recession. Whereas Sweden, Poland and Germany substantially increased government spending, the austerity measures adopted in the UK (expenditure cut of about £245 per capita) ranked the third largest for spending cuts in Europe after Greece and Luxemburg. Greece, Spain and Portugal adopted strict fiscal austerity and restricted health budget and a rise in prevalence of suicides and infection disease were evident in these countries. In the contrast, Iceland had little or no negative effect on health when it rejected austerity and instead increased public expenditure (Karanikolos et al., 2013).

Though health outcomes are influenced by the distribution of social and economic resources between and within countries, high levels of inequality within a country or region further increases the risk to physical and mental health. Virtually all health and social problems are worse in more unequal societies (Wilkinson and Pickett, 2010). The more inequitable a society is, the higher the risk for its population to experience increased stress, anxiety, depression, and in the worst cases suicide and self-harm (Wilkinson and Pickett, 2010): social inequality is bad for mental health. These adverse effects were evident for both individual-level and area-level aggregated analysis: the neighbourhoods with greater unemployment had higher rates of suicide (Hawton et al., 2016). While population mental health usually declines during an economic recession and then recovers, this has not been the case in the current period: 2013 witnessed the highest male suicide rate since 2001 (ONS, 2015). Between 2010 and 2013, the largest increases in poor mental health (measured by suicide rates, self-reported mental health problems and anti-depressant prescriptions) have been in the most deprived neighbourhoods, leading to increasing inequalities in mental health (Barr et al., 2016). These widening inequalities have been attributed to the raft of welfare cuts, and worsening financial situations, of those on the lowest incomes. Deprived areas have been the hardest hit by austerity and this is having an impact on spatial and society inequality (Hastings et al., 2015). A recent study using data from European social study survey observed that there was a negative association with social expenditure and health inequalities in welfare countries in Europe (Álvarez-Gálvez and Jaime-Castillo, 2018). They also found that social expenditure can moderate the relationship between socioeconomic status (SES) and health inequality.

Social inequalities are closely linked to health inequalities, and by having an impact on social inequality, UK austerity policies are likely to further widen the existing north-south divide and health inequalities at the local level (Beatty and Fothergill, 2013; Bambra et al., 2014; Coope et al., 2014; Bambra and Garthwaite, 2015; Clayton et al., 2015; Bambra, 2016). These negative effects will challenge the progress in reaching the United Nations Sustainable Development Goal 10 of making the world a more equitable society (United Nations). Therefore, it is important to assess and understand the impact of austerity, as evidence has shown that the impact of recession may vary depending on responses, such as whether a country chooses austerity over alternative measures on increased public expenditure. It is crucially important that health inequalities are investigated and understood properly, and adequate policy responses are in place.

Explaining inequalities in mental health

There are three key explanatory models for why such health inequalities exist: materialist, psychosocial and behavioural/cultural (Bambra, 2016; Bartley, 2016).

The materialist explanation of health inequalities describes how the distribution of financial and related resources relates to health

(Williams, 2003; Shaw et al., 2006). It focuses on how the various material conditions of life (such as the physical environment, income, housing, nutrition, opportunities for participation and access to health care services) affect health outcomes. An important aspect of the material model is that there is clear negative association between poverty, deprivation and health. Every increase in deprivation is associated with worse health: the higher the level of neighbourhood deprivation, the higher is level of mortality or illness. The effect is twofold: someone with a low income has limited capacity to buy things important for their health, but s/he also has may well live in a deprived neighbourhood which further limits their access to salutogenic factors: the amplification of deprivation (Macintyre, 2007). Dreger et al. (2014), for example, have identified material deprivation, such as ability to pay for basic goods and services, as a significant determinant of mental health and wellbeing.

Psychosocial models of health inequalities focus on how relative deprivation may influence health outcomes: "What matters is where we stand in relation to others in our own society" (Wilkinson and Pickett, 2010: 25). The position held in a social hierarchy can make a person feel frustrated and stressed if they are lower down. This is particularly the case in high income countries (Wilkinson and Pickett, 2010), where people from lower socioeconomic backgrounds cannot afford the range of commodities available and accessible to wealthier households. The psychosocial pathway describes how stress related to low position and feelings of lack of power caused by living in an unequal society act as psychosocial risk factors for mental health (Marmot and Wilkinson, 2001; Bambra, 2011; Marmot, 2017). It emphasises that people's experience and emotions are translated as acute and chronic stress and then cumulatively have an impact on the body and result in adverse physical and mental health outcomes (Marmot and Wilkinson, 2006; Thoits, 2010). The effect of chronic anxiety, low levels of self-esteem and a lack of control at work – or at the community level – can be very damaging to physical and mental health (Brunner and Marmot, 2006). Availability of social support, having control and autonomy at work, being able to balance between home and work and having a balance between efforts and rewards are also included as factors in this model that can affect health (Bartley, 2016).

Behavioural models, on the other hand, suggest that what people do as an individual can be damaging to their health, and that certain groups of people are more likely to demonstrate health damaging behaviours compared to others (Marmot and Bell, 2012). They focus on unhealthy behaviours, such as smoking, drinking alcohol, lack of fruit and vegetable consumption and lack of exercise. These behaviours are more commonly seen in deprived communities. The behavioural model shifts the focus from collective to individual responsibilities for health inequalities. This model attributes health inequalities to the personal characteristics of individuals (that is, their choice of behaviour) (Bartley, 2016). The wider structural determinants of health (and health behaviours) are thereby marginalised in favour of focusing on the individual, and apportioning blame, and the impetus for change, firmly on that person.

Stockton-on-Tees survey

Stockton-on-Tees is an area in the North East of England with high spatial and social inequality (Bambra et al., 2014; Mattheys et al., 2016), which has one of the highest life expectancy gaps of all English local authorities (Schrecker and Bambra, 2015; Bambra, 2016). This chapter examines changes in inequalities in mental health between least and most deprived neighbourhoods of Stockton-on-Tees using a longitudinal household survey that was conducted over 18 months between 2014–16. It investigates the size of the gap in mental health between the least and most deprived areas of Stockton-on-Tees over the study period and assesses the relative contribution of different factors in explaining neighbourhood inequalities in mental health: physical material environment, socioeconomic material environment, and psychosocial and behavioural factors. It also presents a longitudinal analysis of the key factors associated with the mental health outcomes.

We conducted a longitudinal household survey over an 18-month period with participants surveyed at Wave 1 (April–June 2014), Wave 2 (October–December 2014), Wave 3 (April–July 2015) and Wave 4 (October 2015–February 2016). The gap in health between the two areas is examined using a multistage stratified random sampling of adults aged over 18, split between participants from the 20 most and 20 least deprived lower layer super output areas (LSOAs). In order to create a sample for the survey the research team used the 2010 Index of Multiple Deprivation (IMD) to identify the 20 most and 20 least deprived LSOAs in Stockton-on-Tees (DCLG, 2011). The IMD is a summary measure of relative deprivation for each local authority district, unitary authority and LSOA in England. It is published at the level of LSOA and is formed by pulling together 38 individual indicators that are situated within seven broader domains: income deprivation; employment deprivation; health deprivation and disability; education, skills and training deprivation; barriers to housing and services; living environment deprivation; and crime. Figure 6.1 shows the neighbourhoods included in the survey.

Figure 6.1: Maps of Stockton-on-Tees including most and least deprived survey neighbourhoods

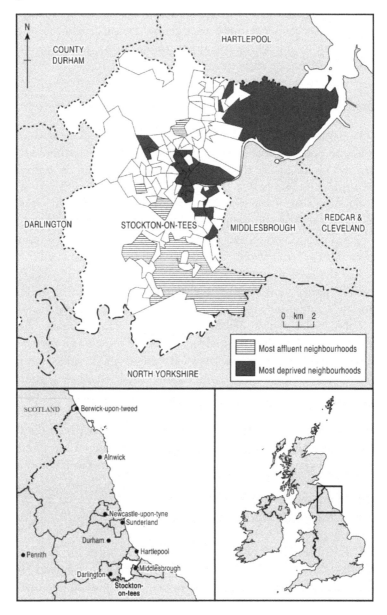

Source: Mattheys et al., 2016

The *scale* at which deprivation is studied can have a really significant impact on the results, as different patterns prevail with different geographical scales. Using larger areas, such as data at the local authority level, can lead to variations within them being smoothed out. As such it is important to use data at as low a level as possible. LSOAs provide the best means of doing this in England (ONS, 2017). LSOAs are small areas of relatively even size (of around 1,500 people in each). There are 32,484 LSOAs in England (DCLG, 2011). It is important to be aware however that although the IMD will identify areas that have characteristics that are associated with deprivation, it does not identify *deprived people* (people who could be considered as deprived may be living in an area that is not considered so). It also should be considered a summary measure; IMD scores are made up of weighted individual domain scores and so the summary score does not tell us how each individual domain is scoring.

Participants were sampled initially by household, and then at the individual level, using a multi-stage sampling strategy. Within this approach, a sample of areas are drawn up (initially larger areas are selected and then progressively smaller ones until a sample of households are randomly selected within the areas) (De Vaus, 1991). A random sample of 200 target households in each of the 40 LSOAs

Figure 6.2: Sampling strategy for the survey

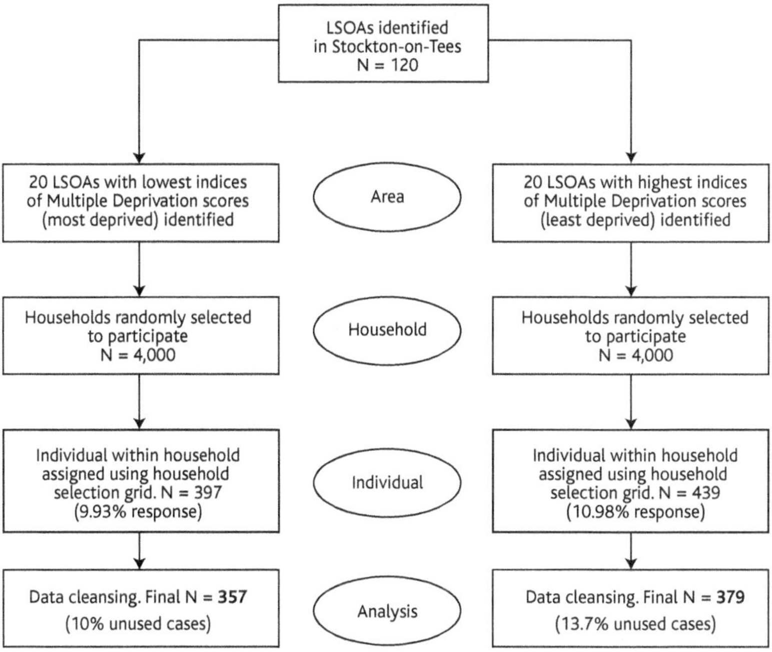

179

was selected resulting in a total of 8000 households (4,000 most and least deprived) who were sent study invitation letters (200 per LSOA) in April and May 2014. This was done assuming a response rate of 10%. In order to avoid bias in the selection of individuals within a household (for instance the person who is not in employment in a household always responding), we followed the selection procedure that is outlined by De Vaus (1991).

Mental health outcomes

Two measures were selected to assess mental health in the survey: the Warwick Edinburgh Mental Wellbeing Scale and the SF8 Mental Health Score. The Warwick-Edinburgh Mental Well-Being Scale (WEMWBS) is a 14-point scale that considers both hedonic and eudaemonic aspects of wellbeing and asks respondents to self-report their experience of each of the statements over the past two weeks. The 14 statements included in WEMWBS each has five possible answers that are scaled from 'none of the time' up to 'all of the time'. The scale gives the individual a total score (up to a maximum of 70), which is used as the dependent variable and is treated as a continuous variable. It has been well validated for use in the general population and has moderate to high levels of construct validity (it measures what it says it is measuring) (Tennant et al., 2007).

The SF8 instrument provides a measure of physical and mental health and provides a separate score for both physical and mental health. It is a condensed version of the SF36 and has eight questions. The individual is asked to report how much each question is applicable to them over the past 30 days. The SF8 tool has two components: Physical Component Summary (PCS) and Mental Component Summary (MCS). The SF8MCS includes questions about social functioning, mental health and emotional role limitation (Roberts et al., 2010). The shorter version of SF8 was used as it was felt that although it is less sensitive than the longer version, on balance it was a more cost effective tool to use within a relatively large survey (Bowling, 2005).

Factors that explain inequalities

To understand how mental health is influenced by various factors, variables were separated into four categories: material socioeconomic variables; material physical environment variables; psychosocial variables and behavioural variables. The group of material socioeconomic variables included questions around how the person occupied their home, whether anyone in the household was in receipt of benefits, receipt of housing benefit, whether the participant was in paid employment, whether the household was a workless household, total household income and highest educational level. The material physical environment variables included questions around living conditions including whether there were problems with damp, whether the house was too dark and not warm enough in winter. It also included questions around the neighbourhood status including problems with crime, pollution/environmental problems and problems with noise. The psychosocial variables included frequency of meeting socially with friends, family or work colleagues; how safe the participant felt walking alone after dark; how often the participant felt they lacked companionship; how often the participant felt left out; how often the participant felt isolated from others; and how happy the person would identify as on a scale of 1–10. Finally, the behavioural questions included whether the participant smoked, whether the participant drank alcohol, weekly alcohol consumption units, daily fruit and vegetable consumption portions and frequency of physical exercise.

Analysis

The study data were initially utilised to produce summary statistics and visualisation aids, which described the changes in demographic, material socioeconomic, material physical, psychosocial and behavioural factors over the study period.

The key analyses are then done in three segments: first, in line with the objective of the survey to investigate neighbourhood inequality in mental health between the most and least deprived LSOAs in Stockton-On-Tees over time, we fitted multilevel models (MLM) for the mental health outcomes with only deprivation indicator and Waves as the predictor variables. The models also included demographic factors (age and gender), so that the results are adjusted for them. MLMs were used to analyse the mental health outcomes so that it will account for correlation between the repeated observations per participant. The study used individual level data collected from the same individual over a period, which means that these repeated measures are likely to be correlated.

Second, in addition to the longitudinal analysis, compositional and contextual analysis of the relative contribution of the different health inequalities factors to the inequality gap was performed on the baseline data. The analysis focused on the gap in the two mental health scores between respondents from the most and least deprived areas. MLMs were used to calculate what percentage of the mental health inequalities between the most and least deprived areas were explained by material, psychosocial and behavioural factors. A similar approach was used with regard to explaining socioeconomic inequalities in health in Norway (Skalická et al., 2009) and with respect to the North–South health divide in England (Bambra et al., 2015).

The reference model for each health outcome is a MLM containing only the indicator for the most and least deprived areas together with age and gender. The percentage reduction on inequality gap due to different health inequalities factors or combinations of them was calculated as the ratio of the difference between the reference model and the model including the compositional and contextual factors. Repeating the same process, percentage reduction in inequality gap was calculated for material socioeconomic; material physical environmental; psychosocial, and behavioural factors. This process allowed calculation of their relative contribution in explaining the health inequality gap.

Finally, MLMs were used to assess which factors were associated with mental health inequality over the study period. Associations were examined using longitudinal data for SF8MCS and WEMWBS outcomes separately. The most parsimonious models were used to explain the outcome that included variables adequately explaining the association.

Further details of the underpinning statistical methods are available in Mattheys et al. (2016) and Akhter et al. (2018).

Results

Demographic characteristics

About 27% of the participants in the most-deprived LSOAs belonged to the age group of 65 years and above at Wave 1, which was slightly higher in the least deprived areas (Table 6.1). In the later waves, the percentages of older participants tended to increase with 38% in most deprived and 46% in the least deprived LSOA's. There was not much change in percentage of females participating to the study in both areas (57%–59% for most deprived; 59%–61% for least deprived LSOAs). Throughout the period, the percentages of single participants were much higher in most deprived areas (35%–39%); whereas it ranged from 11%–17% in least deprived areas. In both areas, over time there was slight increase (6%–8% in most deprived; 1%–2% in least deprived) in participation of those who were married and living with their spouses.

Table 6.1: Summary statistics (mean, standard deviation or %, n/N) for outcome and demographic indicators for least and most deprived areas in Stockton-on-Tees across waves

	Variable	Wave1	Wave2	Wave3	Wave4
Most deprived	SF8MC (mean, SD)	49.5 ± 11.8	49.4 ± 10.8	49.7 ± 10.7	48.7 ± 11.0
	WEMWBS (mean, SD)	49.7 ± 12.6	50.6 ± 11.6	51.7 ± 11.5	50.1 ± 12.5
	Age >=65 (%)	27.5 (109/397)	33.6 (77/229)	35.3 (77/218)	38.1 (67/176)
	Female (%)	59.4 (236/397)	57.2 (131/229)	57.8 (126/218)	56.8 (100/176)
	Single (%)	39.0 (155/397)	28.8 (66/229)	28.4 (62/218)	25.0 (44/221)
Least deprived	SF8MCS (mean, SD)	53.5 ± 8.4	52.4 ± 9.0	53.7 ± 7.7	52.2 ± 8.5
	WEMWBS (mean, SD)	54.8 ± 10.2	55.3 ± 9.2	55.8 ± 11.1	55.8 ± 9.7
	Age >=65 (%)	32.8 (144/439)	40.6 (116/286)	43.2 (112/259)	46.2 (108/234)
	Female (%)	58.8 (258/439)	60.8 (174/286)	61.5 (160/260)	60.3 (141/234)
	Single (%)	17.3 (76/439)	14.0 (40/286)	12.7 (33/260)	10.7 (25/234)

Material socioeconomic characteristics

Table 6.2 shows that at Wave 1, 23% more people living in most deprived areas had no formal education compared to those living in least deprived boroughs (47% vs 24.1). The characteristics of participants in both areas remained very similar over the next waves of data collection and the difference remained static (24%). Similarly, majority (72% at baseline) people in most deprived boroughs rented their house, which was significantly lower for the least deprived areas. Over the period, although percentage of those renting houses dropped a bit for the most deprived areas, at any point it was 58%–60% higher than that of the least deprived LSOAs. In the most deprived areas nearly 90% received any benefit at the Wave 1 and it was 6% less at Wave 4. At Wave 1, it was about 18% less in the least deprived areas and remained unchanged for next one and half years. Almost half of those living in most deprived areas received Housing Benefit during baseline, which was less than 5% for least deprived areas. At Wave 4, it dropped by 13% in most and 3% in least deprived areas. About one quarter of the participants in most deprived areas were employed, which remained similar. For those living in least

Table 6.2: Summary statistics (%, n/N and median) for material socioeconomic indicators across waves for most deprived and least deprived areas of Stockton-on-Tees

	Variable	Wave1	Wave2	Wave3	Wave4
Most deprived	No formal education	46.7 (185/396)	46.1 (105/228)	46.1 (100/217)	46.0 (81/176)
	Tenure-rent	72.0 (286/397)	66.8 (153/229)	65.7 (132/201)	64.1 (109/170)
	Annual income*	£26,916 (377)	£29,716 (222)	£30,657 (208)	£33,413 (170)
	Benefit	88.2 (350/397)	83.0 (190/229)	83.0 (181/218)	81.8 (144/176)
	Housing Benefit	54.7 (217/397)	38.4 (88/229)	46.8 (102/218)	41.5 (73/176)
	Workless household	67.8 (269/397)	–	–	–
	Employed	23.9 (95/397)	25.8 (59/229)	26.6 (58/218)	26.1 (46/176)
Least deprived	No formal education	24.1 (106/439)	22.0 (63/286)	21.9 (57/260)	21.8 (51/234)
	Tenure-rent	11.6 (51/439)	8.7 (25/286)	8.5 (22/260)	6.4 (15/234)
	Annual income*	£110,173 (388)	£111,990 (258)	£106,268 (238)	£94,603 (215)
	Benefit	70.4 (309/439)	66.8 (191/286)	71.9 (187/260)	72.6 (170/234)
	Housing Benefit	4.1 (18/439)	3.1 (9/286)	2.7 (7/260)	1.3 (3/234)
	Workless household	36.7 (161/439)	–	–	–
	Employed	46.9 (206/439)	39.9 (114/286)	40.4 (105/260)	38.5 (90/234)

*Median income

developed areas, it was nearly double at baseline, which then dropped by 9% at Wave 4.

Material physical environmental characteristics

Table 6.3 describes the physical environment of the participants living in most and least deprived areas of Stockton–on–Tees. At Wave 1, double the participants in the most deprived areas responded that their houses were too dark than in least deprived areas (18% vs. 9%).

Table 6.3: Summary statistics (%, n/N) for material physical environmental indicators among households from most deprived and least deprived areas in Stockton-on-Tees across waves

	Variable	Wave1	Wave2	Wave3	Wave4
Most deprived	Dark	18.1 (72/397)	18.3 (42/229)	19.9 (40/201)	6.8 (12/176)
	Damp	25.4 (101/397)	21.8 (50/229)	18.9 (38/201)	13.6 (24/176)
	Warmth	80.3 (318/396)	78.2 (179/229)	76.6 (154/201)	86.9 (153/176)
	Noise	22.9 (91/397)	22.7 (52/229)	20.4 (41/201)	17.6 (31/176)
	Pollution	13.1 (52/397)	14.8 (34/229)	13.9 (28/201)	12.5 (22/176)
	Crime	28.0 (111/397)	31.9 (73/229)	31.3 (63/201)	24.4 (43/176)
Least deprived	Dark	9.3 (41/439)	8.4 (24/286)	9.2 (24/260)	2.1 (5/234)
	Damp	2.3 (10/438)	1.4 (4/285)	0.8 (2/259)	0.9 (2/234)
	Warmth	93.4 (410/439)	89.9 (257/286)	85.4 (222/260)	97.4 (228/234)
	Noise	10.5 (46/439)	11.5 (33/286)	10.8 (28/260)	6.0 (14/234)
	Pollution	3.4 (15/439)	4.5 (13/286)	4.2 (11/260)	1.7 (4/234)
	Crime	6.4 (28/439)	6.3 (18/286)	6.5 (17/260)	5.1 (12/234)

The situation remained similar all through, except that fewer people from both areas reported this at the last wave. About one quarter to the participants from most deprived areas mentioned in Wave 1 that they experienced having damp in their households. Over period, this percentage tended to be smaller and at Wave 4 it was about 11% less. However, in the least deprived areas it was only 1%–2% who mentioned having damp at any point of the study.

Psycho-social characteristics

Similarly, differences existed for those living in most deprived areas with 8%–11% more of them experiencing their houses not warm enough, or noise and pollution in the area. This difference was larger in terms of crime which was 19%–22% higher in most deprived areas. Only 5%–6% households in least deprived areas experienced crime within the period of survey. Table 6.4 shows the profile of households from most deprived and least deprived LSOAs in Stockton-on-Tees. Nearly double the participants in the most deprived areas reported that they often felt lack of companionship. In the least deprived areas, about 5%–8% participants often felt lack of companionship. At Wave 1, 11% participants from most-deprived areas reported often feeling left out and there was slight decrease to 8% at Wave 4. However, only 3%–4% participants in the least deprived areas had such experience. Similar difference was evident for often feeling isolated, which was reported by small percentage (3%–4%) among

Table 6.4: Profile of psychosocial indicators (%, n/N or mean, standard deviation) for households in most and least deprived areas of Stockton-on-Tees across waves

	Variable	Wave1	Wave2	Wave3	Wave4
Most deprived	Often lack companion	12.1 (48/397)	14.1 (33/229)	15.1 (33/218)	10.2 (18/176)
	Often felt left out	11.1 (44/397)	10.9 (25/229)	8.7 (19/218)	8.0 (14/176)
	Often felt isolated	11.8 (47/397)	11.8 (27/229)	10.6 (23/218)	10.8 (19/176)
	Social meeting	24.7 (98/397)	21.0 (48/229)	22.5 (49/218)	13.1 (23/176)
	Feels unsafe walking	34.0 (130/382)	35.7 (79/221)	34.8 (73/210)	25.6 (40/156)
	Happiness	7.4 ± 2.1	7.4 ± 2.0	7.4 ± 2.0	7.5 ± 1.9
Least deprived	Often lack companion	6.4 (28/438)	8.0 (23/286)	6.9 (18/260)	4.7 (11/234)
	Often felt left out	3.9 (17/438)	2.8 (8/286)	2.7 (7/260)	3.0 (7/234)
	Often felt isolated	4.1 (18/438)	3.8 (11/286)	2.7 (7/260)	4.3 (10/234)
	Social meeting	15.3 (67/438)	15.4 (44/286)	14.6 (38/260)	9.0 (21/234)
	Feels unsafe walking	2.7 (29/435)	6.4 (18/283)	6.6 (17/258)	7.6 (17/225)
	Happiness	7.9 ± 1.6	7.8 ± 1.5	7.9 ± 1.4	8.0 ± 1.4

participants from least developed areas. About 20%–30% more participants from most deprived areas also felt their area was unsafe. Social meeting, however was more common in most deprived areas but average happiness score remained roughly 0.4–0.5 point lower than those living in least deprived areas.

Behavioural characteristics

In terms of behavioural aspect, consumption of alcohol was much lower (19%–16%) among participants in the most-deprived areas (Table 6.5). About 57% in least deprived areas drank alcohol at Wave 1, which was somewhat lower in Wave 2 and Wave 3. At Wave 4, half the participants there were drinking alcohol. On the contrary, higher percentage of study participants in most deprived areas were doing exercise every day. The difference was 6% at Wave 1 and halved at Wave 4, but was bigger in Wave 2 and Wave 3. On average,

Table 6.5: Summary statistics for behavioural factors (%, n/mean, SD) among most and least deprived areas of Stockton-on-Tees

	Variable	Wave1	Wave2	Wave3	Wave4
Most deprived	Drink alcohol	57.2 (227/397)	41.0 (94/229)	41.7 (91/218)	50.6 (89/176)
	Exercise everyday	34.5 (137/397)	41.5 (95/229)	45.0 (98/218)	31.8 (56/176)
	Fruits & Veg	2.9 ± 2.0	2.9 ± 2.1	2.9 ± 2.0	2.9 ± 1.9
	Smoking	36.8 (146, 3970	28.8 (66, 229)	28.0 (61, 218)	25.6 (45, 176)
Least deprived	Drink alcohol	75.9 (333/439)	67.1 (192/286)	65.0 (169/260)	70.1 (164/234)
	Exercise everyday	28.9 (127/439)	31.1 (89/286)	34.2 (89/260)	28.6 (67/234)
	Fruits & Veg	4.0 ± 2.0	3.8 ± 1.8	3.8 ± 1.8	3.9 ± 1.8
	Smoking	9.8 (43, 439)	7.0 (20, 286)	7.7 (20, 260)	5.6 (13, 234)

consumption of fruits and vegetables among participants from most deprived areas was about one portion less and it remained static.

Changes in neighbourhood inequalities in mental health

The average profiles presented in Figure 6.3 shows a significant gap in mental health outcomes between the least and most deprived areas at baseline and that this remains more or less constant during the 18-month study period. As expected, for both WEMWBS and SF8MCS participants living in least deprived areas have better mental health scores than those living in the most deprived areas.

The MLMs also showed that the neighbourhood inequality in mental health in Stockton did not change during the study period. The results show that people living in the most deprived areas are much worse at baseline than those living in the least deprived areas. The difference in scores for the participants from the most deprived areas were on average 3.71 (confidence intervals: 2.26, 5.15) and 5.16 (confidence intervals: 3.55, 6.77) unit lower than the participants from the least deprived areas as measured by SF8MCS and WEMWBS, respectively (Figure 6.3). However, the gap in mental health did not change significantly over time. The average difference between the most and least deprived at Wave 1 is not statistically different from the mean difference between the most and least deprived areas at Waves 2, 3 and 4 for both the SF8MCS and WEMWBS. In general, average

Figure 6.3: Mean Warwick Edinburgh Mental Wellbeing Score (WEMWBS) and SF8 Mental Component Summary (SF8MCS) for study participants in most and least deprived areas across waves

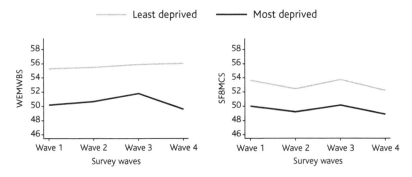

mental health scores were constant over the study period, independent of the neighbourhood of the participants. The longitudinal analysis results confirm that the difference in health outcomes between the least and most deprived areas identified at baseline remained constant over the study period.

Contribution of different factors in explaining the mental health gap

Using the baseline data, we explored the relative contribution of different material, psychosocial and behavioural factors to the gap in mental health between the least and the most deprived areas. Table 6.6 presents the relative contribution of the different factors to gap in mental scores between the least and most deprived areas. Among the material factors, socioeconomic factors explained 32% of the health inequality while the material physical environment factors explained 5% based on WEMWBS. For this outcome, material factors contributed the most to explaining the estimated inequality gap while behavioural factors contributed the least. Psychosocial factors appear to contribute 54% of the gap in SF8 MCS score in Stockton-on-

Table 6.6: Percentage contribution of direct and indirect effects SF8-MCS and WEMWBS

Direct effects	SF8-MCS	WEMWBS
Material (combined)	17.38	36.51
Material socioeconomic	7.62	32.00
Material physical environment	9.45	4.56
Behavioural	4.91	1.61
Psychosocial	54.07	7.61

Tees, while material factors were secondary in importance (17%) to psychosocial factors. The combination of the different factors is also likely to be important as, for example, people often experience both psychosocial and material factors simultaneously (Mattheys et al., 2016).

The MLMs for the longitudinal analysis of the factors associated with SF8MCS and WEMWBS outcomes found that among material factors, employment and income had statistically significant positive association with SF8MCS and WEMWBS, respectively. On average, those with employment are likely to have 1.61 (confidence intervals: 0.58, 2.65) unit higher score for SF8MCS than those without an employment. On the other hand, having one or more dark rooms in their house had a statistically significant negative association. Those living an accommodation with one or more dark room had on average −2.65 (confidence Intervals: −4.36, −0.94) unit lower SF8MCS score than those who did not have such room in their houses.

Figure 6.4 shows the psychosocial factors that were statistically significantly associated with mental health outcomes. Those who felt lacking in companionship, felt left out, felt isolated or did not feel safe walking home at night had significantly lower SF8MCS score than their counterparts. Except for the lack of companionship variable, similar negative associations were also evident for WEMWBS. Those who felt left out had on average −1.50 (confidence intervals: −2.33, −0.67) unit lower score for SF8MCS, whereas the difference was larger for WEMWBS (−1.88 unit lower, confidence intervals: −2.71, −0.93). Happiness was positively associated with both SF8MCS

Figure 6.4: Longitudinal analysis of association between psychosocial factors and mental health outcomes, estimates from multilevel models

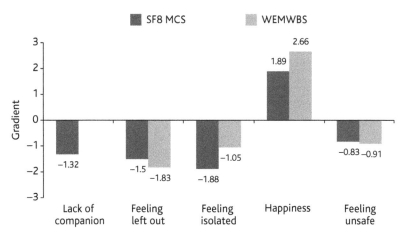

and WEMWBS. The happier a participant was, the better was their SF8MCS and WEMWBS score – regardless of which neighbourhood they lived in.

In terms of behavioural factors associated with mental health outcomes over the study period, consumption of alcohol was significantly positively associated with both outcomes. Those who had less frequent exercise or physical activity also had significantly lower (−0.40 unit, confidence intervals: −0.62, −0.18) WEMWBS scores those that exercised more frequently.

Discussion

This chapter explored the mental health gap between people from the most and least deprived areas of Stockton-on-Tees, during austerity. It also examined the contribution of different type of factors to explaining these inequalities. The longitudinal analysis showed that there was a large inequality gap at baseline, which remained constant during the study period. Over the study period, material factors such as employment and income were positively associated with inequalities in mental health. Similarly, from a psychosocial perspective, people who did not lack companionship, did not feel left out or isolated, felt safe walking at night or were happier had better mental health. In terms of behavioural factors, people who regularly exercised had better mental health outcomes.

At the beginning of the study there was a large gap in mental health between those from the most and the least deprived areas. We did not observe any increases or decreases in this gap over time. There could be several reasons for not observing any further widening of gap over the period. First, the gap was already big at baseline, which shows that the people living in most deprived areas were already living a difficult life and had much worse mental health. The potential of further changes in their context reflecting on the gap could have been limited. In most cases, the MLMs used in this study to longitudinally examine factors associated with mental health did not observe significant changes. It is therefore reasonable that without significant changes in the underlying factors, that the outcome remained unchanged. However, the IMF suggests that there will be significant rise in the implementation of austerity starting in 2017. This could exacerbate the existing inequalities in mental health that we found in Stockton.

The second reason is that it may be that a longer period of assessment would identify further changes to the gap in mental health between people from the most and least deprived areas, as the incomes of those in the most deprived areas are further stretched. Our study was only 18 months' duration. The programme of 'welfare reform' has been a regressive programme that has almost exclusively targeted those of working age on the lowest incomes, leading to a worsening financial situation for the poorest members of society (Belfield et al., 2014, 2016). As shown in Chapter Five, this has had a chronic impact on the lives and mental health of those who are forced to deal with the effects of these policies. Current moves towards rolling out Universal Credit are likely to have an additional financial and emotional toll. This study may have underestimated the inequality gap due to timing of the survey. Data were collected between 2014–16, a post-recession period when the acute phase of the recession had already passed and *after* the implementation of the first wave of austerity. Ruckert and Labonte (2017) noted that austerity and budget cuts enacted between 2012–15 were at a much slower rate.

Assessment of changes in Stockton-on-Tees between 2010–16 using public health data is in keeping with the observation of Ruckert and Labonte (2017). The negative trends in self-harm and long-term unemployment were much less evident during 2013–16, compared to the earlier period. For example, the unemployment rate in Stockton-on-Tees between 2014–16 was lower than the rate between 2009–13 (Figure 6.5). However, increasing rates of employment in the study period has not led to improved mental health for people living in the more deprived areas of Stockton-on-Tees. This suggests that rising employment is not having a protective mental health impact. Although employment may have risen in Stockton-on-Tees, the figures do not incorporate the quality of that employment, for instance whether that is precarious, low paid or zero hours employment. This type of work has been found to be as damaging to mental health as unemployment (Kim and von dem Knesebeck, 2015). In-work poverty has also increased nationally since 2009, with over half of all people in poverty now either in work or living with a working adult (Belfield et al., 2016).

The composition of our survey sample may have also affected this results, as comparison with census results showed that our sample were generally older than general population of the Stockton-on-Tees. Since austerity measures were more protective of pensioners and older people, it might partially explain why we did not see further deterioration in mental health in our study. It is important to note that, the universal state pension and other universal allowances for the elderly (including winter fuel allowances) were unchanged and in some cases were increased (Green et al., 2017). Our findings are therefore

Figure 6.5: Unemployment prevalence in Stockton-on-Tees 2004–17 in comparison to North East England and Britain

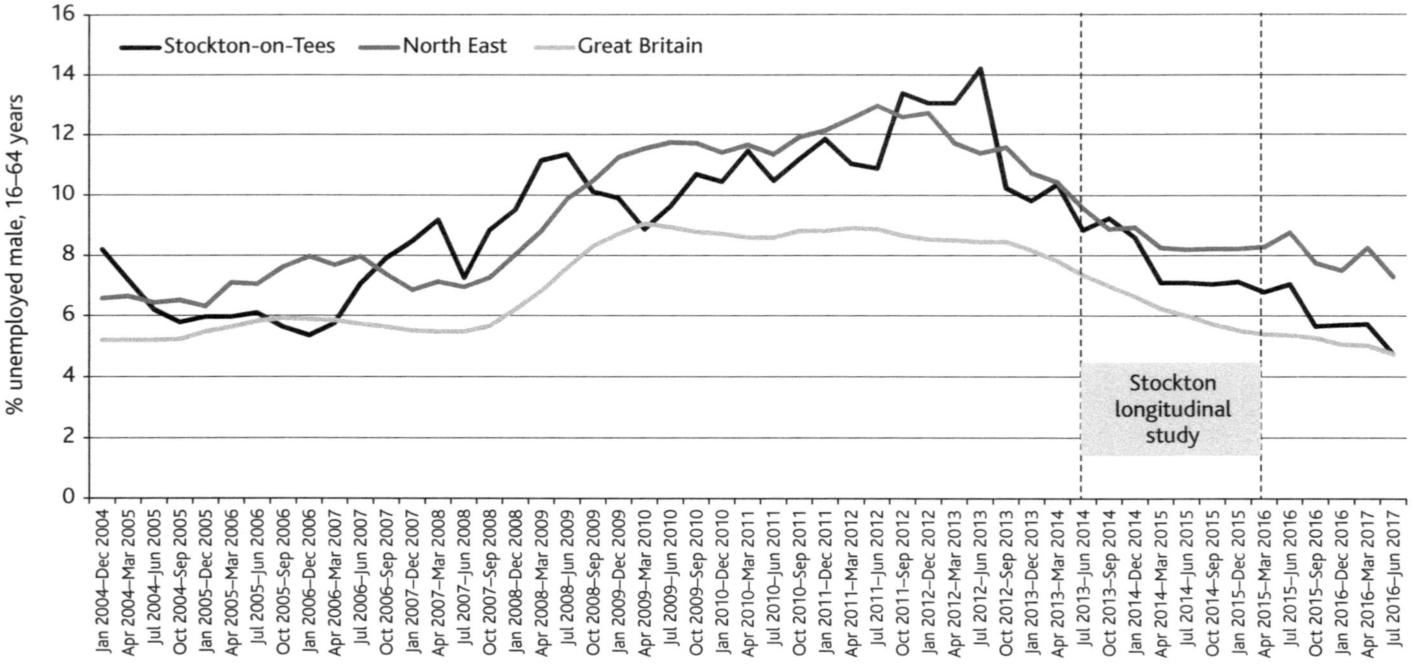

Source: Public Health England, 2017 data

likely to have underestimated the effects of austerity measures, which were implemented from 2010 onwards by the incoming coalition government. Some of the austerity measures were already in place by the first wave of the survey (in 2014), although cuts to social security and to public spending have continued since. It is possible that some of the mental health harm caused by austerity, as identified by national studies finding widening mental health inequalities between 2010–13 (Barr et al., 2015), was already reflected in the baseline gap.

A social determinants model was applied to explore the relative contribution of material (incorporating material physical environment and material socioeconomic), psychosocial and behavioural determinants of mental health and wellbeing. We have demonstrated the importance of material factors in explaining the gap in mental health in Stockton-on-Tees. A continuation of measures that lead to worsening finances for those on the lowest incomes (while those at the other end of the income spectrum remain largely unaffected) is likely to have an impact on spatial inequalities in mental health. Living in less deprived areas affords considerable protection towards mental health and mental wellbeing, and people who live in these areas are likely to score significantly higher on mental health measures (SF8-MCS and the WEMWBS). This is consistent with the substantial research base evidencing inequalities in mental health (Marmot and Bell, 2012). Consistent associations have been found between mental ill health and low income, low education; low social status; unemployment; and poorer material circumstances (Fryers et al., 2004). The literature suggests that it is not only individual factors (such as having a higher income or better housing) that have an impact on the relationship between living in a more affluent area and better mental health, but also the context of the area itself which could be protective including such things as the physical environment (for example, there is better access to green space in more affluent areas), opportunity structures (for example, better access to health care services or education or childcare), or the economic environment (for example, availability of better jobs) (Bambra, 2016).

The baseline analyses showed that material and psychosocial factors are the most important determinants of the divide in mental health and wellbeing in Stockton-on-Tees. With the SF8 score, psychosocial factors contributed most to the gap (54%), whereas in the WEMWBS it was material factors that took precedence (37%). Psychosocial variables, such as social isolation was particularly important in the SF8. Participants in the most deprived areas, who tended to be slightly younger, seemed more isolated and lacking in companionship than those in the least deprived areas. These are social problems that are often associated with the mental health of older people (Cattan et al., 2005). As such, our findings suggest that either deprivation is strongly associated with social isolation in addition to age, or that the older participants in the most deprived areas were feeling much more isolated than their counterparts in the least.

Our results have also shown that behavioural indicators are the least important of the categories determining the inequality gap in mental health and wellbeing. This is important, as many public health activities focusing on reducing health inequalities tends to lean towards behavioural interventions and individual behaviour change. This shift towards a focus on the individual has been labelled as 'lifestyle drift'. This finding should be a wakeup call to policy makers that focusing on the individual (Hunter et al., 2009) alone will not reduce the inequality gap in mental health. Health is socially determined, and approaches that avoid a consideration of the contexts in which people live will not succeed in addressing health inequalities (Bambra, 2018).

Conclusion

Our study used detailed longitudinal data to examine the effect of austerity on inequalities in mental health. We found a significant gap in mental health at baseline. However, no statistically significant change in the gap was observed over the 18-month, post-recession period of austerity. We found that material factors (most notably income and employment) and psychosocial factors contributed the most to explaining the mental health gap while behavioural factors contributed the least. Over the study period, employment, companionship, feeling included, not feeling isolated, safety, happiness and exercise were positively associated with mental health. Psychosocial factors such as feeling left out, isolated or not feeling happy or safe were commonly associated with decreased mental health. However, this effect could be a combination of the direct and indirect effects of material deprivation. Overall, the factors associated with mental health are interrelated and have combined effects on the mental health gap.

References
Akhter, N., Bambra, C., Mattheys, K., Warren, J. and Kasim, A. (2018). Inequalities in mental health and well-being in a time of austerity: Follow-up findings from the Stockton-on-Tees cohort study. *SSM-Population Health*, 6: 75–84

Álvarez-Gálvez, J. and Jaime-Castillo, A. M. (2018). The impact of social expenditure on health inequalities in Europe. *Social Science & Medicine*, 200, 9–18, doi:https://doi.org/10.1016/j.socscimed.2018.01.006

Bambra, C. (2011). Health inequalities and welfare state regimes: theoretical insights on a public health 'puzzle'. [10.1136/jech.2011.136333]. *J Epidemiol Community Health*

Bambra, C. (2016). *Health divides: where you live can kill you.* Bristol: Policy Press

Bambra, C. (2018). First do no harm: Developing interventions that combat addiction without increasing inequalities. *Addiction*, 113: 787–788

Bambra, C. and Garthwaite, K. (2015). Austerity, welfare reform and the English health divide. *Area*, 47(3), 341–343, doi:10.1111/area.12191

Bambra, C., Barr, B. and Milne, E. (2014). North and South: addressing the English health divide. *Journal of Public Health*, 36(2), 183–186, doi:10.1093/pubmed/fdu029

Bambra, C., Cairns, J. M., Kasim, A., Smith, J., Robertson, S., Copeland, A., et al. (2015). This divided land: An examination of regional inequalities in exposure to brownfield land and the association with morbidity and mortality in England. *Health Place*, 34, 257–269, doi:https://doi.org/10.1016/j.healthplace.2015.05.010

Barnes, M. C., Donovan, J. L., Wilson, C., Chatwin, J., Davies, R., Potokar, J., et al. (2017). Seeking help in times of economic hardship: access, experiences of services and unmet need. *BMC Psychiatry*, 17(1), 84, doi:10.1186/s12888-017-1235-0

Barr, B., Kinderman, P. and Whitehead, M. (2015). Trends in mental health inequalities in England during a period of recession, austerity and welfare reform 2004 to 2013. *Social Science & Medicine*, 147 (Supplement C), 324–331, doi:https://doi.org/10.1016/j.socscimed.2015.11.009

Barr, B., Taylor-Robinson, D., Stuckler, D., Loopstra, R., Reeves, A. and Whitehead, M. (2016). 'First, do no harm': are disability assessments associated with adverse trends in mental health? A longitudinal ecological study. [10.1136/jech-2015–206209]. *Journal of Epidemiology & Community Health*, 70(4), 339

Bartley, M. (2016). *Health inequality: An introduction to concepts, theories and methods*, 2nd Edition. Cambridge: Polity Press

Beatty, C. and Fothergill, S. (2013). Hitting the poorest places hardest: the local and regional impact of welfare reform. Sheffield: Sheffield Hallam University

Beatty, C. and Fothergill, S. (2016). The uneven impact of welfare reform: The financial losses to places and people. Sheffield: Sheffield Hallam University

Belfield, C., Cribb, J., Hood, A. and Joyce, R. (2014). *Living standards, poverty and inequality in the UK: 2014* (vol. R96). IFS Reports, Institute for Fiscal Studies. London: The Institute for Fiscal Studies

Belfield, C., Cribb, J., Hood, A. and Joyce, R. (2016). *Living standards, poverty and inequality 2016*. London: The Institute for Fiscal Studies

Blakely, T., Tobias, M. and Atkinson, J. (2008). Inequalities in mortality during and after restructuring of the New Zealand economy: repeated cohort studies. *BMJ: British Medical Journal*, 336(7640), 371–375

Bowling, A. (2005). Measuring health outcomes from the patient's perspective. *Handbook of Health Research Methods*, 428–444

Brunner, E. and Marmot, M. G. (2006). 'Social Organization, Stress, and Health'. In M. G. Marmot and R. G. Wilkinson (Eds.) *Social Determinants of Health*, 2nd Edition. Oxford: Oxford University Press

Cattan, M., White, M. Bond, J. and Learnmouth, A. (2005). Preventing social isolation and loneliness among older people: a systematic review of health promotion interventions. *Ageing Society*, 25, 41–67

Chang, S.-S., Stuckler, D., Yip, P. and Gunnell, D. (2013). Impact of 2008 global economic crisis on suicide: time trend study in 54 countries. *BMJ*, 347, doi:10.1136/bmj.f5239

Clayton, J., Donovan, C. and Merchant, J. (2015). Emotions of austerity: Care and commitment in public service delivery in the North East of England. *Emotion, Space and Society*, 14: 24–32

Coope, C., Gunnell, D. and Hollingworth, W. (2014). Suicide and the 2008 economic recession: who is most at risk? Trends in suicide rates in England and Wales 2001–2011. *Social Science and Medicine*, 117, doi:10.1016/j.socscimed.2014.07.024

Corcoran, P., Griffin, E., Arensman, E., Fitzgerald, A. P. and Perry, I. J. (2015). Impact of the economic recession and subsequent austerity on suicide and self-harm in Ireland: An interrupted time series analysis. *International Journal of Epidemiology*, 44(3), 969–977, doi:10.1093/ije/dyv058

DCLG (Dept for Communities and Local Government) (2011). English Indices of Deprivation 2010 www.gov.uk/government/uploads/system/uploads/attachment_data/file/6871/1871208.pdf

Delgadillo, J., Asaria, M., Ali, S. and Gilbody, S. (2016). On poverty, politics and psychology: the socioeconomic gradient of mental healthcare utilisation and outcomes. [10.1192/bjp.bp.115.171017]. *The British Journal of Psychiatry*, 209(5), 429

De Vaus, D. A. (1991). *Surveys in social research*. London: UCL Press

Dreger, S., Buck, C. and Bolte, G. (2014). Material, psychosocial and sociodemographic determinants are associated with positive mental health in Europe: a cross-sectional study. *BMJ Open*, 4(5): e005095

Frasquilho, D., Matos, M. G., Salonna, F., Guerreiro, D., Storti, C. C., Gaspar, T., et al. (2016). Mental health outcomes in times of economic recession: a systematic literature review. *BMC Public Health*, 16(1), 115

Friedli, L. (2009). *Mental health, resilience and inequalities.* Denmark: World Health Organization Regional Office for Europe

Fryers, T., Jenkins, R. and Melzer, D. (2004). *Social inequalities and the distribution of the common mental disorders.* Psychology Press

Gamble, A. (2009). *The spectre at the feast: capitalist crisis and the politics of recession.* Basingstoke: Palgrave

Green, JM., Buckner, S., Milton, S., Powell, K., Salway, S. and Moffatt, S. (2017). A model of how targeted and universal welfare entitlements impcat on material, psycho0social and structural determinants of health in older adults. *Social Science & Medicince*, 187: 20–28

Hastings, A., Bailey, N., Bramley, G., Gannon, M. and Watkins, D. (2015). *The cost of the cuts: the impact on local government and poorer communities.* York: Joseph Rowntree Foundation

Hawton, K., Bergen, H. and Geulayov, G. (2016). Impact of the recent recession on self-harm: a longitudinal ecologic and patient level investigation from multicentre study of self-harm in England. *Journal of Affective Disorders*, 191, doi:10.1016/j.jad.2015.11.001

Hunter, D. J., Popay, J., Tannahill, C., Whitehead, M. and Elson, T. (2009). *Lessons learned from the past. Shaping a different future.* Marmot Review Working Committee 3 Cross-cutting sub-group report. www.instituteofhealthequality.org/projects/the-marmot-review-working-committee-3-report/working-committee-3-final-report.pdf

Karanikolos, M., Mladovsky, P., Cylus, J., Thomson, S., Basu, S., Stuckler, D., et al. (2013). Financial crisis, austerity, and health in Europe. *The Lancet*, 381(9874), 1323–1331, doi:https://doi.org/10.1016/S0140-6736(13)60102-6

Kim, T. J. and von dem Knesebeck, O. (2015). Is an insecure job better for health than having no job at all? A systematic review of studies investigating the health-related risks of both job insecurity and unemployment. *BMC Public Health*, 15(1), 985

Kitson, M., Martin, R. and Tyler, P. (2011). The geographies of austerity. *Cambridge Journal of Regions, Economy and Society*, 4(3), 289–302, doi:10.1093/cjres/rsr030

Knapp, M. (2012). Mental health in an age of austerity. [10.1136/ebmental-2012-100758]. *Evidence Based Mental Health*, 15(3), 54

Macintyre, S. (2007). Deprivation amplification revisited; or, is it always true that poorer places have poorer access to resources for healthy diets and physical activity? *International Journal of Behavioral Nutrition and Physical Activity*, 4(32), 1–7

Marmot, M. (2017). Social justice, epidemiology and health inequalities. *European Journal of Epidemiology*, 32(7), 537–546

Marmot, M. and Bell, R. (2012). Fair society, healthy lives. *Public Health*, 126, S4–S10

Marmot, M. and Wilkinson, R. G. (2001). Psychosocial and material pathways in the relation between income and health: a response to Lynch et al. *British Medical Journal*, 322(7296), 1233.

Marmot, M. and Wilkinson, R. (2006). *Social determinants of health*. Oxford: Oxford University Press

Mattheys, K., Bambra, C., Warren, J., Kasim, A. and Akhter, N. (2016). Inequalities in mental health and well-being in a time of austerity: Baseline findings from the Stockton-on-Tees cohort study. *SSM – Population Health, 2* (Supplement C), 350–359, doi: https://doi.org/10.1016/j.ssmph.2016.04.006

Murali, V. and Oyebode, F. (2004). Poverty, social inequality and mental health. [10.1192/apt.10.3.216]. *Advances in Psychiatric Treatment*, 10(3), 216

O'Donoghue, D. (2016). No end in sight for austerity – the North East set to weather hundreds of millions of more cuts. ChronicleLive, 4 October. www.chroniclelive.co.uk/news/north-east-news/no-end-sight-austerity-north-11979128

ONS (Office for National Statistics) (2015). Suicides in the United Kingdom, 2013 Registrations

ONS (2017). Measuring socioeconomic inequalities in avoidable mortality in England and Wales: 2015

Public Health England (2017) Stockton-on-Tees Health Profile 2017. https://fingertips.phe.org.uk/search/employment#page/4/gid/1/pat/6/par/E12000001/ati/101/are/E06000004/iid/91126/age/164/sex/4

Reeves, A., Basu, S., McKee, M., Marmot, M. and Stuckler, D. (2013). Austere or not? UK coalition government budgets and health inequalities. *Journal of the Royal Society of Medicine*, 106(11), 432–436, doi:10.1177/0141076813501101

Reiss, F. (2013). Socioeconomic inequalities and mental health problems in children and adolescents: a systematic review. *Social Science & Medicine*, 90, 24–31

Roberts, B., Damundu, E. Y., Lomoro, O. and Sondorp, E. (2010). The influence of demographic characteristics, living conditions, and trauma exposure on the overall health of a conflict-affected population in Southern Sudan. *BMC Public Health*, 10(1), 518, doi:10.1186/1471-2458-10-518

Ruckert, A. and Labonté, R. (2017). Health inequities in the age of austerity: The need for social protection policies. *Social Science & Medicine*, 187: 306–311

Schrecker, T. and Bambra, C. (2015). Inequality: How politics divides and rules us. In: *How Politics Makes Us Sick*. London: Palgrave Macmillan (pp. 87–111)

Shaw, C., Blakely, T., Atkinson, J. and Crampton, P. (2005). Do social and economic reforms change socioeconomic inequalities in child mortality? A case study: New Zealand 1981–1999. *Journal of Epidemiology & Community Health*, 59(8), 638–644

Shaw, M., Dorling, D. and Smith, G. D. (2006). Poverty, social exclusion and minorities. In M. Marmot and R. Wilkinson (Eds) *Social Determinants of Health*. Oxford: Oxford University Press

Skalická, V., van Lenthe, F., Bambra, C., Krokstad, S. and Mackenbach, J. (2009). Material, psychosocial, behavioural and biomedical factors in the explanation of relative socio-economic inequalities in mortality: evidence from the HUNT study. *International Journal of Epidemiology*, 38(5), 1272–1284, doi:10.1093/ije/dyp262

Stuckler, D. and Basu, S. (2013). *The Body Economic. Why Austerity Kills*. London: Penguin Books Ltd

Tennant, R., Hiller, L., Fishwick, R., Platt, S., Joseph, S., Weich, S., Parkinson, J., Secker, J. and Stewart-Brown, S. (2007). The Warwick-Edinburgh mental well-being scale (WEMWBS): development and UK validation. *Health and Quality of Life Outcomes*, 5(1), 63

Thoits, P. A. (2010). Stress and health: major findings and policy implications. *Journal of Health and Social Behavior*, 51(1_suppl), S41-S53, doi:10.1177/0022146510383499

United Nations. *Sustainable Development Goals* (Webpage). www.un.org/sustainabledevelopment/sustainable-development-goals/

Wilkinson, R. and Pickett, K. (2010). *The spirit level: Why equality is better for everyone*. London: Penguin

Williams, G. H. (2003). The determinants of health: structure, context and agency. *Sociology of Health & Illness*, 25(3), 131–154.

WHO (World Health Organization) (2001). *The world health report: 2001: mental health: new understanding, new hope*. Geneva: WHO.

WHO (2003). *Investing in mental health*. Geneva: WHO

SEVEN

Mothers in Austerity

Amy Greer Murphy

Introduction

This chapter provides an overview of research conducted with mothers living in Stockton-on-Tees. The research is concerned with understanding the impact that austerity and welfare reform are having on mothers, families and their communities in an area of wide health inequalities. Such austerity reforms include the withdrawal of local services, the ongoing precaritisation of the labour market, reduced incomes from reforms to benefit payments, and the general reform of the social security landscape. The chapter begins by setting out the context of austerity in Stockton, a place experiencing many different inequalities – health, spatial, economic. It then discusses the repercussions of austerity for women in particular. Next there is a discussion of the research design and methods employed in this study: qualitative longitudinal interviewing and ethnography. It emphasises the importance of conducting qualitative research with those affected by austerity as women, particularly mothers, face a set of distinct risks. The research takes an intersectional perspective in understanding how gender interacts with other factors such class, age, disability and place. Intersectionality is the consideration of 'multiple, co-constituted differences' and is an important but underutilised way of framing the social context of health. It views social positions as relational and acknowledges the 'multiple positionings that constitute everyday life' (Dhamoon, 2011: 230).

There is then a discussion of three key themes from the research findings. The first theme relates to the role respondents saw themselves playing as mothers. They found the value attributed to their roles as mothers and carers lessened by welfare reforms. The expectation that caring work should be provided by the market and that they should seek formal work as a primary source of income did not fit with their sense of self. Welfare conditionality applied to those claiming benefits of various kinds was felt to be punitive and unhelpful when it came to raising their children. The pressure to demonstrate legitimacy and perform responsibility in the eyes of the state was enacted through the push to be financially autonomous. This was to be enacted through wage labour (albeit low-wage work), or for those out of work, 'actively seeking work' or being 'work focused' was essential, and reinforced the inequalities many of the mothers experienced by exerting excess pressure on them. They felt quality work was unavailable in their areas, childcare was unaffordable, and an important source of identity formation, their role as carers and mothers was of diminished value under austerity.

The second set of findings relates to experiences of health, and specifically to mental health issues. There was a clear indication that austerity was having a negative impact on the mental health and wellbeing of participants. Most respondents had experienced depression and anxiety, and many had taken medication or attended counselling to help deal with these issues. For many mothers in the study, life had 'always been' tough but they felt that austerity was a compounding factor contributing to depression, anxiety and more severe mental health issues. The experience of being mothers in a context of financial insecurity, shouldering emotional burdens, emerging health issues with their children or themselves, as well as the struggles of everyday life under austerity led to poor mental health experiences. The intersectional dimensions of this are discussed with specific reference to financial insecurity, living in poor quality housing, welfare reform and feelings of living in a stigmatised place.

The third theme discusses women's experiences of 'invisible inequality'. This argument is threefold and incorporates economic, political and social factors. First, the effects of austerity on women are multidimensional and relate to a combination of service cuts, labour market reforms and welfare reforms – the 'triple jeopardy' described by the Fawcett Society (2014). The impact is a women's issue because women, on the whole, have less recourse to earn a formal wage and are less able to move around for work (with acknowledged variations based on age, availability of resources and dependents). Second, it is mostly women who engage in the 'non-economic' work of social reproduction. This work takes up a huge amount of time and energy, leaving them unable to engage in public life to the same extent as men. Policy making and government is organised and controlled largely without their input, putting them at a structural disadvantage. Third, the inequalities women experience manifest through higher rates of depression, anxiety and more extreme mental illness (Verbrugge, 1976, 1980). The chapter argues that this situation is not unique to low-income women, although for them the inequality is greater. Rather, that this inequality is due to a combination of different factors, which are not all to do with economic resources, and are played out in all strata of society in different ways at different times.

Context of austerity

Austerity in the UK has been an explicit feature of all national budgets since 2010. It was originally introduced as a set of economic and social policies to reduce the budget deficit post–2008 financial crisis (Konzelmann, 2014). Public overspend was cited as a major cause of individual countries economic failings across European Union states. In the UK it was argued by then-Prime Minister David Cameron that welfare spending had reached unsustainable levels and a period of austerity would be needed to balance the budget. The cuts have had a negative impact on many groups and undermined the health and capacities of certain communities across the country. This chapter contributes to a growing literature on the impacts of austerity in such areas as the voluntary sector (Milbourne and Cushman, 2015), adult social care (Power, 2014) and early childhood education (Lewis and West, 2016), and the everyday lived experiences of welfare reform (Patrick, 2014) as well as the literature on health inequalities in particular parts of the UK, such as Stockton (Bambra and Garthwaite, 2015; Mattheys et al., 2016; Garthwaite and Bambra, 2017).

Different places across the UK have been affected differently by austerity measures. There have been varying degrees of service provision and cuts, labour market changes and local council service provision (Watts et al., 2014). This has in turn played a part in shaping the experiences and practices of individuals, such as mothers, who live in different places and occupy spaces in different ways. For example, those with fewer financial resources rely more on state services such as children's centres for family support services, community centres for advice services and libraries for internet access. Notably, it is often those areas already experiencing disadvantage which are most likely to experience larger cuts. In England, the most deprived local authorities have seen cuts of more than £220 per head in contrast to £40 per head in the least deprived (Hastings et al., 2015). Local government has enacted a huge amount of cuts, as the responsibility for carrying them out has been transferred from central government by HM Treasury. Recent benefit changes are having a cumulative effect on many households across Stockton – housing benefit has not increased since 2010 and other changes, such as the 'bedroom tax' (or under-occupancy penalty) are affecting those who have children living with them on a shared basis or have other housing needs, such as those with a disability who cannot share a bedroom with a partner (Beatty and Fothergill, 2016).

However, Beatty and Fothergill (2018) have emphasised that the biggest financial losses for claimants have come, not from the measures that have attracted the most public attention, such as the 'bedroom tax' and Benefit Cap, but from the 'overall jigsaw of welfare reform' and specifically changes to tax credits (£4,210 million a year), Child Benefit (£3,030 million) and the 1% uprating (£2,700 million) which have all had a huge impact (Beatty and Fothergill, 2018: 954). In Stockton there will be a projected overall reduction in government funding of 61% by 2019/2020 (Stockton-on-Tees Borough Council, 2016). In England, local authorities were forecast to spend 11.8% less on children's centres in 2016/17 than in 2015/16, from £763.9m to £673.9m (DfE, 2016). Budgetary responsibility for the provision of a range of core crucial services (for example, old-age social care and children's centres) has been gradually devolved to local governments, who have in turn had their budgets for providing such services severely reduced.

Differences in life expectancy, experiences of health and wellbeing, and years of life lived in good health vary enormously within the borough of Stockton-on-Tees. The gap in life expectancy between most and least deprived words stood in 2017 at 15.7 for men and 12.7 for women (Public Health England, 2017), an improvement for men from 17.3 years in 2015, but a deterioration for women from 11.4 (Public Health England, 2015). At the time of conducting research, this was the largest gap of any local authority in England. As a significant example, Stockton's spending on children's centres fell from £404 million to £276 million between 2011 and 2014 (ONS, 2016a). This is coupled with post-2015 welfare reforms that were predicted to have an impact on families with dependent children (notably lone parents) most of all (Beatty and Fothergill, 2016). The consequences for children's health, wellbeing and development are stark (Bradshaw and Main, 2016) as economic and social policies put in place since austerity began represent a reduction in support for low-income children and their families, something which has been shown to cause anxiety and worry for children and inhibit their life chances (Ridge, 2013). This evidence indicates that 'the poorest places and the poorest people are being the hardest hit' by austerity (Beatty and Fothergill, 2013; Hastings et al., 2015).

Austerity and women

Austerity's effects on women have been considerable. Recent reports calculate that 85% of tax and benefit changes have affected women's incomes directly. Women in deprived, low-income areas are particularly affected. The restructuring of the public sector and major changes to local authority budgets have contributed to this. This is because women rely to a larger extent on a broad array of public sector services and are employed in the public and voluntary sector in higher numbers than men. Their greater reliance on part-time and low-wage work, and more sustained engagement with the benefit system to top-up incomes is leading women to experience a 'triple jeopardy' of cause and effect, from public sector service cuts, job losses and welfare cuts (Fawcett Society, 2014; Craddock, 2017). At present, there are less economically inactive women in the UK than at any other time in history (ONS, 2016b), but much labour market growth in recent years, particularly in the North East, has come largely from part-time, temporary work, and self-employment often in low-wage, feminised sectors of the economy (ONS, 2017). This new age of insecure work and financial insecurity in spite of increased economic activity, when coupled with increasingly conditional social welfare reforms, has numerous knock-on effects, particularly for women (Fawcett Society, 2014).

Literature on time and motherhood has indicated that extended periods of mothers' lives are shaped by reproduction, caring work and as a consequence, interrupted engagement with the labour market over time with differing experiences of caring work depending on how they negotiate 're-entry' (Crompton, 2006; Thomson et al., 2011). Furthermore, changes are taking place within the welfare state and labour market challenging greater gender equality achieved in recent decades. In this context, welfare reforms such as the under-occupancy penalty known as the 'bedroom tax' (Moffatt et al., 2016), different experiences of chronic physical and mental health issues (Carter et al., 2013), cuts to services for women, and a reliance on low-paid work affect women in particular ways. These factors all influenced the research. In contrast to respondents' own views about the importance of their caring and other non-waged ('social reproduction') work, and bolstered by the literature which emphasises this (Fraser, 1989), neither the state, particularly the neoliberal austerity state, nor wider society, affords their work a high level of value. Fraser (2016) has described the capitalist economy as 'freeriding' on social reproduction, not affording it a significant level of value. The chapter acknowledges the centrality of social reproduction to maintaining society, and how neoliberalism, with austerity as an intensification of this is undermining it (Fraser, 2013).

Close attention is also given to the impact of austerity on health inequalities for women and for children. Emerging findings suggest that the gap between richer and poorer children in the UK is beginning to widen. In 2015 this gap widened for the first time in a decade (ONS, 2015). As Taylor-Robinson and Barr (2017) have noted, since 2010 the rate for the poorest children has been increasing while continuing to decline for more advantaged groups. What this means is that health inequalities affecting infants, a telling and accurate indicator of the consequences of socioeconomic inequality affecting children, are widening. Child poverty is rising as budget cuts to support services have directly affected children, and indirectly hit them through their families falling incomes (Taylor-Robinson et al., 2014). At the same time it has been recorded that there has been a gendered aspect to this – the gap in life expectancy between the poorest and wealthiest females in England is now at a record high (ONS, 2018).

Research methods: longitudinal and ethnographic methods

The research discussed in this chapter examined qualitatively how life is changing under austerity for mothers living in an area in the North East of England. This chapter draws on qualitative longitudinal interviews (QLR) with 15 women, as well as ethnographic encounters over an 18-month period (March 2015–September 2016). The key research aims and questions underpinning this study were to understand the everyday effects that austerity measures such as welfare reform, public service cuts, and labour market reforms, were having on mothers in Stockton-on-Tees and to examine how these experiences varied across class, income and geographical contexts, and the intersectionality of these. The responses of all participants and respondents were anonymised and ethical considerations respected throughout the research. The research sought to address a lack of empirical qualitative studies on the lived experience of mothers under austerity and highlight the value of women's 'everyday' perspectives on health, life, choices and value making. The research sought to emphasise the importance, for policy making, of considering the everyday lived experiences and narratives of those affected by welfare reform and austerity (Patrick, 2014; Hall, 2015; Garthwaite, 2016; Holloway and Pimlott-Wilson, 2016; Jupp, 2017).

Two qualitative methods were employed: ethnography and qualitative longitudinal interviewing. Ethnography, or participant observation, involves immersing oneself in a particular cultural context to generate 'thick data', concerned with the meaning attributed to both the actions undertaken and the world they take place within (Geertz, 1973). Ethnographic fieldwork was conducted for 18 months. It consisted of becoming a participant in a women's group run by a charity and meeting at a community centre in the town centre. The women's group met weekly and there were numerous other opportunities to engage with the members and the organisation; from training days, workshops, events we attended and informal meet ups for coffee and a chat.

The second method employed was qualitative longitudinal interviews (QLR). Fifteen women, 14 mothers, were interviewed in total. Interviews took place from September 2015 to September 2016. Mothers ranged in age from late teens to mid-sixties. Two interviews were conducted with each to explore everyday lived experiences of austerity. Having respondents from across socioeconomic groups within the borough emphasised classed differences of experience. The method emphasised how experiences evolved over time (Neale, 2012).

Figure 7.1: Home baking from women's group

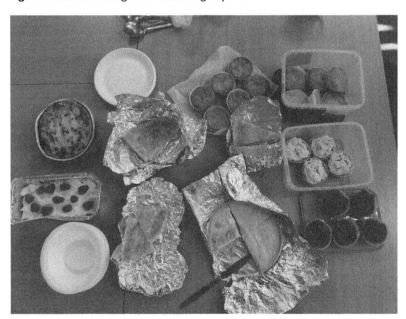

Source: author's photograph

Our discussions of imagined futures (Adam and Groves, 2007; Patrick, 2017) provided insight into hopes, fear, and alternative versions of life respondents envisaged. This is particularly important in the context of austerity, when cumulative waves of cuts and reforms are taking place in quick succession, swiftly changing lives in the midst of the normal parts of life; relationship breakdown and beginning, parenthood, job loss, dealing with death, illness or growing up.

Researching with mothers

The decision to research with mothers was based on the fact that both they and their families are particularly vulnerable to the effects of austerity measures. It was also hoped that mothers would have unique insights into how their everyday lives and families might be shaped by this phenomenon. Women experience subtly different levels of structural disadvantage and in many ways lead different lives from men. This is even more so for mothers. The research employed purposive sampling and snowball sampling (Strauss and Corbin, 1998). As part of the sampling process mothers who had a wide range of experiences were recruited. This included lone mothers, mothers with disabilities and children with disabilities, BAME (black and minority ethnic) women, women who worked in the public sector and third sector; and women of ages ranging from late-teens to mid-sixties. Mothers were recruited through the women's group I attended, Facebook, the local Sure Start centres and through snowballing.

A thematic framework for analysis was derived in part from the study objectives and partly by identifying themes from ongoing analysis of transcripts. Analysis was conducted in several stages. First, the documentation of the data and the process of data collection took place. The data was then organised and categorised into concepts and themes. Next, the data was presented to demonstrate how concepts influenced and related to each other. Following on from that was the process of corroboration or legitimisation, broadly speaking, to find explanations or alternative meanings behind the narratives presented. Finally, the findings were compiled (Schutt, 2012). A combination of NVivo and Microsoft Word were used for coding, classification and grouping. Microsoft Word was used for ordering texts, quotes and themes. Pen and paper was used for highlighting and drawing charts. This multi-modal method allowed the data to be viewed from a variety of angles. Eventually, themes and key concepts began to consistently emerge. There was an ongoing revisiting of assumptions and themes throughout the writing period.

Findings I: Being a mam, juggling paid work and care

For respondents, three key themes emerged in relation to their experience of motherhood, work and care. First, many respondents, particularly those from lower income households, stated that they desired to be first and foremost mothers. Second, while their ideal role was as 'just a mam', they were clear that the stay at home mother (SAHM) role was not available to them as low-income/working-class women. Some needed to work to top up the household income. Benefits no longer covered their cost of living and had conditionality attached to their receipt. This welfare conditionality was a new experience. Intensified since reforms in 2012, sanctions represented the possibility of an entire loss of income for a period of time. There were also historical accounts given of mothers and grandmothers who worked as cleaners, bar staff and child minders to earn crucial money for their household, even though they were considered first and foremost mothers. Finally, for those in work, there was a prevalence of part-time and often also low-paid work – with underemployment cited by many. These experiences of low-paid, part-time work, underemployment and precarity of work (Shildrick et al., 2012) were felt to be increasing as a consequence of austerity.

Desire to be 'just a mam'

Ethnographic findings indicated that engaging in caring work was immensely important for the participants at the women's group. This was reinforced during subsequent interviews. Constant and non-negotiable facets of interviewees' everyday lives were tasks like caring for children, for partners, and managing the home. These tasks form what is broadly characterised as 'social reproduction' and include acts of provisioning, care-giving and interaction that produce and maintain social bonds (Fraser, 2016). To a large extent they shape the everyday experiences of women (and mothers more so) in distinct ways. For many of the women, caring duties were a lifelong job; they didn't finish when children began school, or even when children grew up. Anne, a pensioner, had her own children and grandchildren living with her at various times and she was still very much involved in their day-to-day care. Here she states:

> 'I've started to say no. I don't feel guilty because my family have said no to me before, without giving it a thought. I'm taking me life back. I think its mothers [that can't say no]

actually. I think mother will tend to look after the kids more; it's a natural basic instinct. But you can't do everything. My 38 year old still relies on me; he wants me to solve all his problems he can't solve.' (Anne, Wave II)

Many participants also felt that they were responsible entirely for the household; paying bills, getting the food shopping in, and cooking. If they became unwell, they needed to micro-manage this work, as their partners or husbands wouldn't necessarily know what to do, or how to do it right:

'I can't get sick. I had the flu mind, and I just had to keep going. I have to go out and do the shopping even when I'm sick. I gave him the money once to go shopping … I was trying to tell him what he needed to do, rent, gas, electric. When he come home I said "What did you get for my tea?" He said "Oh, nowt." He'd done no shopping for me for a full week and I thought "I'm gonna be starving." Cos like I said, we've all got different tastes. He didn't have a clue what I liked. Like it doesn't matter if I'm dying I still have to get up, so it doesn't matter, you get used to it.' (Pat, Wave II)

Many respondents felt their roles as carers was not only given a less important place in society under reform, but the emphasis on paid work devalued their endeavours. The type of work constituting 'social reproduction' was highly valued by respondents. This was felt to be at odds with shifts in policy and society at large whereby women are increasingly obliged to engage in wage-labour, while care is not adequately commodified (Lewis and West, 2016) and there was a growing prevalence of low-paid, insecure work (Holloway and Pimlott-Wilson, 2016).

The following extract from fieldwork illustrates an oft-repeated issue the women at the group had with the position of women.

FIELD NOTES

13 October 2015

'When did women have to start going out to work? Mams used to go and do cleaning jobs at night, or bar work but they were at home during the day to do housework and cook meals. Families are different now. Mothers are not given the choice to choose. Being a woman is a 24-hour job. Being a man is a 16-hour job and you get to go to the pub.' (Anne)

Under neoliberalism, and increased during austerity, there has been a distinct rise in 'workfare' policies. These consist of linking the receipt of benefits to labour market engagement or training to become 'work-ready', emphasising individual responsibility of citizens and minimal state supports (Peck, 2001). In this way, work has become a major source of legitimacy in the eyes of the state (Allen and Taylor, 2012). In contrast to the views respondents held about the importance of their caring and other non-economic work, the state does not afford their work the same level of value, nor does wider society. Fraser (2016) has described the capitalist economy as 'freeriding' on social reproduction while affording it no significant level of value. Welfare conditionality explicitly links benefit receipt to 'moving towards' the world of work, and work to legitimacy (Fletcher et al., 2016). As a consequence it diminishes the value of unpaid caring work. Furthermore, the value of benefits was decreasing and low-wage work failed to provide adequate income so respondents found themselves in a bind – expected to find work in order to avoid being labelled a 'scrounger', but destined to work in low-paid jobs that would not cover living expenses.

'Stay at home mother' role: out of reach for many

Those on lower incomes felt the idea of the 'stay at home mother' was a middle-class notion and out of their reach, as the following field note illustrated.

FIELD NOTES
16 June 2015

They acknowledged that working-class women did not have the luxury of being stay at home mams like middle-class women, but that they were very much present in the home and managed the home. They saw it as a middle-class thing to be able to choose unpaid leave to take care of kids. Middle-class relatives ask 'why don't you work' (to women who are unemployed with children) while they themselves are staying at home with their children as their husbands can afford it with their salaries.

The significant factor separating the SAHM from non-working or unemployed respondents was the amount of leisure time and disposable income available to them. In one such instance, Lucy described running into a group of middle-class SAHMs and feeling the contrast with her own position. Lucy had, in the past, lived in a different area with her ex-husband. They had been financially comfortable and her life with her new husband felt a world away, socially and financially:

> 'There were all these yummy mummies in, in all their stuff and it was just like, I was aching with jealousy. And I was "I remember being you. In a different life, I was you." So I'd drop my kids off at school, then I'd go out and have lunch and I'd think that my day was really full, and I'd talk about my budget, in a way that I really believed. That was back when my mortgage was almost paid off, a four-bedroom house. And now, I was sat there on the other side of it.' (Lucy, Wave II)

To give another example, working-class women have, to a greater extent, historically engaged in more sustained periods of low-paid factory, shop or domestic work, as Pat's quote illustrates:

> 'My mam had to work. There was six of us. I'm the youngest; my life was like "Go to the park with your big sisters." That was lucky. Bread and jam, you know, taking sandwiches up, you know. But I had no option. She worked all the time. And me dad did. Six mouths to feed.' (Pat, Wave I)

Respondents were keen at all times to emphasise that a women should have the right to choose whether they would engage in wage labour or not. They also noted that the true ability to be a full-time SAMH was really not available to them and other low-income families. They saw it as a possibility only for middle-class mothers who could spend money on leisure activities and hire a cleaner or a babysitter to go out. The mantra that women now 'have it all' does not reflect the everyday lives of many women, particularly working-class women, who are subject to the 'sociocultural artefacts of class, nation and gender' (Mannay, 2015: 159).

Combining low-wage or part-time work with being a mother

Respondents were critical of the push to engage in paid work they felt from both the state and their partners, amid the pervasiveness of low-paid and insecure work in the area. Anne noted how there were not a lack of jobs, but it was the type of jobs that was an issue:

'Low-paid jobs, that's all there is. You can walk into a job, and it's social caring, cleaning houses, in nursing homes.' (Anne, Wave I)

Five respondents were in paid work. They all worked part time, although the reasons for this were diffuse and not always out of choice – underemployment was an issue for public and third sector workers, as well as the expense of childcare. Of the remaining respondents, some were far removed from the labour market, economically 'inactive', some were taking care of young children and all were in receipt of various benefits as an important source of income. All parents noted the difficulty in finding quality work and adequate childcare.

'They've reduced the age at which mothers have to go out and find work. And they want to be a mam, and they want to stay at home and be a role model to their children in that way. But they can't cos now they're forced to look for a job. The cuts in tax credits, the benefit cap, all of these things, financially have an impact on women. And the lack of services in the local area to support women.' (Jill, Wave I)

There was also an important distinction to be made between paid and voluntary work. Many of the mothers were involved in their local Sure Start centres and volunteered there. It was also a place they could finish their school education, improve literacy and learn new skills. This voluntary work was important to them and added structure to their days and value to their experience as mothers. However, they did not express an interest in doing this work in a paid capacity.

'I haven't thought 'bout a career. In the Star centre we do voluntary. So I'm looking on doing that next year when me daughter goes to the nursery properly and I was hoping since she was going to the nursery I wouldn't have to look after her and can help out with the volunteering.' (Trish, Wave I)

There was also a general consensus among respondents that working as a social care worker or being paid to care for children in a nursery would not be a desirable job, given the zero hour contracts and low pay. One mother stated:

'My partner keeps going "'Oh you've got to get a job soon, even if it's just in a care home," and I go "I don't want to work in a care home. I'll be miserable." I'm not going to just go out and get a job because he says I need to get a job. I'm not doing it. Plus the work wouldn't fit around her because it can be late at night or in the middle of the day or whatever. I want a job to fit around what she's doing and he doesn't understand that … I'm a full-time mum and he just comes and goes. He doesn't understand how much it takes to look after her.' (Jody, Wave II)

It is important to note that these experiences and perspectives run contrary to wider policy context and media discourse and are part of a historical preoccupation with working-class habits, values and practices (Skeggs, 2005a). There is an enduring and entrenched attitude that those in receipt of benefits and those not actively engaged in the labour market, particularly women such as white working-class mothers, get pregnant 'as a career option' and are lazy and work-shy (Tyler, 2008).

Class, mothers and respectability: policy and politics

Evans' (2016) work on women, poverty and the 'politics of respectability' has highlighted that under austerity women's 'respectability' is increasing being linked to their participation in the labour market. This is in part perpetuated through negative media stereotypes which have a historical legacy (Skeggs, 2005a, 2005b; Hayward and Yar, 2006; Tyler, 2008). In the austerity era this rhetoric has centred on such categories as large families and families on out-of-work benefits being framed as 'welfare problems' (Jensen and Tyler, 2015: 11). By framing those not engaged in formal wage labour in this way, and the corresponding withdrawal of benefits, a distinction between 'deserving' and 'undeserving' female poverty is being created. Women who live on a low income with more than two children, those engaged in low-paid work, living in social housing, or not living with partners are some of those groups framed as 'undeserving' (Jensen and Tyler, 2015).

   The contemporary discourse around work and active participation in the labour market is highly gendered and classed; discussion of gender equality and women's participation in the labour market so often centres around the struggles and gains of middle-class women, and their future-oriented career trajectories (Allen and Taylor, 2012: 17).

This is due, in part, to a sociological and economic tradition which has taken the family or the household as the unit of analysis. The result was a screen which effectively prevented gender from coming into view as an axis of inequality. Thus, the tradition of social-class analysis based on male occupation created 'a whole genus of work which was restricted to class as a male concept' (Oakley, 1993: 217). In the contemporary austerity context emerging literature indicates that poorer families, those from working-class communities and young mums experiencing are at the receiving end of an ongoing process of normalisation, individualisation of their problems and stigmatisation by the state and media (Jensen and Tyler, 2015; Wenham, 2015).

Working-class women (such as in the anecdote shared by Pat about growing up) have been engaging in low-paid work for much longer than the period in which middle-class women have been entering into higher education and professional work in large numbers. This is obscured by not only dividing up economic and non-economic work, but of discounting this low-paid women's work entirely. The following fieldwork extract elaborates on this point.

FIELD NOTES
16 June 2015

Working-class women had to be either factory workers or barmaids, and that was that. Anne said that her mam was a 'stay at home mam', but when we delved a little deeper we learned that in fact she had always worked in jobs as well as being the main carer in the family. The members of the group came to an agreement that working-class women had 'always worked', they did not have the luxury of being a stay at home mam like middle-class [women], but that they were very much present in the home and managed the home.

The desire to be first and foremost a mother was felt to be at odds with shifts in government policy, and society at large. There is a pervasive theme of valorising being in paid work (in opposition to being 'on benefits') running strongly through social policy in recent decades (Jupp, 2017). Women are increasingly obliged to engage in wage-labour without the requisite provision for childcare or accommodation for time off due to having a baby. As well as this, parents are increasingly held accountable for the social mobility of their children and themselves in the gradual removal of a safety net. The government reinforce these ideas through linking claiming out-of-work benefits with behaving irresponsibly and lazily (Cameron, 2011; Jensen and

Tyler, 2015). Lisa's experience represents this situation very clearly, and also illustrates the valuable insight to be gained from longitudinal research as her circumstances changed considerably between Wave I and Wave II. When Lisa split with her partner, she found herself and her two sons, both with autism, on the sharp edge of the cuts. Lisa's mental wellbeing worsened due to the stress of financial insecurity and of her relationship coming to an end. The family, who already struggled with money, risked getting into further debt. They risked being unable to run the car (which the boys needed as they did not find it easy to use public transport) and not being able to properly heat their home. The uncertainty of when her stopped benefit payments might resume, coupled with the perceived unfairness of this when caring for two children with complex needs and issues, weighed heavily on Lisa:

> 'I'm now on my own with the boys. Waiting for my Housing Benefit, my tax credits, everything got stopped for me. My partner's claim continued, mine all stopped. They classed his change as a change of circumstances, mine as a new claim. So my money got suspended. Until that's sorted you can't get any Housing Benefit. So even though I haven't actually moved out of the house, that's been stopped. Because it's a new claim, with no date as to when it's going to start again. Even though the tax credits are for the children, that's been stopped. We're in limbo now. And I have to have a work-focused interview at the job centre every six months. Or whenever they call me in. He never has to have one.' (Lisa, Wave II)

Respondents did not agree with classed forms of 'placed parenthood' (Allen and Taylor, 2012) – self-regulating, future-oriented subjects who should earn money and not rely on the state for benefits or services. They also resented the notion that women should aspire first and foremost to be 'skilled' workers, rather than mothers and carers.

FIELD NOTES
4 August 2015

Pat felt pressured by her husband to go into caring work at a hospital, because it was some job, any job. She doesn't want to care for old people in a hospital, and is quite adamant about that. She already does more than enough caring work in her own home.

Respondents indicated that they valued caring for their families, having enough money to live a reasonably comfortable life, and to have the ability to have time for themselves, either to do hobbies or leisure activities, or to do training or further education. They wanted to be involved in building stronger and more cohesive communities. They challenged the notion that their worth was located primarily in the job they might do.

Findings II: Mental health of respondents compromised by austerity

Mental health issues emerged as a strong theme throughout the research. Most respondents had experienced depression and anxiety, and many had taken medication or attended counselling for these issues. Experiences of post-natal depression, anxiety, and depression were common. More extreme manifestations of poor mental health, such as suicidal tendencies and self-harm were also discussed. It is very important to emphasise that for many mothers in the study, life had 'always been' tough. However, austerity was a compounding factor and something which was characterised out as having clear impacts on some respondents' mental health. One respondent, Lucy discussed the very sad circumstances surrounding the death of her child in this era of austerity, stating that the lack of state support and lack of a safety net for her family made managing much harder:

> 'The tax credits one [proposed reforms in 2015] were genuinely terrifying. This was the first time in a long time that we'd been eligible. Because he'd earn quite a lot in a short period, the knock-on effect when he lost his job was we'd lost our entitlement to them when we needed them most. One year they massively overpaid us, about six years ago, and they're still clawing it back off us. In fact, we got a letter from them just a couple of months ago saying "We're going to change the way that we're taking back overpayments by taking more out of your tax credits." And that was it, no when, how much, nothing. And I was like "What? Is that on purpose just to intimidate people?" When we came out of the hospital after losing our son, and you need to rest and you just can't function anyway. Without my buffer [of income] we were absolutely buggered, like within a month. It was a disaster. We weren't paid, people were angry, what we were entitled to was really confusing.

> I lost him in April, and I had to go back to work in early July. I really wasn't ready, it was absolutely horrible. It was so brutal, and this is what we've come to.' (Lucy, Wave I)

To emphasise the difference more generous welfare provision could have on mental wellbeing, at our second interview Lucy was in a great mood. She explained that a chunk of money had arrived in her bank account – the tax credits which had been taken off the family (which, it transpired, was due to an administrative error). She said her physical health and that of her husband's was improving and their confidence had increased enormously after a bad few months.

The main factors attributed to the experience of poor mental were related to financial insecurity (not having enough money and benefit cuts), the stress of dealing with a reforming benefit system, anti-social behaviour on estates and poor quality housing. For respondents, their experience of being mothers in a context of financial insecurity, heavy emotional burdens, emerging health issues with their children or themselves, as well as the struggles of everyday life under austerity in Stockton-on-Tees led to poor mental health experiences. As Mattheys et al. (2016) found, living in more deprived areas increased the likelihood of experiencing mental ill health. Public Health England (2017) data has also indicated a widening in the gap in life expectancy for women in Stockton, up to 12.7 years from 11.4 years in 2015.

Mental health is crucial for general wellbeing, and to live a happy and productive life. Psychosocial stress is of huge significance; chronic low-level stress 'gets under the skin' and makes this difficult to achieve (Garthwaite and Bambra, 2017). Discussions of mental health issues arose in interviews with all but one participant. Jackie, the mother with the highest income, a husband working in a professional job, and a mortgage, never mentioned struggling with mental health issues (that is not to say she did not experience any, of course). The lived experience of social depletion (the pressure of combining caring work with the additional pressures of austerity including mounting debt, a feeling of the deteriorating in the quality of community life and worsening mental health) (Rai et al., 2013) may have led to the stress or mental ill-health that was reported by others. For respondents, their experience of being mothers in a context of financial insecurity, heavy emotional burdens, emerging and evolving health issues with their children, as well as the struggles of everyday life such as poor quality housing and living in places where anti-social behaviour was prevalent, led to poor mental health experiences.

Financial insecurity and ill health

Personal over-indebtedness and financial vulnerability can have a huge impact on physical and mental health (GCPH, 2016). It can also generate knock-on consequences for families and exacerbate levels of exclusion. Glasgow Centre for Population Health have argued that being in debt, especially to high cost lenders, represents a public health risk as it can lead to increased stress levels and mental health issues (GCPH, 2016). Mental wellbeing was being affected through increased feelings of insecurity and disempowerment and struggling with money. Pat's family, for example, were living on less and less money all the time. She found juggling increasingly difficult. She said, 'it does worry me, yeah. And I'll tell you the truth. Today I've walked in cos I've got 30p in me purse and that's gotta last me til … next week. Cos it's the only time I get paid' (Pat, Wave I).

Brenda, who was struggling through multiple austerity reforms and ill health, had been very negatively affected. She had been hit by the bedroom tax and had to move, had been denied disability benefits and won them on appeal, and had mounting priority debts (unpaid rent and council tax) and high-interest debt. Here, she describes her situation:

> 'Because the rent arrears were accumulating, a welfare rights adviser was put on to help us. She put me through for PIP [Personal Independence Payment] and I got it. I was absolutely dreading it, and when that letter came I cried. Although my health has deteriorated since I was put on PIP, I was put on the lowest rate, but it wasn't about that. I phoned my welfare rights adviser and she said "You can appeal this, you should be on a higher rate," but I said "I'm not doing it." With Carer's Allowance, when my husband was found eligible for that, he got a letter, they said "Yeah, but you're not getting it until eight weeks' time."' (Brenda, Wave I)

In Wave II Brenda was living in new accommodation and, while she was feeling much better the day I spoke to her, her mood had not been good overall. She said:

> 'The doctor at the hospital accepts that I am in pain, but says there's nothing more they can do for me. Nothing shows up on the scans. Even morphine doesn't touch me. I'm on three lots of medication for pain. When I went to see the psychologist there I said I feel like I've got two

depressions – one is for me physical health and the other's for the … the mental stuff. The emotional things. I said I wanted to concentrate on the emotional things first, which I've been trying to do with no success. I'm still fighting the depression and all of this. I've come to the point where I feel like there's nothing more I can do, everyone's just waving me away …' (Brenda, Wave II)

Place, austerity and mental health

The places you live in, come from and spend time in affect your health. The work of Cummins and colleagues is useful here in conceptualising the 'relational' ways place affects health – 'through complex relational spatial interdependencies which exist between people and places' (Cummins et al., 2007: 1835). Many respondents lived in areas with multiple and complex issues of deprivation, clustered around a few specific estates. Dee had been told to remove the name of her estate from job applications, to only use the postcode as the estate had a bad reputation. This is a pertinent example of how certain places are rendered tainted or blemished – 'territorial stigma' (Wacquant et al., 2014). Trish explained the situation on her estate, which was the same place where quite a few respondents lived or had lived at some point:

'It can be nice round here but … lately, it's different. Things are different from when I first moved in. It was horrible when I first moved in. Police round every night. Then things quietened down. And then last couple of months it's changed, really. Young guys on motorbikes round the streets. Where I live on the corner on a morning you get drug dealing. On the corner. And they're there every morning. The atmosphere's not the same anymore. There's a community centre but it's not open. Becky went to a meeting with the housing association a fortnight ago, she brought it up that there is a community centre there and to do something with it cos it's just getting ruined.' (Trish, Wave I)

Respondents detailed anti-social behaviour in their areas, such as drug dealing, which made day-to-day life that bit more challenging. Jody said on her estate "most people will keep to themselves. There's some dealing going on. There's about three or four drug dealers in one block of flats. It's very hard from that sense because I don't want [daughter] to go outside" (Jody, Wave I). As Shildrick et al. (2012: 163) stated, 'living and growing up in neighbourhoods of multiple and concentrated deprivation meant that the interviewees faced wider disadvantage beyond their difficulties in accessing decent, lasting employment'.

Many respondents spoke negatively about their houses. Both the location of poorer-quality housing, on specific estates in specific parts of the borough, and the houses themselves which were described as being damp and breezy, reinforce a set of inequalities for those living in certain places. Lisa's experience relates to multiple issues – an insecure tenancy in unsuitable housing, dealing with her children's disabilities and negotiating the welfare system in a period of major reforms to the social security system:

> '... It's better [now] than what we were living in before. We were living in a two-bedroom bungalow that was cold, it had damp, I had a bad chest the whole time we lived there. We're lucky we've managed to move on. We got the boys'

Figure 7.2: Row of terraced housing in Town Centre ward

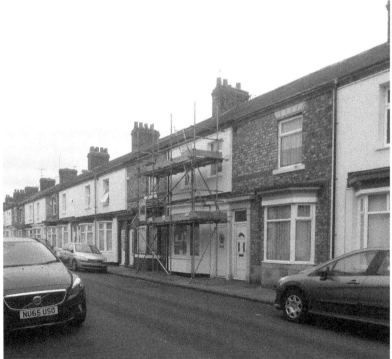

Source: author's photograph

diagnosis, and I managed to get Carer's Allowance. It was because of that that we could move. Before, when your children still have something different about them, you still have to look after them but you don't get Carer's Allowance. I couldn't get Job Seeker's [Allowance], I couldn't get any Income Support, I could get nothing. I was being a carer, but that wasn't being recognised.' (Lisa, Wave I)

'The sense of social indignity that has come to enshroud certain urban districts ... has implications for residents in terms of employment prospects, educational attainment, and receipt of social assistance' (Slater, 2017: 8). It led Dee to report, as stated previously, that her Jobcentre Plus adviser had told her to avoid putting her estate on her CV, and to opt for the postcode instead. Dee refused; she wasn't ashamed of where she came from (Wave I). These mechanisms place those in poorer areas at a disadvantage and have a significant impact on mental health. Pearce (2013: 1924) has found that austerity will have implications for future health inequalities as 'one of the likely implications of reducing investment into communities with a multitude of social problems is that such places will become increasingly stigmatised, which is likely to be detrimental to the health of local residents'.

Findings III: Intersectionality and invisible inequalities

Experiences of inequality are mediated through the intersections of disability, place, socioeconomic status and gender. The intersections of these inequalities both create the conditions for, and exacerbate lived experiences of poor health, debt, and multiple disadvantages. There is a lack of insight into the intersecting nature of gendered and spatial inequalities stemming from austerity (Greer Murphy, 2016). Gender is an important determinant of health because gender inequality leads to different experiences of health for women, rooted in imbalances of power and societal roles and expectations. Stein has argued that health has been perceived as having a single, dominant determinant but to more adequately understand women's health it might be more sensible to view it as having multiple determinants or as 'an intricate, non-linear, tangled web of factors, some of which are socio-political' (Stein, 1997: 89). This can be enhanced by an intersectional perspective (Hill, 2016) wherein characteristics of individuals or groups represent 'reciprocally constructing phenomena' which combine to affect how inequalities are experienced (Collins, 2015).

Brenda's experience illustrates the intersectionality of inequality. Brenda was in her late forties at the time of our interviews. She had two children and had remarried. In Brenda's childhood she was a victim of abuse, and suffered from post-traumatic stress disorder as a result. Her first marriage was conflictual. From it she had two children, a daughter who lived with her, and a son who was homeless and addicted to drugs, living in Newcastle. She had suffered from post-natal depression with her first baby, and again with her second. With her second, she used to take her temper out on her eldest all the time without being able to control it. In her own words, she "would have knocked her across the room if the bed hadn't been there". She told her midwife this straight away and reported feeling bad about her behaviour. She was glad she divulged this when she did and got the help she needed (Wave II). Brenda suffered from osteoarthritis and at times had been confined to a wheelchair. She reported suffering from very poor mental health, had depression and sometimes felt suicidal. She was taking numerous pain killers, including morphine, for chronic pain. Our second interview highlighted how her mental health had deteriorated in a few short months:

> 'Me health's been up and down. I had the crisis team involved with me because I'm suicidal. They said they'd contacted somebody the first time they were out in September but nobody had contacted me for counselling. But they got them out the same day for me. They referred me to a local counselling service and I thought "Yes, I'm finally going to get some help." Not once were any of my issues broached. I had a couple of sessions and then either, I think I cancelled one. She cancelled a few of them and when I cancelled the last one she went "Well do you want us to just close your file?" and I went "You might as well." And I was devastated.' (Brenda, Wave II)

Brenda's mental health and debt issues were intertwined, as she explained:

> 'Last year, we asked for help, we went to the housing for help, all these people for help, and nobody would help us. I suffer from serious depression, so my mental state was just on the floor. All these things they put into place, you get with one hand and it's taken with the other. I hate not being mobile and not being able to work. I wasn't bothered

by the rent and that when we were both working, d'you know what I mean? We could do that. Even though we struggled.' (Brenda, Wave I)

Women's lives frequently feature what could be characterised as an 'invisible inequality' whereby economic, political and social factors intersect to amplify the aspects of women's lives which reinforce gender-based inequality and which are subsumed under dominant beliefs rooted in biological determinism and gender roles. Under austerity some of these effects are magnified. Women are being affected to a great extent by service cuts, labour market and social security reforms. The Women's Budget Group have recently produced an important report highlighting the intersectionality of inequalities for women under austerity (Hall et al., 2017) highlighting that low-income families, lone parent-headed households and BAME households have been particularly affected. As women are the main group carrying out social reproduction, their diminishing financial capacities coupled with more pressure to carry out such work with fewer supports places them at a further disadvantage and may increase levels of stress, anxiety and worry. It is of enduring importance that women, particularly women on low incomes, living in poverty, with disabilities and in vulnerable situations, are heard and that policy is formed taking their experiences into account.

Figure 7.3: Town centre on market day

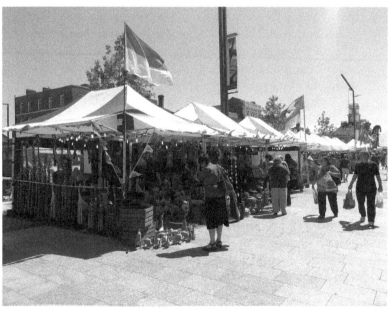

Source: author's photograph

Conclusion

This chapter introduced the significance of austerity's effects on Stockton and on women in a context of growing inequality. It discussed research findings relating to the specific experiences of mothers in Stockton – their experiences of being a mother, of low-paid work, of caring duties, and the desire for many to be first and foremost a mother. It illustrated some of the inequalities respondents face – the desire to be a stay at home mother in a time of diminishing incomes, and mounting pressure leading to anxiety, depression and other mental health issues. I have argued that there is a need to acknowledge the role of social reproduction and how ongoing austerity measures are exacerbating the deeply gendered dynamics of the politics of inequality in the UK. Articulations of austerity which critique welfare state retrenchment without focusing on its gendered structure and an intersectionality of advantages and disadvantages are limited. In this context of worsening mental health, decreased incomes, diminished value of the roles of carers, the experience of women, especially in an intersectional context, warrants ongoing investigation. Future research which explores the everyday lived experiences of those groups specifically targeted by welfare reforms (women, those with disabilities, minority ethnic groups) is therefore of great importance. Longitudinal research has the added benefit of being able to explore how these experiences change over time.

The central arguments of this chapter were threefold. First, it was argued that there is an inherent interplay between macro level policies such as national politics and policy making and the micro experiences of these. Second, the everyday experiences of austerity, particularly relating to experiences of health, require ongoing academic investigating. Qualitative investigation such as this piece of research is well suited to drawing out the nuances of the lived experience of austerity. Finally, the experiences of women, particularly the 'invisible inequalities' of women's lives discussed in the previous section, constitute a negative outcome of austerity, and one which needs further investigation and to be challenged. These experiences represent an intersectionality of inequality whereby the way gender roles operate place women at a structural disadvantage. This disadvantage is being increased under austerity.

References

Adam, B. and Groves, C. (2007) *Future Matters: action, knowledge, ethics.* Brill, Leiden and Boston

Allen, K., and Taylor, Y. (2012) Placing parenting, locating unrest: failed femininities, troubled mothers and riotous subjects. *Studies in the Maternal*. Volume 4, Issue 2, pp. 1–25

Bambra, C. and Garthwaite, K. A. (2015) Austerity, welfare reform and the English health divide. *Area*. Volume 47, Issue 3, pp. 341–343

Beatty, C. and Fothergill, S. (2013) Hitting the poorest places hardest: The local and regional impact of welfare reform. Centre for Regional Economic and Social Research, Sheffield Hallam University. www4.shu.ac.uk/research/cresr/sites/shu.ac.uk/files/hitting-poorest-places-hardest_0.pdf

Beatty, C. and Fothergill, S. (2016) *The Uneven Impact of Welfare Reform: The financial losses to places and people*. Sheffield/York/London: Sheffield Hallam University Centre for Regional Economic and Social Research, Joseph Rowntree Foundation and Oxfam. http://policy-practice.oxfam.org.uk/publications/the-uneven-impact-of-welfare-reform-the-financial-losses-to-places-and-people-604630

Beatty C. and Fothergill, S. (2018) Welfare Reform in the United Kingdom 2010–16: Expectations, outcomes, and local impacts. *Social Policy Administration*. Volume 52, pp. 950–968. https://onlinelibrary.wiley.com/doi/epdf/10.1111/spol.12353

Bradshaw, J. and Main, G. (2016) Child poverty and deprivation. In Bradshaw, J. Ed. *The well-being of children in the UK*. Policy Press, Bristol

Cameron, D. (2011) 'Speech on Welfare Reform Bill'. www.number10.gov.uk/news/speeches-and-transcripts/2011/02/pms-speech-on-welfare-reform-bill-60717

Carter, B., Danford, A., Howcroft, D., Richardson, H., Smith, A., Taylor, P. (2013) 'Stressed out of my box': employee experience of lean working and occupational ill-health in clerical work in the UK public sector. *Work, Employment and Society*. Volume 27, Issue 5, pp. 747–767

Collins, P. H. (2015) Intersectionality's definitional dilemmas. *Annual Review of Sociology*. Volume 41, Issue 1, pp. 1–20

Craddock, E. (2017) Caring about and for the cuts: a case study of the gendered dimension of austerity and anti-austerity activism. *Gender, Work and Organization*. Volume 24, Issue 1, pp. 69–82

Crompton, R. (2006) *Employment and the family: the reconfiguration of work and family life in contemporary societies*. Cambridge University Press, Cambridge

Cummins, S. Curtis, S. Diez-Roux, A. V. Macintyre, S. (2007) Understanding and representing 'place' in health research: a relational approach. *Social Science and Medicine*. Volume 65, Issue 9, pp. 1825–1838

DfE (Department for Education) (2016) Planned LA and school expenditure: 2016 to 2017 financial year. Department for Education. Darlington

Dhamoonm R. K., (2011) Considerations on Mainstreaming Intersectionality. *Political Research Quarterly* Volume 64, Issue 1, pp. 230–243

Evans, M. (2016) Women and the politics of austerity: New forms of respectability. *British Politics*. Volume 11, Issue 4, pp. 438–451

Fawcett Society (2014) The changing labour market 2: women, low pay and gender equality in the emerging recovery. Fawcett Society, London

Fletcher, D. R., Flint, J., Baty, E., McNeill, J. (2016) Gamers or victims of the system? Welfare reform, cynical manipulation and vulnerability. *Journal of Poverty and Social Justice*. Volume 24, No 2, pp. 171–85

Fraser, N. (1989) *Unruly practices: power, discourse and gender in contemporary social theory*. Polity Press, Oxford

Fraser, N. (2013) *Fortunes of feminism. From state-managed capitalism to neoliberal crisis*. Verson, London and New York

Fraser, N. (2016) Contradictions of capital and care. *New Left Review*. Volume 100

Garthwaite, K. (2016) *Hunger pains: Life inside foodbank Britain*. Policy Press, Bristol

Garthwaite, K. and Bambra, C. (2017) 'How the other half live': Lay perspectives on health inequalities in an age of austerity. *Social Science & Medicine*. Vol 187, pp. 268–275

GCPH (Glasgow Centre for Population Health) (2016) Public Health Implications of Payday Lending. Briefing Paper 48. Glasgow Centre for Population Health, Glasgow

Geertz, C. (1973) Thick description: Toward an interpretive theory of culture. In Geertz, C. *The Interpretation of Cultures: Selected Essays*. Basic Books, New York

Greer Murphy, A. (2016) Austerity in the United Kingdom: the intersections of spatial and gendered inequalities. *Area*. Volume 49, Issue 1

Hall, S. M. (2015) Personal, relational and intimate geographies of austerity: ethical and empirical considerations. *Area*. Volume 49, Issue 3, pp. 303–310

Hall, S., McIntosh, K., Neitzert, E., Pottinger, L., Sandhu, K., Stephenson, M. A., Reed, H. and Taylor, L. (2017) *Intersecting inequalities: The impact of austerity on black and minority ethnic women in the UK*. Women's Budget Group, London

Hastings, A., Bailey, N., Bramley, G., Gannon, M. and Watkins, D. (2015) *The cost of the cuts. The impact on local government and poorer communities*. Joseph Rowntree Foundation, York

Hayward, K. and Yar, M. (2006) 'The 'chav' phenomenon: consumption, media and the construction of a new underclass'. *Crime, Media, Culture*. Volume 2, Issue 1, pp. 9–28

Hill, S. (2016) Axes of health inequalities and intersectionality. In Smith, K. E., Hill, S., Bambra, C. *Health inequalities: Critical perspectives*. Oxford University Press, Oxford

Holloway, S. and Pimlott-Wilson, H. (2016) New economy, neoliberal state and professionalised parenting: mothers' labour market engagement and state support for social reproduction in class-differentiated Britain. *Transactions of the Institute of British Geographers*. Volume 41, Issue 4, pp. 376–388

Jensen, T. and Tyler, I. (2015) Benefits broods: the cultural and political crafting of anti-welfare commonsense. *Critical Social Policy*, Volume 35, Issue 4, pp. 470–491

Jupp, E. (2017) Families, policy and place in times of austerity. *Area*. Volume 49, Issue 3, pp. 266–272

Karlsen, S. and Nazroo, J. Y. (2006) 'Measuring and analysing 'race', racism and racial discrimination'. In Oakes, J. M. and Kaufman , J. S. Eds. *Methods in Social Epidemiology*. Jossey-Bass, San Francisco

Konzelmann, S. (2014) The political economics of austerity. *Cambridge Journal of Economics*. Volume 38, Issue 4, pp. 701–741

Lewis J. and West, A. (2016) Early childhood education and care in England under austerity: continuity or change in political ideas, policy goals, availability, affordability and quality in a childcare market? *Journal of Social Policy*. Volume 46, Issue 2, pp. 1–18

Mannay, D. (2015) Achieving respectable motherhood? Exploring the impossibility of feminist and egalitarian ideologies against the everyday realities of lived Welsh working-class femininities. *Women's Studies International Forum*. Volume 53, pp. 159–166

Mattheys K., Bambra C., Warren J., Kasim A., and Akhter N. (2016) Inequalities in mental health and well-being in a time of austerity: Baseline findings from the Stockton-On-Tees cohort study. *Social Science and Medicine: Population Health*. Volume 2, pp. 350–359

Milbourne, L., and Cushman, M. (2015) Complying, transforming or resisting in the new austerity? Realigning social welfare and independent action among English voluntary organisations. *Journal of Social Policy*. Volume 44, Issue 3, pp. 463–485

Moffatt, S., Lawson, S., Patterson, R., Holding, E., Dennison, A., Sowden, S., Brown, J. (2016) A qualitative study of the impact of the UK 'bedroom tax'. *Journal of Public Health*. Volume 38, Issue 2, pp. 197–205

Neale, B. (2012) *Qualitative longitudinal research: an introduction.* Timescapes Methods Guides Series. No. 1. Timescapes, Leeds

Oakley, A. (1993) *Essays on women, medicine and health.* Edinburgh University Press, Edinburgh

ONS (Office for National Statistics) (2015) *Childhood Mortality in England and Wales: 2015*. London: ONS, www.ons.gov.uk/ peoplepopulationandcommunity/birthsdeathsandmarriages/deaths/ bulletins/childhoodinfantandperinatalmortalityinenglandandwales/ 2015

ONS (2016a) How is the welfare budget spent? http://visual.ons.gov. uk/welfare-spending/

ONS (2016b) UK Labour Market: June 2016. www.ons.gov.uk/ employmentandlabourmarket/peopleinwork/employmentand employeetypes/bulletins/uklabourmarket/june2016

ONS (2017) Statistical bulletin: UK labour market: August 2017. Estimates of employment, unemployment, economic inactivity and other employment-related statistics for the UK. ONS, London. www.ons.gov.uk/employmentandlabourmarket/peopleinwork/ employmentandemployeetypes/bulletins/uklabourmarket/ latest#main-points-for-april-to-june-2017

ONS (2018) Statistical bulletin: Health state life expectancies by national deprivation deciles, England and Wales: 2014 to 2016. Life expectancy and years expected to live in 'good' health using national indices of deprivation to measure socio-economic inequalities. London: ONS, www.ons.gov.uk/peoplepopulationandcommunity/ healthandsocialcare/healthinequalities/bulletins/healthstatelife expectanciesbyindexofmultipledeprivationimd/englandandwales 2014to2016

Patrick, R. (2014) Working on welfare: Findings from a qualitative longitudinal study into the lived experiences of welfare reform in the UK. *Journal of Social Policy*. Volume 43, Issue 4, pp. 705–725

Patrick, R. (2017) *For whose benefit? The everyday realities of welfare reform.* Policy Press, Bristol

Pearce, J. (2013) Commentary. *Environment and Planning A: Economy and Space.* Volume 45, Issue 9, pp. 2030–2045

Peck, J. (2001) *Workfare states.* Guilford Press, New York

Power, A. (2014) Personalisation and austerity in the crosshairs: government perspectives on the remaking of adult social care. *Journal of Social Policy.* Volume 43, Issue 4, pp. 829–846

Public Health England, (2015) Stockton-on-Tees Unitary Authority Health Profile 2015. http://fingertipsreports.phe.org.uk/health-profiles/2015/e06000004.pdf

Public Health England (2017) Stockton-on-Tees Unitary Authority Health Profile 2017. http://fingertipsreports.phe.org.uk/health-profiles/2017/e06000004.pdf

Rai, S., Hoskyns, C., and Thomas, D. (2013) Depletion – the cost of social reproduction. *International Feminist Journal of Politics.* Volume 16, Issue 1, pp. 86–105

Ridge, T. (2013) 'We are all in this together'? The hidden costs of poverty, recession and austerity policies on Britain's poorest children. *Children and Society.* Volume 27, Issue 5, pp. 406–417

Schutt, R. K. (2012) *Investigating the social world: the process and practice of research.* Sage Publications, California and London

Shildrick, T., MacDonald, R., Furlong, A., Roden, J. and Crow, R. (2012) *Are 'cultures of worklessness' passed down the generations?* Joseph Rowntree Foundation, York

Skeggs, B. (2005a) *Class, self and culture.* Routledge, London

Skeggs, B. (2005b) The making of class and gender through visual moral subject formation. *Sociology.* Volume 39, Issue 5, pp. 965–982

Slater, T. (2017) Territorial stigmatization: Symbolic defamation and the contemporary metropolis. in Hannigan, J. and Richards, G. Eds. *The Handbook of New Urban Studies.* Sage Publications, London

Stein, J. (1997) *Empowerment and women's health: Theory, methods, and practice.* Zed Books, London

Stockton-on-Tees Borough Council (2016) Council takes on 'monumental' budget task. www.stockton.gov.uk/news/2016/february/council-takes-on-monumental-budget-task/

Strauss, A. and Corbin, J. (1998) *Basics of qualitative research techniques and procedures for developing grounded theory* (2nd edition). Sage Publications, London

Taylor-Robinson, D., and Barr, B. (2017) Gap in health between rich and poor death rate now rising in UK's poorest infants. *British Medical Journal,* 357, www.bmj.com/content/357/bmj.j2258

Taylor-Robinson, D., Whitehead, M. and Barr, B. (2014) Great leap backwards. *British Medical Journal*, 349, www.bmj.com/content/349/bmj.g7350/rapid-responses

Thomson, R., Kehily, M. J., Hadfield, L., and Sharpe, S. (2011) *Making modern mothers*. Policy Press, Bristol

Tyler, I. (2008) 'Chav mum chav scum'. *Feminist Media Studies*. Volume 8, Issue 1, pp. 17–34

Verbrugge, L. M. (1976) Females and illness: recent trends in sex differences in the United States. *Health, Society and Behaviour* Volume 17, pp. 387–403

Verbrugge, L. M. (1980) Sex differences in complaints and diagnoses. *Journal of Behavioural Medicine*. Volume 3, pp. 327–355

Wacquant, L., Slater, T. and Pereira, V. B. (2014) Territorial stigmatisation in action. *Environment and Planning* Issue 46, Volume 6, pp. 1270–1280

Watts, B., Fitzpatrick, S., Bramley, G. and Watkins, D. (2014) *Welfare Sanctions and Conditionality in the UK*, York: Joseph Rowntree Foundation

Wenham, A. M. (2015) 'I know I'm a good mum – no-one can tell me different': Young mothers negotiating a stigmatized identity through time. *Families, Relationships and Societies*. Volume 5, Issue 1, pp. 127–144

EIGHT

Conclusion: Health in Hard Times

Clare Bambra

In this concluding chapter, I bring together the main themes of the previous chapters highlighting the key contributions which the Stockton-on-Tees project has made to the wider social science and health inequalities literature; specifically, our understanding of geographical inequalities in health during austerity. The following three key contributions that the research project has made are discussed: (1) The value of taking a case study, mixed methods approach to the exploration of place-based health inequalities; (2) The contribution made by the project to understanding health inequalities and the relationship between health and place by localising the study of health inequalities; and (3) what the project found in terms of the effects of austerity on health inequalities. The chapter concludes by outlining the research, policy and practice implications of the project emphasising how our case study shows the need to integrate political economy perspectives into geographical research; the importance of universal social policy safety nets especially for women, those with disabilities and health conditions, and older people; and for practitioners to look beyond health behaviours when designing public health interventions.

Revitalising the case study approach

Our project has contributed to the literature methodologically by resurrecting the case study approach in UK social science. The case study approach has a long tradition in UK social research, arguably dating back to the work of Charles Booth in the late 19th century (1889–97). Other prominent early research in this tradition includes Joseph Rowntree's studies of poverty in York in the early 20th century (1901) as well as the Marienthal town study in Austria (Jahoda et al., 1971 [1930]). In the post-war period, the case study method was elaborated by the Chicago School of urban ethnography (for example, Whyte, 1993 [1944]), while in the UK, there was more of a focus on particular occupational settings or occupational groups with the intention of examining the dynamics of social class such as *Coal is*

Our Life (Dennis et al., 1956), *Working for Ford* (Beynon, 1973) or *The Affluent Worker* (Goldthorpe, 1963). However, the popularity of the case study method declined in recent decades in UK social science, partly as a result of an increased contestation of the concepts of 'place' and 'community' in social science research (Studdert, 2006; Agnew, 2011). Methodologically though the case study approach has many advantages – many of which have been demonstrated in the previous chapters – it encourages the combination of quantitative and qualitative data and methods of analysis and interpretation, it is interdisciplinary – drawing on the insights of different disciplines within and beyond the health and social sciences.

In our case study of health inequalities in Stockton-on-Tees during a period of austerity, we have produced an example of an intensive, longitudinal, triangulated study. This has enabled the production of a rich, multi-faceted and detailed explanatory account. This is in stark contrast with the majority of health inequalities research which has traditionally been dominated by quantitative approaches and the broad-level analysis of a large number of cases or places. This reflects the dominance of epidemiological methods in the study of health and of health inequalities conventionally being viewed from a public health rather than a social science perspective. In applying an intensive, mixed methods case study approach, we have instead demonstrated how different methodological approaches (including ethnographic, qualitative and archival research) and different disciplines (including anthropology, sociology, social policy, geography, history alongside social epidemiology) can also contribute to and advance our understandings of health inequalities. The methodological and disciplinary diversity of the case study approach enabled the research to take a long view on the nature of health inequalities, anthropological and sociological approaches meant that the project could engage with issues of intersectionality and the fluid nature of place and community, while the social policy and geography traditions were fundamental throughout the project in thinking through the impacts on geographical inequalities in health of austerity and welfare reform. Our project has therefore shown how research into health inequalities can be methodologically reshaped and the perspectives from different disciplines incorporated. In doing so, we hope that we have shown how a broader range of social scientists and even humanities scholars can engage with health inequalities and enhance understandings of their causes within a period of austerity.

Nonetheless, it also needs to be noted that a case of approach obviously has some limitations. First, by only examining one place

– Stockton-on-Tees – albeit in an intensive manner, and research findings are not easily generalisable to other locations. Data only relates to one place and the uniqueness of Stockton-on-Tees in terms of the scale of its health inequalities also means that it may be that specific issues affect Stockton that might not affect other localities. However, we are still able to expand knowledge of the complex causal factors involved in the aetiology of health inequalities and the theoretical and empirical insights from our case study will still have implications for research and practice in other localities and nationally. Second, by taking a mixed methods approach, the findings from the different methodologies are sometimes complementary but on other occasions they contradict one another. It's difficult therefore to tease out universal findings even within the specific case study area. Finally, the contested nature of community within social science and place is also something encountered within this project. Different parts of the project conceived community and place in different ways. For example, the quantitative analysis in Chapters Three and Six used a more traditional, bounded and fixed conception of place that used administrative geographical boundaries to define which neighbourhoods of Stockton-on-Tees – and therefore which people – were sampled for the survey (Pahl, 2005). In contrast, the qualitative research in Chapters Four, Five and Seven and the historical research in Chapter Two took more fluid approaches to the conceptualisation of place and community. For example, in Chapter Seven, Amy Greer Murphy's sampling approach emphasised the importance of social networks (Savage, 2008), while the relational nature of community was evident in the sampling frame taken by Kate Mattheys and Kayleigh Garthwaite in Chapters Four and Five (Studdert, 2006). The role of affect in communal being-ness is very apparent within all of the qualitative chapters (Walkerdine and Jimenez, 2012). The project therefore incorporated developments in the social scientific understanding of place and community into the case study.

Advancing understanding of health inequalities

There is a long history in the UK of research into health inequalities and the relationship between health and place, arguably dating back over three hundred years (Macintyre, 2003; Smith et al., 2016). For example, records from the 1840s show that gentry and professional men residing in Bath had a life expectancy which was more than double that of labourers living in the same area (Chadwick, 1842). A similar socioeconomic health divide was visible in Liverpool, although life expectancies for both occupational groups were lower than for the equivalent groups in Bath – demonstrating spatial as well as socioeconomic inequalities in health (Chadwick, 1842). Despite significant increases in life expectancy for all-population groups over the last two centuries, socioeconomic and spatial inequalities in health remain with gaps in life expectancy between the most and least deprived neighbourhoods of England amounting to nine years for men and seven years for women (ONS, 2015). Health inequalities also remain higher in the North of England than in the South (Bambra et al., 2014). Gender and ethnic inequalities also exist, operating in an intersectional way (Gkiouleka et al., 2018).

Historically, there have been intermittent UK government attempts to tackle socioeconomic health inequalities. For example, Chadwick's work on sanitary conditions underpinned the 1848 Public Health Act (Golding, 2006). Concerns over inequalities in health also contributed to the establishment of the post-war welfare state and the National Health Service (NHS). The persistence though of health inequalities in the post-war period led to the government-commissioned Black Report (1980) on inequalities in health, which examined aetiology and made policy recommendations on reduction. In more recent decades, health inequalities have managed to sustain a more consistently high policy profile with, for example, the 1997–2010 Labour governments commissioning two further reports (Acheson, 1998; Marmot, 2010) and putting into place the first national reduction strategy in Europe (Barr et al., 2014; Bambra, 2016; Barr et al., 2017). The strategy included 'upstream' interventions such as the national minimum wage and higher benefits and pensions, as well as more targeted initiatives, such as the Sure Start programme and increased NHS spending as well as 'downstream', more behavioural interventions (such as nicotine replacement therapy) (Mackenbach, 2011). Over time, the policy suffered from 'lifestyle drift' – whereby the government moved from a commitment to dealing with the wider structural, social determinants of health to instigating narrow, lifestyle interventions focused on individual behaviour change (Hunter et al., 2010). However, arguably as a result of this 'lifestyle drift' (and the curtailing of the policy by the economic crisis and the change to austerity under the Conservative led governments since 2010) the New Labour approach was only partially successful, there were small reductions in health inequalities in terms of life expectancy and infant mortality rates but these were not on the scale anticipated (Mackenbach, 2011; Bambra, 2012; Barr et al., 2014; Bambra, 2016; Barr et al., 2017). Subsequent Conservative-led governments since 2010, have focused exclusively on lifestyle interventions while also implementing austerity

(Bambra, 2016). The lack of success of the New Labour approach may have been as a result of the 'lifestyle drift' (discussed below) or because interventions were nationally conceived and delivered on a 'one size fits all' policy basis despite evidence that 'standard issue' public health and social policy interventions may not work in every context (Chow et al., 2009; Joyce et al., 2010). Within this context, our case study of Stockton-on-Tees aimed to provide a more *localised* understanding of health inequalities and particularly the impact of a major economic, social and policy 'system shock' in the form of austerity on health inequalities in the local authority.

The UK has also long been at the forefront of research into health inequalities with a considerable body of work – largely situated in the public health and epidemiological literature – which outlines patterns of health by socioeconomic factors and considers their causes (Smith et al., 2016). However, while there has been much UK and international research into the causes of health inequalities, the aetiology is still unclear particularly when examined at the local level. This is especially the case in terms of examining geographical health inequalities where there are additional debates about the importance of place in shaping people's health (Dorling et al., 2001). There are competing explanations for inequalities in health between socioeconomic groups: cultural-behavioural (inequalities result from health-related behaviours), materialist (inequalities result from income, access to goods and services including health care, as well as exposures to material conditions such as housing or the physical work environment), psychosocial (inequalities result from exposure to feelings of inferiority and subordination particularly in the workplace), life course (inequalities result from the accumulation of social, psychological, and biological advantages and disadvantages over time) (Bartley, 2004). However, the majority of studies tend to privilege the behavioural explanation over the others, even though the importance of the social determinants of health (access to essential goods and services, housing and the living environment, access to health care, unemployment and social security, and working conditions) is almost universally accepted (Marmot, 2010). This is mirrored in public health practice and policy responses to the 'wicked issue' of health inequalities (Blackman et al., 2011) which, with some notable exceptions such as the New Labour government policies of the late 1990s (discussed above), have almost exclusively tried to tackle health inequalities (if they have tried at all) through behavioural or health service means.

Our research project *localised* the examination of the multi-faceted causality of socioeconomic health inequalities in Stockton-on-Tees

–qualitatively, quantitatively and historically. In contrast to much previous research and policy trends though, we found little evidence that behavioural factors were the most important determinants of socioeconomic and spatial health inequalities in Stockton. Indeed, we found that material and psychosocial factors mattered far more for the health divides found between the most and least deprived neighbourhoods of Stockton-on-Tees. This was a consistent finding across the different methodological and disciplinary approaches as shown in the previous chapters. This suggests that a research focus on examining health behaviours – particularly in isolation from the wider social and economic environment – as the main cause of health inequalities is at best misguided and at worst it lends support to the continuation of behavioural interventions and individualised policy solutions (of 'lifestyle drift') which are unlikely to be effective in the long term (Hunter et al., 2010).

Through qualitative work, our project has also examined how socioeconomic status and locality intersects with gender in the aetiology of health inequalities (Arber and Cooper, 1999; Hill, 2016; Gkiouleka et al., 2018). Intersectionality was initially developed by Black critical thinkers and activists as a way to conceptualise multiple disadvantage (like that experienced by Black women) as an oppressive experience that could not be captured by approaches that disregarded power relations and treated race and gender as distinct entities (Crenshaw, 1991). Since then, intersectionality has influenced scholarship in various fields (Crenshaw, 2001) – most recently it is beginning to influence health inequalities research. Intersectionality can be defined as an analytical strategy in which social categories like gender, race, socioeconomic status, or sexuality are mutually constructed and underlie intersecting systems of power that foster social formations of complex social inequalities (Gkiouleka et al., 2018). Individuals, groups and places are differentially located within the intersecting systems of power and their location shapes their experience – including their health (Hill, 2016). In Chapter Seven, Amy Greer Murphy draws on intersectionality to show how the health of women – and particularly of mothers – living in deprived neighbourhoods is particularly affected by austerity and the cuts to social safety nets and social services that this entailed. This considerably advances the use of intersectionality as an analytical frame within health inequalities – where research into gender and health, ethnicity and health, or socioeconomic status and health have traditionally emerged as distinct and separate fields of research. Indeed, the sizeable health inequalities literature has had a predominant (and arguably excluding) emphasis on socioeconomic status as the key axis of inequality. In the UK for example, the term 'health inequalities' refers almost exclusively to socioeconomic status with little reflection on how that is stratified by other factors such as gender. Our project has therefore added to the growing interest in intersectionality in health inequalities research by highlighting empirically – not just theoretically or discursively – the gendered implications of austerity for health (Gkiouleka et al., 2018). It has also shown that fears raised by women's groups and poverty charities about the unequal gendered effects of austerity were well founded (MacLeavy, 2011).

Our project has also engaged with and advanced a key debate in the geographical literature about the relationship between health and place. Specifically, and as outlined in the introductory Chapter One and in Chapter Three, this concerns the relative health impacts of the composition (socioeconomically disadvantaged people live in socioeconomically disadvantaged areas) versus the context (socioeconomically disadvantaged places may suffer from having poor economic, social and physical environments) (Macintyre et al., 1993). There have been theoretical moves away from this dualism towards a more relational approach that recognises the 'mutually reinforcing and reciprocal relationship between people and place' (Cummins et al., 2007: 1826). A consensus is beginning to emerge that acknowledges that different contexts have different health effects on different individuals: that place matters (Dorling, 2001). However, little attention has previously been made to factors that sit above the individual (composition) or the local (contextual) such as the role of macro political economy factors. Context has also been shown to be important in terms of the success – or not – of public health interventions (Chow et al., 2009). However, to date, much of our knowledge of geographical inequalities in health in England comes from national-level datasets that are unable to account for the specificities of particular places or use proximal area-level deprivation indicators which are themselves the aggregate of individual characteristics (Cummins et al., 2007). Our project provided the opportunity for a more detailed and multi-faceted investigation into how geographical inequalities in health develop, are subsequently shaped and experienced at the local level during a period of substantial changes in political-economy – austerity.

Our case study of Stockton-on-Tees empirically demonstrated the importance of a relational understanding of health and place – that it is not either context or compositional factors that matter for health but their interaction. Most notably in Chapter Three, Ramjee Bhandari's quantitative analysis demonstrated that the interaction of individual, compositional factors (behavioural, material and psychosocial) with contextual place-based environmental factors accounted for the greatest amount of the inequality gap in physical health. This was further emphasised in Chapter Six where Nasima Akhter and colleagues noted the importance of the interaction of environmental-material factors with individual factors in explaining geographical inequalities in mental health during austerity. The qualitative chapters by Amy Greer Murphy, Kayleigh Garthwaite and Kate Mattheys also highlighted how individual factors interacted with the wider context to produce different lived experiences of austerity and health. For example in Chapter Five, Kate Mattheys interviews with people with mental health issues showed that the effects of austerity varied both by place and individual circumstances. The relational approach was also demonstrated in Mike Langthorne's historical research in Chapter Two whereby the contextual social determinants of health in 1930s Stockton interacted with compositional factors. Most significantly though, through focusing on the effects of austerity, the whole project has demonstrated the importance for research into the relationship between health and place to take political economy factors into account. Our findings in relation to austerity and health inequalities are explored further in the next section.

Health inequalities in an age of austerity

An important aspect of our project was examining local health inequalities in Stockton during austerity. Austerity was an important meta-contextual factor or political economy backdrop for our study. The political economy approach to explaining health inequalities focuses on the social, political and economic structures and relations that may be, and often are, outside the control of the individuals (compositional) or the local areas (contextual) they affect (Krieger, 2003). In this sense, geographical patterns of health and disease are produced by the structures, values and priorities of political and economic systems (Krieger, 2003). Area-level health – be it local, regional or national – is determined, at least in part, by the wider political, social and economic system and the actions of the state (government) and international-level actors (supra-national government bodies such as the European Union, international trade agreements such as the Transatlantic Trade and Investment Partnership, as well as the actions of large corporations) in shaping the compositional and contextual determinants of health (Bambra,

2016). Political choices are seen as the causes of the causes of the causes of geographical inequalities in health (Bambra, 2016). The effects of recessions and austerity on the social determinants of health and the resulting effects on health inequalities is a clear example of the importance of macro political and economic factors – an example that was the focus of our project and this edited collection.

The global economic downturn which followed the widespread financial collapse of 2007 and 2008 (Gamble, 2009) was followed in the UK by the implementation of a wrath of austerity policies (reducing budget deficits in economic downturns by decreasing public expenditure and/or increasing taxes). As outlined in the Introduction Chapter, economic downturns are characterised by instability (in terms of inflation and interest rates) and sudden reductions in production and consumption with corresponding increases in unemployment. In terms of the general population health effects of economic downturns, the fairly large international research literature suggests that while all-cause mortality – as well as deaths from cardiovascular disease and motor vehicle accidents – decreases during economic downturns, deaths from suicides among men, psychological ill health, limiting long-term illness and poor self-rated health all appear to increase (Bambra, 2011). The evidence base also suggests that health behaviours improve during downturns, especially among heavy alcohol and tobacco consumers (Bambra, 2011). However, the effects of downturns on health inequalities are less clear with far fewer studies in this area. For example, a Japanese study found that economic slowdown increased relative occupational inequalities in self-rated health among men but not women (Kondo et al., 2008), while a Finnish study found that it slowed down the trend towards increased inequalities in mortality (Valkonen et al., 2000), and a series of Scandinavian studies of morbidity concluded that there were no significant effects of the 1990s recession on inequalities in morbidity in these countries (Lahelma et al., 2002). The health effects of downturns are also unequally distributed geographically with some areas doing better than others (so called 'resilient' areas) (Cairns and Bambra, 2013).

An important aspect of the economic crisis of 2007/08 was the policy response in the UK where austerity measures were applied with public expenditure on health, education and welfare as well as local authority budgets, which were radically decreased in order to reduce the public deficit. Commentators have called the austerity measures in the UK (which include welfare benefit cuts and caps, restrictions on benefit entitlements, and freezes or reductions to health, education and local authority budgets – as outlined in the Introduction Chapter) 'unprecedented' in scale (Taylor-Gooby, 2012). They were predicted to have the most negative impact on those with the lowest incomes or in receipt of benefits (especially those on incapacity-related benefits), and on women (MacLeavy, 2011). Our project was designed to explore if this was the case in one particular place – Stockton-on-Tees.

Further, we focused on exploring the effects of austerity on health inequalities as, although there is a long-standing British tradition of poverty research examining unemployment, benefit receipt, living on a low income and the effects on communities of de-industrialisation, such studies have seldom engaged with the implications for health (for example, Townsend, 1979). Further, there had been little research before our project which examined the effects of large-scale welfare state retrenchment on health inequalities and the limited research that did exist in this area was very macro in scale, often examining the impacts of welfare state changes on national or cross-national trends in inequalities in mortality (Fawcett et al., 2005; Blakely et al., 2008; Kreiger et al., 2008). Additionally, little attention had been paid to changes in the social determinants of health as a result of rapid welfare state contraction although data from cross-national studies suggest that differences in the generosity of out-of-work benefits and conditionality could well have important impacts on inequalities in health (Bambra and Eikemo, 2009). Further, until our Stockton project, studies of the effects of economic downturns and austerity on health inequalities tended to either be conducted on a large national scale, with little ability to account for differences at the local level, or focused only on the health of specific groups such as the unemployed rather than on the whole community (Bambra, 2011). Differential health effects by gender were also lacking despite considerable changes in the labour market participation of women (Bambra, 2010). So we set up a localised study which explicitly examined the links between changes in macro political economy factors (austerity) and health inequalities.

Through using different methodological approaches and drawing on different disciplinary perspectives, we examined the effects of austerity on health inequalities in Stockton-on-Tees in a multi-faceted way. In Chapter Two, Mike Langthorne's historical research found important changes in inequalities in health in Stockton during the 1930s – the other key example of a period of deep economic recession and subsequent government cut backs. In his study of Stockton during the Great Depression, he found evidence of the detrimental health effects of poverty and unemployment with the poorest areas of Stockton suffering disproportionately high infant and overall mortality rates. In Chapter Three, Ramjee Bhandari's analysis of household survey data found mixed effects of the current period of austerity on health inequalities in Stockton – with increases in the gap between the most and least deprived neighbourhoods of Stockton in terms of physical health, but no change in the gap in terms of general health. He also found that there were no changes in the effects on the gap of the underlying compositional and contextual factors – with material and psychosocial factors and their interaction remaining the most important determinant of the health gap in Stockton-on-Tees both at the beginning and the end of the 18-month survey period. In Chapter Four, long-term ethnographic research by Kayleigh Garthwaite found growing external and internal stigma in people's everyday lives at a time of austerity and that experiences of place, social networks and communities, were all affected by austerity and cuts to the social security safety net. This was further reinforced by Kate Mattheys' qualitative research in Chapter Five into the lived experiences during austerity of people with mental health issues. She found that there were clear inequalities in experience based on where people lived and their own individual resources. People with mental health issues living in the most deprived neighbourhoods of Stockton particularly adversely affected by cuts to their welfare benefits and this is exacerbated their mental health conditions. However, in contrast, in Chapter Six, Nasima Akhter and colleagues' analysis of trends in inequalities in mental health using the household survey found that there was no significant increase in health inequalities during austerity in Stockton-on-Tees. Further, there were no changes in the underpinning social determinants. Throughout the study period, a large gap in mental health existed between the most and least deprived neighbourhoods of Stockton and this was as a result of the interaction of psychosocial and material factors. In her analysis of the specific experiences of mothers in one of the deprived neighbourhoods of Stockton-on-Tees, Amy Greer Murphy (Chapter Seven) found that these low-income women particularly negatively affected by changes to the welfare system and that this increased their stress and isolation and she also noted emerging mental health problems. Overall then we found mixed effects of austerity on health inequalities in Stockton-on-Tees – while there was little evidence from the quantitative survey of increases in health inequalities in Stockton during austerity, the qualitative research suggested that key groups – most notably mothers and people with mental health issues were particularly adversely affected.

The results of our qualitative research is therefore in keeping with broader research into the effects of austerity on health inequalities in the UK and internationally where studies suggest that austerity has increased existing health inequalities such as that between the North and the South of England and between deprived and affluent neighbourhoods. For example, Barr et al. (2015a) found that geographical inequalities in mental health and wellbeing increased at a higher rate between 2009 and 2013. Further, people living in more deprived areas have seen the largest increases in poor mental health (Barr et al., 2015b) and self-harm (Barnes et al., 2017). It has also been shown that austerity is having a disproportionate impact on the health of vulnerable groups especially those individuals and families, including children, on the lowest incomes or in receipt of welfare benefits (MacLeavy, 2011). Internationally, Niedzwiedz et al. (2016) found that reductions in spending levels or increased conditionality may have adversely affected the mental health of disadvantaged social groups. Our qualitative results are also therefore in keeping with research into welfare state retrenchment in the 1980s and 1990s. These studies found that reductions in the social safety net increased inequalities in premature mortality and infant mortality rates in the US (for example, Kreiger et al., 2008), all-cause mortality in New Zealand (for example, Pearce and Dorling, 2006), and life expectancy and mortality rates in the UK (for example, Scott-Samuel et al., 2014). Our qualitative research therefore adds weight to this international evidence base showing that social safety nets matter for health inequalities (Bartley and Blane, 1997). Reductions in the provision of welfare benefits for people who are experiencing poverty – either by being out of work (due to unemployment, lone parenthood or ill-health) or having low wages (in work poverty) – have negative health effects, particularly in terms of mental health and other related measures such as psychosocial stress. Because the reduction in welfare benefits and key local services (such as social services or leisure facilities) particularly affect people from more deprived neighbourhoods, austerity therefore has very negative implications for health inequalities by reducing the resources available to people in the most deprived communities to live a healthy life.

However, the findings from our quantitative analysis of the household survey data – that health inequalities remained fairly stable during austerity is in contrast with other national and international research. This may be as a result of some of the limitations of the survey (such as timing and sampling – as discussed further in the relevant chapters) but it may also be because participants in the survey were generally older than the general population with a higher proportion of people who were retired. This has important implications for how we interpret the results of the household survey as austerity measures particularly with regards to welfare reform, were targeted at working age people as well as children. Pensioners were largely protected (with the exception of reductions in social care which had the biggest impact on those over 85 years (Hiam et al., 2017). Most notably, the universal state pension and other universal allowances for older people such as the winter fuel allowance (Green et al., 2017) were either left untouched during austerity or were enhanced (for example, the pensions 'triple lock') while working-age and child-related benefits were cut (Green et al., 2017). Arguably, then, the survey findings are actually in keeping with the wider literature as the fact that the gap in mental health among an older group did not change over time potentially shows the importance of maintaining social safety nets. This is in keeping with other studies of the importance of pensions for health and health inequalities, including pan-European research by Lundberg and colleagues (2008) who found that increased expenditure on pensions improved older age mortality; Beckfield and Bambra (2016) who highlighted the importance of pensions for post-65 life expectancy; and Copeland and colleagues (2015) who noted the importance of social safety nets for stabilising health inequalities during times of recession.

Implications for research, policy and practice

Our study has major implications for research, policy and practice: first it shows the need for research into geographical inequalities in health to integrate political economy perspectives; second, for policy makers, it highlights the importance of universal social policy safety nets for health inequalities particularly in terms of vulnerable groups such as low-income women and mothers, those with mental health conditions and older people; and third, for public health practitioners to look beyond their focus on health behaviours when designing interventions to reduce health inequalities.

Research into geographical inequalities in health and the role of place in shaping health has focused almost exclusively on examining the effects of compositional and contextual factors and their inter-relationship (Cummins et al., 2007). Traditionally, geographical inequalities in health have been explained in terms of the effects of compositional and contextual factors (Bambra, 2016). More recently, it has been acknowledged that these two approaches are not mutually exclusive and that the health of places results from the interaction of people with the wider environment – the relational perspective (Cummins et al., 2007). While this body of work has advanced our understanding of the effects of local neighbourhoods on health considerably, and re-established an awareness of the importance of place for health, it has arguably done so by privileging horizontal influences and at the expense of marginalising and minimising the influences of vertical, macro political and economic structures on both place and health (Cummins et al., 2007; Bambra, 2016). Our study has overtly set out to examine health inequalities during a period of rapid economic change and it has important implications for geographical research, not just in terms of understanding the causes of geographical inequalities in health but also for theorising and implementing policy solutions. In their seminal paper on the relational nature of health and place, Cummins and colleagues highlighted the importance of vertical place-based influences on health, stating that researchers should 'incorporate scale into the analysis of contexts relevant for health …. For the local to the global' (Cummins et al., 2007: 1832). Further, Macintyre and colleagues (2002) note the importance of incorporating scale and into the analysis of contexts. Elsewhere in epidemiology, other commentators have asserted the importance of political economy approaches for understanding health inequalities (for example, Schrecker and Bambra, 2015; Beckfield, 2018). In this project, we built on the analytical space opened up by these authors by outlining what one example of such a scaled up political economy approach to understanding the relationship between health and place looks like – looking beyond individual and local factors to thinking through the health implications of the wider political and economic context. We urge other researchers to build on our work so that they can make a contribution to political and policy efforts to reduce place-based health inequalities, by identifying the policy levers with the most potential to reduce health inequalities, at both local and national levels.

In terms of policies to reduce health inequalities, then, our project has further highlighted the importance of universal social policy safety nets for health inequalities particularly in terms of vulnerable groups such as low-income women and mothers, those with mental health conditions, and older people. Austerity has led to severe and rapid decreases in social security benefits for working age people in and out of work and reduced the support available to children growing up in low-income neighbourhoods or families. Our study has shown that this has had negative implications for health – particularly among the most vulnerable groups. Relatedly, our research has also suggested that the maintenance of social safety nets for pensioners may have protected their health – and prevented health inequalities in Stockton increasing. This is in keeping with a wider body of research into the effects of social policies on health and health inequalities and suggests that a basic social security safety net is essential for preventing an increase in health inequalities. It suggests that the effects of austerity have not been shared equally – people in the UK were not 'all in it together' as Prime Minister David Cameron claimed (Cameron, 2010) – but that certain groups have been more adversely affected than others. Health inequalities are not just an issue though for those most affected, but also for our wider society. For example, an European Union-level analysis suggested that the costs of health inequalities amounted to EUR 980 billion per year, or 9.4% of gross domestic product (GDP) – as a result of lost productivity and health care and welfare costs (Mackenbach et al., 2011). Similarly, in England, over 250,000 excess hospitalisations were associated with health inequalities (Cookson et al., 2018) with an estimated cost to the English NHS of £4.8 billion per year (Asaria et al., 2016). Analysis has also suggested that increasing the health of the lowest 50% of the European population to the average health of the top 50% would improve labour productivity by 1.4% of GDP each year – meaning that within five years of these improvements, GDP would be more than 7% higher (Mackenbach et al., 2011). So austerity has negative implications health care spending, productivity and competitiveness – the latter are becoming particular concerns for the UK in light of Brexit.

In terms of more day-to-day public health practice, our project has shown the need for practitioners to look beyond their long-term focus on health behaviours when designing interventions to reduce health inequalities. We found that inequalities in health behaviours were the least important determinant of the health gap between the most and least deprived neighbourhoods of Stockton-on-Tees-health behaviours did matter when they interacted with psychosocial, material and contextual place-based factors. Our study therefore suggests two things, first that practitioners need to look beyond just focusing on health behaviours if they want to reduce health inequalities; and second, that behavioural change interventions need to understand the wider context within which they are taking place (Bambra, 2018). Evidence suggest that behavioural interventions – however well intended – (such as smoking cessation or health education interventions (Lorenc et al., 2013; Thomson et al., 2018) – are unlikely to reduce health inequalities – and might actually increase them (Bambra, 2018) unless they also address the contextual determinants of health such as by using regulatory (for example, age restrictions, standardised packaging, fast food marketing restrictions) or fiscal approaches (e.g. tobacco pricing; food subsidy programmes) (Lorenc et al., 2013; Thomson et al.,

2018). So our study suggests that a more context driven approach is required that combines behavioural interventions with more place-based interventions. An example of a successful set of interventions which combined 'upstream' and 'downstream' approaches to reduce health inequalities is the English Health Inequalities strategy that ran from 1997 to 2010 (outlined earlier in this chapter) and which led to some reductions in inequalities in life expectancy and infant mortality rates (Mackenbach, 2011; Bambra, 2012; Barr et al., 2014; Bambra, 2016; Barr et al., 2017). However, our project, in highlighting the importance of political and economic factors most notably austerity – means that it must be acknowledged that the efforts of local public health practitioners are likely to only have limited effects on health inequalities when they are fighting against the tide of austerity.

References

Acheson, D. (chair) (1998) *Independent inquiry into inequalities in health.* London: TSO

Agnew, J. (2011) Space and place, in *The SAGE handbook of geographical knowledge*, J. Agnew and D. Livingstone, Editors. Sage: London. p. 316–330

Arber, S. and Cooper, H. (1999) Gender differences in health in later life: the new paradox? *Social Science & Medicine*, 48: 61–76

Asaria M., Doran T., Cookson R. (2016) The costs of inequality: whole-population modelling study of lifetime inpatient hospital costs in the English National Health Service by level of neighbourhood deprivation. *Journal of Epidemiology and Community Health*, 70(10): 990–6

Bambra, C. (2010) Yesterday once more? An analysis of unemployment and health in the 21st century. *Journal of Epidemiology and Community Health*, 64: 213–215

Bambra, C. (2011) *Work, worklessness and the political economy of health.* Oxford University Press

Bambra, C. (2012) Reducing health inequalities: New data suggests that the English strategy was partially successful. *Journal of Epidemiology and Community Health*, 10.1136/jech-2011-200945

Bambra, C. (2016) *Health inequalities: where you live can kill you*, Bristol: Policy Press

Bambra, C. (2018) First do no harm: Developing interventions that combat addiction without increasing inequalities. *Addiction*, 113: 787–788

Bambra, C. and Eikemo, T. (2009) Welfare state regimes, unemployment and health: A comparative study of the relationship between unemployment and self-reported health in 23 European countries. *Journal of Epidemiology and Community Health*, 63: 92–98

Bambra, C., Barr, B. and Milne, E. (2014) North and South: addressing the English health divide, *Journal of Public Health*, 36: 183–186

Barnes, M. C., Donovan, J. L., Wilson, C., Chatwin, J., Davies, R., Potokar, J., et al. (2017) Seeking help in times of economic hardship: access, experiences of services and unmet need. *BMC Psychiatry*, 17: 84

Barr, B., Bambra, C., and Whitehead, M. (2014) The impact of NHS resource allocation policy on health inequalities in England 2001–2011: longitudinal ecological study. *BMJ*, 348: g3231

Barr, B., Kinderman, P., and Whitehead, P. (2015a) Trends in mental health inequalities in England during a period of recession, austerity and welfare reform 2004–2013. *Social Science & Medicine* 147: 324–331

Barr, B., Taylor-Robinson, D., Stuckler, D., Loopstra, R., Reeves, A., Whitehead, M. (2015b) 'First, do no harm': are disability assessments associated with adverse trends in mental health? A longitudinal ecological study. *Journal of Epidemiology and Community Health*, 70: 1–7

Barr, B., Higgerson, J., Whitehead, M. (2017) Investigating the impact of the English health inequalities strategy: time trend analysis, *BMJ*, 358: j3310

Bartley, M. (2004) *Health inequality: An introduction to theories, concepts and methods*. Cambridge: Polity Press

Bartley, M. and Blane, D. (1997) Health and the lifecourse: Why safety nets matter. *BMJ*, 314:, 1194–1196

Beckfield, J. (2018) *Political sociology and the people's health*, Oxford, New York

Beckfield, J and Bambra, C. (2016) Shorter lives in stingier states: Social policy shortcomings help explain the US mortality disadvantage, *Social Science & Medicine*, 170: 30–38

Beynon, H. (1973) *Working for Ford*. Milton Keynes, Open University Press.

Black, D. (chair) (1980) *Inequalities in health: The Black Report*. London: Pelican

Blackman, T., Wistow, J., and Byrne, D. (2011) A qualitative comparative analysis of factors associated with trends in narrowing health inequalities in England. *Social Science & Medicine*, 72: 1965–1974

Blakely, T., Tobias, M. et al. (2008) Inequalities in mortality during and after restructuring of the New Zealand economy: repeated cohort studies. *Brit Med J*, 336: 371–375

Booth, C. (1889–97) *Life and labour of the people of London vols 1–9*. London, Macmillan

Cairns, J. M. C. and Bambra, C. (2013) Defying the odds: A mixed-methods study of health resilience in deprived areas of England. *Social Science & Medicine*, 91: 229–237

Cameron, D. (2010) Big Society Speech, www.gov.uk/government/speeches/big-society-speech

Chadwick, E. (1842) *Report on the sanitary conditions of the labouring classes in Britain*. London: HMSO

Chow, C. K., Lock, K., Teo, K., et al. (2009) Environmental and societal influences acting on cardiovascular risk factors and disease at a population level: a review. *Int J Epidemiol*. 38: 1580–1594

Cookson, R., Asaria, M., Ali, S., Shaw, R., Doran, T., Goldblatt, P. (2018) Health equity monitoring for healthcare quality assurance. *Social Science & Medicine*, 198: 148–56

Copeland, A., Bambra, C., Nylen, L., Kasim, A. S., Riva, M., Curtis, S., and Burstrom, B. (2015) All in it together? The effects of recession on population health and health inequalities in England and Sweden, 1991 to 2010. *International Journal of Health Services*, 45: 3–24

Crenshaw, K. (1991) Mapping the margins: Intersectionality, identity politics, and violence against women of color. *Stanford Law Review*, 1241–1299

Crenshaw, K. (2001) First decade: critical reflections, or a foot in the closing door. *UCLA Law Re-View*, 49, 1343–1394

Cummins, S., Curtis, S., Diez-Roux, A. et al. (2007) Understanding and representing 'place' in health research: A relational approach. *Social Science & Medicine*, 65: 1825–1838

Dennis, N., Henriques, F., and Slaughter, C. (1956) *Coal is our life*. London, Routledge

Dorling, D. (2001) Anecdote is the singular of data. *Environment and Planning A*, 33: 1335–1340

Dorling, D., Smith, G., Noble, M. et al. (2001) How much does place matter? *Environment and Planning A*, 33: 1335–1369

Fawcett, J., Blakely, T. and Kunst, A. (2005) Are mortality differences and trends by education any better or worse in New Zealand? A comparison study with Norway, Denmark and Finland, 1980–1990s. *European Journal of Epidemiology*, 20, 683–691

Gamble, A. (2009) *The spectre at the feast: Capitalist crisis and the politics of recession*. Basingstoke: Palgrave

Gkiouleka, A., Huijts, T., Beckfield, J., Bambra, C. (2018) Understanding the micro and macro politics of health: inequalities, intersectionality and institutions – a research agenda, *Social Science & Medicine*, 200: 92–98

Golding, A. M. B. (2006) Sir Edwin Chadwick and inequalities. *Public Health*, 120: 474–476

Goldthorpe, J. (1963) *The affluent worker: Political attitudes and behaviour*. Cambridge: Cambridge University Press

Green, JM, Buckner, S., Milton, S., Powell, K., Salway, S. and Moffatt, S. (2017) A model of how targeted and universal welfare entitlements impact on material, psycho-social and structural determinants of health in older adults. *Social Science & Medicine*, 187: 20–28

Hiam, L., Dorling, D., Harrison, D., and McKee, M. (2017) Why has mortality in England and Wales been increasing? An iterative demographic analysis, *Journal of the Royal Society of Medicine*, 110: 153–162

Hill, S. (2016) Axes of health inequalities and intersectionality, in *Health inequalities: Critical perspectives*, K. E. Smith, S. Hill and C. Bambra, Editors. Oxford University Press: Oxford

Hunter, D., Popay, J., Tannahill, C. and Whitehead, M. (2010) Getting to grips with health inequalities at last? *BMJ*, 340: c684

Jahoda, M.,Lazarsfeld, P., Zeisel, H. (1971 [1930]) *Marienthal: The sociography of an unemployed community*. New Brunswick, NJ, Transaction

Joyce, K. E., Smith, K. E., Bambra, C. et al. (2010) 'Most of industry's shutting down up here...': employability initiatives to tackle worklessness in areas of low labour market demand. *Social Policy and Society*, 9: 337–353

Kondo, N., Subramanian, S., Kawachi, I., Takeda, Y. and Yamagata, Z. (2008) Economic recession and health inequalities in Japan: analysis with a national sample, 1986–2001. *Journal of Epidemiology and Community Health*, 62: 869–875

Krieger N. (2003) 'Theories for social epidemiology in the twenty-first century: an ecosocial perspective', in: R. Hofrichter (ed) *Health and social justice: Politics, ideology, and inequity in the distribution of disease – a public health reader*. San Francisco: Jossey-Bass, pp. 428–450

Krieger, N., D. H. Rehkopf, et al. (2008) The fall and rise of US inequities in premature mortality: 1960–2002. *PLoS Medicine*, 5: 227–241

Lahelma, E., Kivela, K., Roos, E., Tuominen, T., Dahl, E., Diderichsen, F. et al. (2002) Analysing changes of health inequalities in the Nordic welfare states. *Social Science & Medicine*, 55: 609–25

Lorenc T., Petticrew M., Welch V., Tugwell P. (2013) What types of interventions generate inequalities? Evidence from systematic reviews. *J Epidemiol Community Health*, 67: 190–93

Lundberg, O., Yngwe, M., Kölegård Stjärne, M., Elstad, J., Ferrarini, T., Kangas, O. (2008) The role of welfare state principles and generosity in social policy programmes for public health: an international comparative study. *Lancet*, 372: 1633–40

Macintyre, S. (2003) Before and After the Black Report: Four Fallacies. In V. Berridge and S. Blume (eds) *Poor health: Social inequalities before and after the Black Report*. London: Frank Cass: 198–219

Macintyre, S., Maciver, S. et al. (1993) Area, class and health: should we be focusing on places or people? *Journal of Social Policy*, 16: 213–234

Macintyre, S., Ellaway, A. and Cummins, S. (2002) Place effects on health: How can we conceptualise, operationalise and measure them? *Social Science & Medicine*, 55(1): 125–139

Mackenbach, J. P. (2011) Can we reduce health inequalities? An analysis of the English strategy (1997–2010) *J Epidemiol Community Health*, 65: 568

Mackenbach, J. P., Meerding, W. J. and Kunst, A. E. (2011) Economic costs of health inequalities in the European Union. *Journal of Epidemiology & Community Health*, 65(5):412–419

MacLeavy, J. (2011) A 'new politics' of austerity, workfare and gender? The UK coalition government's welfare reform proposals. *Cambridge Journal of Regions, Economy and Society*, 4: 355–367

Marmot, M. (2010) *Fair society, healthy lives: the Marmot review*. London: University College

Niedzwiedz, C. L. Mitchell, R. J. Shortt, N. K. and Pearce, J. R. (2016) Social protection spending and inequalities in depressive symptoms across Europe. *Social Psychiatry and Psychiatric Epidemiology*: 1–10

ONS – Office for National Statistics (2015) Inequality in healthy life expectancy at birth by national deciles of area deprivation: England, 2011 to 2013

Pahl, R. (2005) Are all communities in the mind? *Sociological Review*, 53: 621–40

Pearce, J. and Dorling, D. (2006) Increasing geographical inequalities in health in New Zealand, 1980–2001. *International Journal of Epidemiology*, 35(3): 597–603

Rowntree, J. (1901) *Poverty: A study of town life*. London, Macmillan

Savage, M. (2008) A note on the ancestoral Toronto home of social network analysis. *Connections*, 18: 15–19

Schrecker, T and Bambra, C. (2015) *How politics makes us sick: Neoliberal epidemics*, London: Palgrave Macmillan

Scott-Samuel, A., Bambra, C., Collins, C., Hunter, D., McCartney, G., and Smith, K. (2014) The impact of Thatcherism on health and well-being in Britain, *International Journal of Health Services*, 44(1): 53–71

Smith, KE., Bambra, C and Hill, S. (2016) Chapter 1: Background and introduction: UK experiences of health inequalities, in K. E. Smith, S. Hill, and C. Bambra (eds) *Health inequalities: Critical perspectives*, Oxford, Oxford University Press

Studdert, D. (2006) *Conceptualising community: Beyond the state and the individual*. Basingstoke, Palgrave

Taylor-Gooby, P. (2012) Root and branch restructuring to achieve major cuts: The social policy programme of the 2010 UK coalition government. *Social Policy and Administration*, 46: 61–82

Thomson, K., Hillier-Brown, F., McNamara, C., Huijits, T., Todd, A and Bambra, C. (2018) The effects of public health policies on health inequalities in European welfare states: umbrella review, *BMC Public Health*, 18(1): 869

Townsend, P. (1979) *Poverty in the United Kingdom*. London, Pelican

Valkonen, T., Martikainen, P., Jalovaara, M., Koskinen, S., Martelin, T. and Makela, P. (2000) Changes in socioeconomic inequalities in mortality during an economic boom and recession among middle-aged men and women in Finland. *European Journal of Public Health*, 10, 274–80

Walkerdine, V. and Jimenez, L. (2012) *Gender, work and community after de-industrialisation: A psychosocial approach to affect*. Basingstoke, Palgrave

Whyte, W. (1993 [1944]) *Street Corner Society: The social structure of an Italian slum*. Chicago, University of Chicago Press

Index

Note: page numbers in *italic* type refer to Figures; those in **bold** type refer to Tables.

A
Affordable Homes Programme 64
air pollution 6, 7, 98
  see also pollution
alcohol consumption 3, 80, 97, 122–3,
    134, 161, 177, 181, 186, 190, 241
  Stockton-on-Tees health inequalities
    comparative study 89, 93
  see also behavioural factors in health
    inequalities
anger, among benefits claimants 153–4
asylum seekers 128
austerity 12–13
  and diet and nutrition 16–17, 19,
    58, 59–60
  and family life 109, 129–34, 136
  and health inequalities 18–21,
    82–3, 233, 240–5
  and mental health 82, 141–65, 171,
    174–5
  and middle classes 131–4, 136
  and mothers 26–27, 201–3, 225,
    243
    background and context 203–6
    employment 205, 210, 212–14,
      215
    intersectionality and invisible
      inequalities 201, 202–3, 206,
      222–4, *224*, 225, 238
    mental health issues 202,
      217–22, *221*
    mothers' roles 201–2, 209–17,
      225
    research methodology 206–8,
      207
  Stockton-on-Tees ethnographic
    study 129–35

UK 13, **14**, 15–18, *16*, *17*, 35–6,
    82–3, 99–100, 172, 174, 175,
    191, 203–6, 241–2
  see also Great Recession
Australia 98

B
Baltimore, USA 6
Bath, UK 235
Bay Street, Stockton-on-Tees 44
bedroom tax (under-occupancy charge)
    13, **14**, 96, 147, 204, 205, 219
'behavioural-cultural' theory 80
behavioural factors in health inequalities
    4, 80, 176–7, 237, 238, 240,
    247, 248
  Stockton-on-Tees:
    ethnographic study 114–16, 134
    health inequalities comparative
      study **92**, **94**
    mental health longitudinal
      household survey comparative
      study 171, 180, 181, 186–7,
      187, 188, **188**, 190, 193, 194
Benefit Cap 204
'Benefits Britain: Life on the Dole'
    television programme 144
benefits sanctions 17, 58–9, 130,
    152–3, 209
'Benefits Street' television programme
    119, 121, 144, 154
Black Report (1980) 236
Blackpool, UK 15
Booth, Charles 233
brownfield land 6

C
CAB (Citizens Advice Bureau) 111,
    127, 129, 145, 146, 154, 160–1,
    164, 165

Cameron, David 13, 203, 247
'Cancer Alley' Mississippi, USA 6
capitalist economy, and social
    reproduction 205, 211
Care and Support Specialised Housing
    Fund 64
Carer's Allowance 219, 222
case study approach to research 233–5
Chadwick, Edwin 236
Chamberlain, Neville 40
Chicago School of urban ethnography
    233
Child Benefit 204
child poverty 16, 206
Citizens Advice Bureau (CAB) 111,
    127, 129, 145, 146, 154, 160–1,
    164, 165
class issues:
    and place-based case studies
        233–4
    and women 214–17
coalition government 2010–2015
    (Conservatives and Liberal
    Democrats) 13, 236–7
    see also Cameron, David
collective resources model 7
collective social functioning 5–6
Committee on National Expenditure
    1931 (May Committee) 39, 40
community, contested nature of 235
community networks, Stockton-on-
    Tees 126–8
Community Right to Build 64
compositional factors in health
    inequalities 2–4, 7–8, 24–5, 77,
    78, 80, 81, 87, **88–9**, 91, **92**,
    93–4, **94**, *94*, 95, 96, 98–9, 100,
    109–10, 239, 240, 243, 245
conditionality **14**, 19, 82, 151, 152,
    201–2, 209, 211, 242, 244
    see also welfare reforms
Conservative government 2010–present
    13, 236–7
    see also Cameron, David; coalition
    government 2010–2015
    (Conservatives and Liberal
    Democrats)

contextual factors in health inequalities
    2, 4–8, 24–5, 77, 78, 80, 81, 89,
    89, 91, **92**, 93–4, **94**, *94*, 95, 96,
    97–8, 98–9, 100, 109–10, 239,
    240, 243, 245, 247–8
Copeland, West Cumbria 6
cost of living 146, 149
costs, of health inequalities 247
council housing, Stockton-on-Tees
    47–8
County Durham, Great Depression,
    1930s 37–8
credit, cost of 148–9
crime 89, 95, 161, 181
    see also material factors in health
        inequalities

D

debt 172, 219
deindustrialisation, Stockton-on-Tees
    23
demography 80
Denmark 11, 12
deprivation amplification 7, 96, 176
'deserving' cases 51–2
diet and nutrition 3, 5, 80, 134, 148,
    177, 181, 187
    and austerity policies 16–17, 19,
        58, 59–60
    and mental health 173
    Stockton-on-Tees 58–9, 65, 66
        Great Depression 1930s 41, 48,
            52–3, 57–8, 65–6
    see also behavioural factors in health
        inequalities
disabilities, people with 155–6, 233
DLA (Disability Living Allowance)
    130, 145
drug abuse 3, 80, 117, 120, 122–3, 161

E

East of England 15
economic stimulus policies 18, 174
Education Maintenance Allowance
    (EMA) 147

EMA (Education Maintenance
Allowance) 147
'empathetic ethnographers' 136–7
employment:
    barriers to 159
    and mental health 142, 154–9
    precarity 129, 131–2, 142, 155
    psychosocial working environment
        79, 158–9
    as social determinant of health 79
    Stockton-on-Tees:
        health inequalities comparative
            study 93, 95
        longitudinal household survey
            comparative study 183, 189,
            191
        and women/mothers 205, 210,
            212–14, 215
    voluntary reduction in 150
Employment and Support Allowance
    (ESA) 129, 130, 145, 147,
    151–2
England:
    austerity policies, impact of 15
    health, impact of recessions on
        11–12
    mental health, impact of recessions
        on 10–11
    see also UK
environment:
    environmental deprivation 7
    material physical environment
        variables, Stockton-on-Tees
        mental health longitudinal
        household survey comparative
        study 180, 181, 184–5, **185**,
        188, **188**, 193
    see also material factors in health
        inequalities
environmental mechanism 81
EQ5D measure 84, 85, 86, 90, **90**, *91*
ESA (Employment and Support
    Allowance) 129, 130, 145, 147,
    151–2
ethnicity/race 80, 238
    racial tension 127–8
    see also intersectionality

European Union 240
exercise and physical activity 3, 5, 80,
    93, 97, 122, 177, 181, 186, 190
    see also behavioural factors in health
        inequalities

F
family life, and austerity 109, 129–34,
    136
Fannie Mae 9
fast food 5, 122
    see also diet and nutrition; obesity
fatalism 113, 116–17
Fawcett Society 202
financial crisis, 2007 see Great
    Recession
Finland 11, 12, 241
food see diet and nutrition
foodbanks 16–17, 19, 58, 59, 82, 111,
    129, 132
France 10
Freddie Mac 9
fuel poverty 17–18

G
gender 12
    see also intersectionality; mothers;
        women
General Health Questionnaire
    (GHQ12) 10–11
gentrification 127
geographical factors in health
    inequalities 80–82
Germany 174
GHQ12 (General Health
    Questionnaire) 10–11
Glasgow Centre for Population Health
    219
gold standard 36, 37
'Great British Benefits Handout, The'
    television programme 144
Great Depression, 1930s 10, 35,
    36–7
    Stockton-on-Tees 23, 24, 35–6, 37,
        65–6, 240, 242

Great Depression, 1930s (CONTINUED)
   comparison with current
      conditions 58–65, *60*, *61*, *62*
   health and healthcare 48, *49*,
      50–2, 66
   housing *42*, 42–8, *43*, *47*, *49*,
      50, *60*, 60–1, *61*, 66
   unemployment 37–42, *38*, *39*, *40*
Great Recession 9, 171–2, 241
   and health inequalities 82–3
   and mental health 11, 174
   suicide rates 11, 174
   unemployment rates 10, 172
   see also austerity policies
Greece 9, 11, 174
   austerity policies 13, 18, 96, 174
green spaces 6–7, 162

H
happiness 96
Hartburn ward, Stockton-on-Tees 1,
   42, 43, 62, 63
   ethnographic study 111–12,
      114–15, 122, 123–4, 125–6,
      126–7, 132–4, 136
health:
   impact of austerity policies on
      18–21
   impact of recessions on 10–12,
      241
   and poverty 115–16
   social determinants of 79–83
   Stockton-on-Tees, Great Depression
      1930s 52–8, *54*, *55*, *56*, *57*, 66
   WHO definition 78
health behaviours 2, 3, 80
   see also behavioural factors in health
      inequalities
health inequalities 1–2
   and austerity 18–21, 82–3, 233,
      240–5
   compositional factors 2–4, 7–8,
      24–5, 77, 78, 80, 81, 87, **88–9**,
      91, **92**, 93–4, **94**, *94*, 95, 96,
      98–9, 100, 109–10, 239, 240,
      243, 245

contextual factors 2, 4–8, 24–5, 77,
   78, 80, 81, 89, **89**, 91, **92**, 93–4,
   94, *94*, 95, 96, 97–8, 98–9, 100,
   109–10, 239, 240, 243, 245, 247–8
costs of 247
geographical factors 80–2
and the Great Recession 82–3
impact of recessions on 10–12
lay perspectives on 109, 110,
   113–20
and place 233, 235–40
political economy factors 2, 8–9,
   24, 239, 240, 245, 246
relational factors 2, 7–8, 25, 77, 80,
   81–2, 98–9, 100, 220, 239–40,
   245
and socioeconomic status 237, 238,
   239
Stockton-on-Tees 234–5
   comparative study 77–8,
      83–100, *84*, **85**, **87**, **88–9**,
      90, **91**, **92**, **94**, *94*, 242–3
   ethnographic study 109, 110–37
   Great Depression 1930s 55–6,
      56, *57*
   see also behavioural factors in health
      inequalities; material factors in
      health inequalities; psychosocial
      factors in health inequalities
healthcare services, Stockton-on-Tees,
   Great Depression 1930s 48, *49*,
   50–2
heart disease, causes of 8
HHSRS (Housing Health and Safety
   Rating System) 64
hobbies 149–50
housing 95
   'decent' housing criteria 64
   and mental health 142, 173, *221*,
      221–2
   as social determinant of health 79
   Stockton-on-Tees 63–5, 66–7, 89
      Great Depression, 1930s *42*,
         42–8, *43*, *47*, 48, *49*, 50, 60,
         60, 60–1, *61*, 66
   see also material factors in health
      inequalities

Housing (Financial Provisions) Act
1933 45
Housing Benefit 13, **14**, 64, 165, 183,
204, 216
Housing Health and Safety Rating
System (HHSRS) 64

I
IB (Incapacity Benefit) 145
Iceland 18, 174
IMD (Index of Multiple Deprivation)
scores 83, 177, 179
IMF (International Monetary Fund) 9,
172
immigrants 128
Incapacity Benefit (IB) 145
Income Support 222
Index of Multiple Deprivation (IMD)
scores 83, 177, 179
Indonesia 18
infant mortality rates 3, 59
Stockton-on-Tees, Great Depression
1930s 54–5, *55*, 56, *56*, *57*,
57–8
institutional mechanism 79, 81
International Labour Organization
172
International Monetary Fund (IMF) 9,
172
intersectionality 201, 202–3, 206,
222–4, *224*, 225, 238–9
Ireland 174
Italy 9, 13, 174

J
Japan 11, 241
JSA (Job Seeker's Allowance) 130, 145,
147, 151, 152, 222
judgemental attitudes 118–20, 134,
135

K
Keynes, John Maynard 36
King Street, Stockton-on-Tees 44

L
Labour governments 1997–2010 236,
237
land pollution 6, 7
see also pollution
'landscapes of risk' 160
lay perspectives on health inequalities
109, 110, 113–20
Lehmann Brothers 9
Liberal Democrats *see* coalition
government 2010–2015
(Conservatives and Liberal
Democrats)
life expectancy 1, 59, 80, 235–6,
244
Stockton-on-Tees 63, 77, 204,
218
'lifestyle drift' 194, 236, 237, 238
Liverpool 235–6
living environment 5
and mental health 159–63, 220–2,
221
as social determinant of health
79
Stockton-on-Tees health inequalities
comparative study 89, 95
living standards decline 147
local authority spending cuts 15, 172,
203, 204
see also austerity
London, UK 18
loneliness 96, 97
Love Canal, New York 6
LSOA (lower super output areas) 83,
86, 177, 179, 180
luck 117
Luxembourg 174

M
MacDonald, Ramsay 36, 37
Malaysia 18
material factors in health inequalities 3,
80, 96, 146, 174–5, 237, 238
Stockton-on-Tees 240, 243
health inequalities comparative
study **92**, **94**

material factors in health inequalities
(CONTINUED)
Stockton-on-Tees (CONTINUED)
mental health longitudinal
household survey comparative
study 171, 180–1, 183–4,
184, 184–5, **185**, 188, **188**,
189, 190, 193, 194
material physical environment variables,
Stockton-on-Tees mental health
longitudinal household survey
comparative study 180, 181,
184–5, **185**, 188, **188**, 193
material socioeconomic variables,
Stockton-on-Tees mental health
longitudinal household survey
comparative study 180–1,
183–4, **184**, 188, **188**, 193
maternity care, Stockton-on-Tees
50–1, 52
May Committee (Committee on
National Expenditure 1931) 39,
40
Mayor's Clothing Bureau 41
Mayor's Committee for the Help of the
Unemployed 3
mental health 97, 244
and austerity 82, 141–65, 171,
174–5
background and context 142–4
concepts of 173
and employment 142, 154–9
Great Recession 11, 174
and housing 142, 173, *221*, 221–2
impact of recessions on 10–11
importance of universal social policy
safety net for 245, 246
inequalities in 19, 173–5
and living environment 159–63,
220–2, *221*
medical models of 142–3
models of causes of inequalities
175–7
and place 159–63, 220–2, *221*
and poverty 142, 146–7, 163–4,
173
and social inequality 174–5

social models of 143
social security system 150–4
and socioeconomic status 142, 173,
175
Stockton-on-Tees 25–6
austerity policies study 141–65,
240, 243
ethnographic study 123, 135
longitudinal household survey
comparative study 171–94,
178, *179*, **183**, **184**, **185**,
186, **187**, *188*, *189*, *192*
and unemployment 79, 142, 175
Merthyr Tydfil 136
M'Gonigle, George 23, 24, 35, 45, 46,
47, 48, 50–1, 52, 53, 57–8, 66
middle classes, and austerity 131–4, 136
Ministry of Health 45, 48, 52
mortality rates:
impact of recessions on 10
Stockton-on-Tees 65, 66
Great Depression 1930s 53–4, *54*
and unemployment 95
mothers 26–7, 201–3, 225, 243
background and context 203–6
and employment 205, 210, 212–14,
215
intersectionality and invisible
inequalities 201, 202–3, 206,
222–4, *224*, 225, 238
mental health issues 202, 217–22,
221
mothers' roles 201–2, 209–17, 225
research methodology 206–8, *207*
SAHM (stay at home mothers) 209,
211–12
social reproduction role of 202,
205–6, 209–11, 224, 225
see also gender; women

N
National Health Service (NHS) 67, 236
National Unemployed Worker's
Movement (NUWM) 41–2
New Labour *see* Labour governments
1997–2010

'new welfare commonsense' 135
New Zealand 19, 20, 244
NHS (National Health Service) 67,
    236
Niedzwiedz, C.L. 19, 82, 244
noise problems 161, 181
    Stockton-on-Tees health inequalities
        comparative study 89, 95, 98
    see also material factors in health
        inequalities
North East of England 15, 16, 18, 172
North of England 1, 15, 18, 19, 236,
    244
North West of England 15–16, 18
Northern Ireland 11
Northern Rock 9
Northumberland and Durham Property
    Owners' and Ratepayers'
    Association 46–7
Norway 11, 12
NUWM (National Unemployed
    Worker's Movement) 41–2

O
obesity 5, 6, 80, 116, 122–3
older people 82, 244–5
    importance of universal social policy
        safety net for 233, 245, 246
opportunity structures 5, 79, 81, 193
Orr, John Boyd 48
'Others' 136
overcrowding 45–8, 47, 66–7
    see also housing

P
pathogenic places 2, 4
pensioner households 15, 245
    see also older people
Personal Independence Payment (PIP)
    145, 219
Personal Service League 41
physical activity see exercise and physical
    activity
PIP (Personal Independence Payment)
    145, 219

place 1–2
    and health inequalities 233, 235–40
    and meaning in Stockton-on-Tees
        109
    and mental health 159–63, 220–2,
        221
    salutogenic and pathogenic 2, 4
place attachment 6
Poland 174
policy:
    research, policy and practice
        implications 233, 245–8
political economy factors in health
    inequalities 2, 8–9, 24, 239,
    240, 245, 246
pollution 181
    Stockton-on-Tees health inequalities
        comparative study 89, 95, 98
    see also air pollution; land pollution;
        material factors in health
        inequalities
Portugal 9, 13, 96, 174
poverty 4
    and health 115–16
    impact of austerity policies on 15–16
    and mental health 142, 146–7,
        163–4, 173
'poverty porn' television programmes
    119, 121, 144, 154
'poverty premium' 148–9
powerlessness 153
practice:
    research, policy and practice
        implications 233, 245–8
Priestley, J.B. 23
psychosocial factors in health
    inequalities 3–4, 80, 96–7, 176,
        219
    Stockton-on-Tees 240, 243
        ethnographic study 116
        health inequalities comparative
            study 92, 94
        mental health longitudinal
            household survey comparative
            study 171, 180, 181, 185–6,
            186, 188, 188–9, 189,
            189–90, 193–4

psychosocial working environment 79,
    158–9
Public Health Act 1848 236

Q
Queen Street, Stockton-on-Tees 44

R
race *see* ethnicity/race
racial tension 127–8
recessions:
    definitions 10, 171
    impact on health and health
        inequalities 10–12, 174, 241
    see also Great Recession
relational factors in health inequalities
    2, 7–8, 25, 77, 80, 81–2, 98–9,
    100, 220, 239–40, 245
rent arrears 165
'resilient' areas 241
Robson Maternity Home 50–1
Rowntree, Joseph 233

S
safety 89, 98, 124–6, 161, 181
    see also material factors in health
        inequalities; psychosocial factors
        in health inequalities
SAHM (stay at home mothers) 209,
    211–12
salutogenic places 2, 4
Salvation Army 41
sanctions 17, 58–9, 130, 152–3, 209
'scroungers' 135, 211
sex work, Stockton-on-Tees 125
SF 8 measure 84, 85, 180, 193
    MCS (Mental Component
        Summary) 86, 180, 182, **183**,
        187, **188**, *188*, 188–9, *189*,
        189–90, 193
    PCS (Physical Component
        Summary) 86, 90, **90**, 91, *91*,
        92, 93, **94**, 98–9, 180
'shirkers' 143

slum clearance, Stockton-on-Tees
    44–5, 47, 48, *49*, 50, 55, *60*,
    60–1, *61*
smoking 3, 80, 89, 97, 116, 117, 134,
    177, 181, 241
    see also behavioural factors in health
        inequalities
social capital 5
social cohesion 5
social inequality, and mental health
    174–5
social-interactive mechanism 81
social networks, Stockton-on-Tees
    126–8
social reproduction role of women
    202, 205–6, 209–11, 224, 225
    see also mothers, and austerity
socioeconomic status 2, 3–4, 80, 87
    and health inequalities 237, 238,
        239
    and mental health 142, 173, 175
South East of England 15, 16, 18
South East ward, Stockton-on-Tees 62
South of England 1, 18, 19, 236, 244
Spain 9, 10, 11, 13, 18, 174
stay at home mothers (SAHM) 209,
    211–12
stigma:
    and benefits claimants 153–4
    and judgemental attitudes 118–20,
        134, 135
    and place 5–6
        Stockton-on-Tees ethnographic
            study 110, 120–8, 135–6
        territorial stigmatisation 135–6,
            220
    and poverty 164
Stockton and Thornaby District
    Women's Association 41
Stockton and Thornaby Surgical
    Hospital 51
Stockton and Thornaby Unemployed
    Workers Association 42
Stockton-on-Tees:
    children's centres spending cuts 204
    community and social networks
        126–8

deindustrialisation 23
ethnographic study 109–13, 134–7
  family life and austerity 129–34
  lay perspectives on health
    inequalities 113–20
  place-based stigma 110, 120–8,
    135–6
Great Depression, 1930s 23, 24,
  35–6, 37, 65–6, 240, 242
  comparison with current
    conditions 58–65, *60*, *61*,
    62
  health and healthcare 48, *49*,
    50–2
  health inequalities 55–6, *56*,
    57
  housing *42*, 42–8, *43*, *47*, *60*,
    60–1, *61*
  infant mortality rates 54–5, *55*,
    56, *56*, *57*, 57–8
  mortality rates 53–4, *54*
  unemployment 37, *40*, 40–2,
    61–2, *62*
health inequalities 55–6, *56*, *57*,
  234–5
  comparative study 77–8,
    83–100, *84*, **85**, **87**, **88–89**,
    90, **91**, **92**, **94**, *94*, 242–3
  ethnographic study 109, 110–37
housing *42*, 42–8, *43*, *47*, 48, *49*,
  50, *60*, 60–1, *61*, 63–5, 66–7,
  89
Leverhulme study overview 23–7
life expectancy 1, 21, 63, 77, 204,
  218
living environment 89, 95
material factors in health inequalities
  92, **94**, 171, 180–1, 183–4, **184**,
  184–5, **185**, 188, **188**, 189, 190,
  193, 194, 240, 243
  material physical environment
    variables 180, 181, 184–5,
    185, 188, **188**, 193
  material socioeconomic variables
    180–1, 183–4, **184**, 188, **188**,
    193
maternity care 50–1, 52

mental health 25–6
  austerity policies study 141–65,
    240, 243
  ethnographic study 123, 135
  longitudinal household survey
    comparative study 171–94,
    178, *179*, **183**, **184**, **185**,
    186, **187**, *188*, *189*, *192*
  mortality rates 53–54, *54*, 65, 66
  noise problems 89, 95, 98
  overview and context 21, *22*, 23
  pollution 89, 95, 98
  regeneration programme 121–4
  safety and fear in 124–126
  slum clearance 44–5, 47, 48, *49*,
    50, 55, *60*, 60–1, *61*
  social networks 126–8
  unemployment 23
Strategic Housing Market Assessment
  (Stockton-on-Tees Borough
  Council) 63
'strivers' 143
stroke, causes of 8
suicides 11, 18, 153, 172, 174, 175,
  241
Sure Start programme 236
Sweden 11, 12, 174

T
tax credits 13, **14**, 204, 216, 217
territorial stigmatisation 135–6, 220
Thailand 18
Thatcher, Margaret 23
Thatcherism 20
'therapeutic landscapes' 160, 162
Town Centre ward, Stockton-on-Tees
  1, 61, 62, 63, 65, 67, 123–4,
  221
  ethnographic study 111, 117,
    119–20, 122–3, 126, 127, 128,
    129, 136
Transatlantic Trade and Investment
  Partnership 240
trauma, and health 115–16, 144
'triple jeopardy' of women 202, 205
Trussell Trust 17, 59, 111

U

UK 10, 18–19, 20–1, 172
  austerity policies and context 13,
    14, 15–18, *16*, *17*, 35–6, 82–3,
    99–100, 172, 174, 175, 191,
    203–6, 241–2
  suicide rates 11, 172, 174
under-occupancy charge (bedroom tax)
  13, **14**, 96, 147, 204, 205, 219
unemployment 4
  Great Depression, 1930s 37–42, *38,
    39, 40*
  Great Recession 10, 172
  impact on suicide rates 11
  and mental health 79, 142, 175
  and morbidity and mortality rates
    95
  as social determinant of health 79
  Stockton-on-Tees:
    Great Depression, 1930s 37, *40*,
      40–2
    longitudinal household survey
      comparative study 191, *192*
unemployment benefits, Great
  Depression, 1930s 37, 38–9, *39*
Unemployment Grants Committee 40
United Nations Sustainable
  Development Goal 10 175
Universal Credit 59, 165, 191
urban regeneration 121–4
US 10, 11, 18, 19–20, 174, 244

W

Wall Street Crash, 1929 36
Warwick-Edinburgh Mental Well-
  Being Scale (WEMWBS)
  180, 182, **183**, 187, *188, 189*,
  189–90, 193
WCA (Work Capability Assessment)
  151, 152
Welfare Reform Act 2012 59
welfare reforms 13, **14**, 15, 24, 26,
  59–60, 65, 96, 99, 100, 141–2,
  143, 147, 152, 165, 171, 172,
  191, 201–2, 203–4, 205, 206,
  218, 225, 234, 242, 244, 245

benefits sanctions 17, 58–9, 130,
  152–3, 209
conditionality **14**, 19, 82, 151,
  152, 201–2, 209, 211, 242,
  244
WEMWBS (Warwick-Edinburgh
  Mental Well-Being Scale)
  180, 182, **183**, 187, *188, 189*,
  189–190, 193
WHO (World Health Organization)
  78
women:
  and austerity 201, 205–6, 224,
    225
  and employment 205, 210, 212–14,
    215
  impact of policy and politics on
    214–17
  importance of universal social policy
    safety net for 233, 245, 246
  and mental illness 202–3
  social reproduction role of 202,
    205–6, 209–11, 224, 225
  structural disadvantage 208
  see also intersectionality; mothers
work and working environment 5, 79,
  142
  psychosocial working environment
    79, 158–9
  see also employment; unemployment
Work Capability Assessment (WCA)
  151, 152
Work Programme 152
'workfare' policies 211
  see also welfare reforms
World Health Organization (WHO)
  78
World Health Report 2001 173

Y

Yorkshire and Humber 16
youth unemployment 9

Z

zero hours contracts 129